Infectious Diseases and Microbiology

nova
New York

Infectious Diseases and Microbiology

Psychological Consequences of the COVID-19 Pandemic on Children, Teenagers and Adults
Jean-Pascal Assailly, PhD (Editor)
2022. ISBN: 978-1-68507-963-5 (Softcover)
2022. ISBN: 979-8-88697-072-2 (eBook)

COVID-19 Contracting: Opportunities, Actions and Reimbursements
Eric Neudorf
2022. ISBN: 978-1-68507-710-5 (Hardcover)
2022. ISBN: 978-1-68507-733-4 (eBook)

The Aviation Industry and COVID-19
Stefan Schneider
2022. ISBN: 978-1-68507-712-9 (Hardcover)
2022. ISBN: 978-1-68507-729-7 (eBook)

Diseases Transmitted by Ticks
Hacer İşler, Metin Özdemir, MD (Editors)
2021. ISBN: 978-1-68507-359-6 (Hardcover)
2021. ISBN: 978-1-68507-383-1 (eBook)

Impacts and Implications of COVID-19: An Analytical and Empirical Study
Anand Sharma, Prateek Agrawal,
Vishu Madaan , and Anuj Agarwal (Editors)
2021. ISBN: 978-1-53619-670-2 (Hardcover)
2021. ISBN: 978-1-68507-081-6 (eBook)

More information about this series can be found at https://novapublishers.com/product-category/series/infectious-diseases-and-microbiology/

Mark N. Frierson
Editor

COVID-19

Vaccines, Testing and Compensation Programs

snova
New York

Library of Congress Cataloging-in-Publication Data

ISBN: 979-8-88697-167-5

Published by Nova Science Publishers, Inc. † New York

Contents

Preface

Over 450,000 Americans have died due to COVID-19 and the deaths continue to climb. We need to be making continuous improvements that will stop this virus. Chapter 1 examine ways to further expand testing, the use of therapeutics, and increasing vaccine confidence while prioritizing quick and efficient distribution of the vaccines.

More than 200 million Americans have received one or more doses of a Coronavirus Disease 2019 (COVID-19) vaccine, along with billions of people worldwide. A very small percentage of inoculated individuals experience serious adverse reactions to a COVID-19 vaccine. Chapter 2 reviews the compensation programs available if a serious reaction does occur.

Chapter 1

Road to Recovery: Ramping up Covid-19 Vaccines, Testing, and Medical Supply Chain*

Committee on Energy and Commerce[1]

Wednesday, February 3, 2021
House of Representatives,
Subcommittee on Health,
Committee on Energy and Commerce,
Washington, DC.

The subcommittee met, pursuant to call, at 11:00 a.m., via Cisco Webex online video conferencing, Hon. Anna G. Eshoo (chairwoman of the subcommittee) presiding.

Members present: Representatives Eshoo, Butterfield, Matsui, Castor, Sarbanes, Welch, Schrader, Ca´rdenas, Ruiz, Dingell, Kuster, Kelly, Barraga´n, Blunt Rochester, Craig, Schrier, Trahan, Fletcher, Pallone (ex officio), Guthrie (subcommittee ranking member), Upton, Burgess, Griffith, Bilirakis, Bucshon, Mullin, Hudson, Carter, Dunn, Curtis, Joyce, and Rodgers (ex officio).

Also present: Representatives Schakowsky and O'Halleran.

Staff present: Jeffrey C. Carroll, Staff Director; Kimberly Espinosa, Professional Staff Member; Waverly Gordon, General Counsel; Tiffany Guarascio, Deputy Staff Director; Perry Hamilton, Deputy Chief Clerk; Stephen Holland, Health Counsel; Mackenzie Kuhl, Digital Assistant; Aisling McDonough, Policy Coordinator; Meghan Mullon, Policy Analyst; Kaitlyn Peel, Digital Director; Tim Robinson, Chief Counsel; Chloe Rodriguez, Deputy Chief Clerk; Kimberlee Trzeciak, Chief Health Advisor; C.J. Young, Deputy Communications Director; Sarah Burke, Minority Deputy Staff Director; Theresa Gambo, Minority Financial and Office Administrator; Nate Hodson, Minority Staff Director; Peter Kielty, Minority General Counsel; Bijan Koohmaraie, Minority Chief Counsel; Clare Paoletta, Minority Policy Analyst, Health; Kristin Seum, Minority Counsel, Health; Kristen Shatynski, Minority Professional Staff

---

* This is an edited, reformatted and augmented version of Virtual Hearing before the Subcommittee on Health, of the Committee on Energy and Commerce, House of Representatives, One Hundred Seventeenth Congress, First Session, Serial No. 117–2, dated February 3, 2021.

[1] Rachel Roubein contributed to this report.

In: COVID-19: Vaccines, Testing and Compensation Programs
Editor: Mark N. Frierson
ISBN: 979-8-88697-167-5

Member, Health; Michael Taggart, Minority Policy Director; and Everett Winnick, Minority Director of Information Technology.

Ms. ESHOO. The Subcommittee on Health will now come to order. Good morning, everyone. Due to COVID–19, today's hearing is being held remotely, obviously, so all Members and witnesses will be participating via video conferencing. As part of our hearing, microphones will be set on mute to eliminate background noise.

Members and witnesses, you will need to unmute your microphone each time you wish to speak. So keep that in mind.

Documents for the record will be sent to Meghan Mullon at the email address that we have provided to your staff, and all documents will be entered into the record at the conclusion of the hearing.

The Chair now recognizes herself for 5 minutes for an opening statement.

Opening Statement of Hon. Anna G. Eshoo, a Representative in Congress from the State of California

I want to welcome everyone to our first Health Subcommittee hearing of the 117th Congress. It is entitled "Road to Recovery: Ramping up COVID–19 Vaccines, Testing, and Medical Supply Chain," all issues that the Members are very familiar with.

A very warm welcome to all of our new Members, both sides of the aisle. We look forward to the contributions that you are going to make. And a very special welcome to Congressman Brett Guthrie, who is the new ranking member of our subcommittee, and I look forward to working with him. We all look forward to working with you, Brett.

Over the past year, our country has undergone truly profound changes due to COVID–19. I think that the veil has really been torn off every system and laid bare, what I call our country's many preexisting conditions, including inequities of care in communities of color and the inability of too many Americans having a lack of access or can afford healthcare. This subcommittee, I think, needs to move quickly and purposefully to correct these wrongs and do the right thing.

We are in a race against death. We have lost nearly 450,000 of our fellow Americans due to the virus, and as deaths continue to climb, Native, Black and Latino Americans face the highest risk. According to the CDC, these communities are nearly three times more likely to die from COVID–19 than White Americans.

The previous administration lacked a national strategy to end the pandemic and administer vaccines to Americans efficiently, equitably, and effectively. And without effective Federal coordination for the vaccination campaign, we clearly are not going to make any progress. I think we are actually tripping at the starting block, and there are many manifestations of that in our States and our local communities.

With a new administration, and a new Congress, and a new commitment, we can optimize a new beginning. The President has put forward his American Rescue Plan, which recognizes that we are in a battle to save American lives. It responds to this crisis with an all-of-government approach, and an all-of-America wartime plan.

First, the American Rescue Plan provides $20 billion for national vaccination strategy to increase the supply and the vaccination sites to fully vaccinate 300 million Americans by the end of this summer. The plan also creates a public health core of 100,000 newly hired public health workers to conduct individual outreach in local communities to address the vaccine hesitancy and misinformation.

Secondly, it invests $50 billion to scale up testing by buying rapid tests, expanding lab capacity, and coordinating the genetic sequencing that is needed to detect the concerning new variants of the virus.

Third, it invests $3 billion in innovative COVID–19 treatments. While we have effective vaccines to prevent people from getting the virus, we don't yet have accessible medicines to treat patients who are sick with it. This plan funds the research and large-scale clinical trials needed to develop therapeutics, such as antivirals and antibodies, to help people recover from the virus.

Fourth, it buys a strong supply of American-made personal protective equipment. I think that is music to all of our ears. The plan invests $10 billion to ensure we have sufficient protective gear by expanding domestic manufacturing.

So together, these public health efforts to crush the virus will cost $160 billion. The health benefits of this plan are abundantly clear, but the measures will also aid our economic recovery.

Last month, President Trump's White House Council of Economic Advisors estimated that every day our country speeds up vaccinations saves $10 billion in health and economic costs. Moody's Analytics found that the American Rescue Plan would create 7.5 million jobs and add 8 points to the GDP this year.

So I think we have the moral and economic duty to invest in this plan for the sake of our country, the people that we represent, and, obviously, our national economy. I hope our subcommittee is prepared—I believe that we are—prepared to hit the ground running to move these emergency actions through our deliberative process.

So I want to thank our very distinguished panel of witnesses today, including a former Governor, a former top scientist of the FDA, a former Director of the Strategic National Stockpile, and the former public health director of the third-largest American city.

Each of you are going to enlighten and guide our subcommittee on the urgent tasks before us.

Prepared Statement of Hon. Anna G. Eshoo

Welcome to the first Health Subcommittee hearing of the 117th Congress and a very warm welcome to the new Ranking Member Brett Guthrie and the new Members of the Health Subcommittee.

Over the past year our country has undergone profound changes due to COVID– 19.

The veil has been torn off every system and laid bare the many "pre-existing conditions" in our country, including inequities of care in communities of color and the inability of many to access or afford needed healthcare.

This subcommittee must move quickly and purposefully to correct these wrongs and do what's right.

We're in a race against death. We've lost nearly 450,000 of our fellow Americans to COVID–19.

As deaths continue to climb, Native, Black, and Latino Americans face the highest risk. According to the CDC, these communities are nearly 3 times more likely to die from COVID–19 than white Americans.

The previous administration lacked a national strategy to end the pandemic and administer vaccines to Americans efficiently, equitably, and effectively.

Without effective Federal coordination for the vaccination campaign, we've seen seniors spending hours in line for vaccinations or wealthier, whiter communities accessing vaccines ahead of communities of color.

We're tripping at the starting block.

With a new administration and a new Congress, we can optimize this new beginning. The President has put forward his American Rescue Plan which recognizes that we're in a battle to save American lives.

It responds to this crisis with an all-of-government and all-of-America wartime plan:

First, the American Rescue Plan provides $20 billion for a national vaccination strategy to increase supply and vaccination sites to fully vaccinate 300 million Americans by the end of this summer. The plan creates a public health corps of 100,000 newly hired public health workers to conduct individual outreach in their local communities to address vaccine hesitancy and misinformation.

Second, it invests $50 billion to scale up testing by buying rapid tests, expanding lab capacity, and coordinating the genetic sequencing needed to detect the concerning new variants of the virus.

Third, it invests $3 billion in innovative COVID–19 treatments. While we have effective vaccines to prevent people from getting COVID–19, we do not yet have accessible medicines to treat patients who are sick with COVID–19. This plan funds the research and large-scale clinical trials needed to develop therapeutics such as antivirals and antibodies to help people recover from COVID–19.

Fourth, it buys a strong supply of American-made personal protective equipment. The plan invests $10 billion to ensure we have sufficient protective gear by expanding domestic manufacturing.

Together the public health efforts in the American Rescue Plan will cost $160 billion.

The health benefits of the American Rescue Plan are abundantly clear, but these measures will also aid our economic recovery.

Last month, President Trump's White House Council of Economic Advisors estimated that every day the Nation speeds up vaccinations saves $10 billion in health and economic costs.

Moody's Analytics found that the American Rescue Plan would create 7.5 million jobs and add 8 points to the GDP in 2021.

We have the moral and economic duty to invest in the American Rescue Plan.

I hope this subcommittee is prepared to hit the ground running to move these emergency actions through our deliberative process.

I thank the distinguished panel of witnesses who are with us today, including a former Governor, the former top scientist of the FDA, the former Director of the Strategic National Stockpile, and the former public health director of the 3rd largest American city.

Each of you will enlighten and guide this subcommittee on the urgent task before us.

Ms. ESHOO. So the Chair now would like to recognize our new ranking member. We are very proud of you, Brett. Brett has been— Brett, for new Members, you need to know that Mr.

Guthrie has been a high-value member of our subcommittee. So I will now call on him in his new capacity as ranking member for 5 minutes for his opening statement.

Please remember to unmute.

Opening Statement of Hon. Brett Guthrie, a Representative in Congress from the Commonwealth of Kentucky

Mr. GUTHRIE. I did, I think so.

Thank you, Chair, for those very kind words. I really appreciate it very much, and welcome to all the new Members. On our side of the aisle, you are going to get to know John Curtis; Neal Dunn, who's a physician; Dan Crenshaw; and John Joyce, who is a physician as well. So I welcome them to the committee and all the new members, and all the members.

I want to thank you for holding this important hearing. My earplugs keeping popping out. Sorry.

Over 441,000 people have died from the COVID–19 pandemic in the United States, which is greater than the number of American servicemembers we lost in World War II. I know that all of us on this committee are committed to stopping this horrible virus. Specifically, I think we must fully evaluate our country's response efforts on what has worked and what lessons we have learned thus far during the COVID–19 pandemic. Our focus needs to be forward looking in order to make continuous improvements that will stop this virus. Each of us has a choice to make. We can stay in our camps and focus on ideological battles, or we can sit at the negotiating table and get work done that the American people expect us to do during these challenging times.

We need to examine ways to further expand testing, use of therapeutics, and increase vaccine confidence. We also need to prioritize quick and efficient distribution of vaccines.

Let me be clear: We are not starting from scratch. Without Operation Warp Speed, we would not have two vaccines that are currently being administered to Americans, nor potentially additional vaccines that may be authorized by the FDA in the near future. The Biden administration has taken credit for a pathway to 100 million vaccines in 100 days. However, 2 weeks into the Biden presidency, there have been around 52 million vaccines distributed and more than 32 million vaccines administered, thanks to the previous administration's efforts.

As we move forward with vaccine distribution, we will find ways to improve, and we should explore those. Let us not forget this is the fastest we have ever had a vaccine move through the development pipeline and come to market. We never cut any safety corners, despite the extraordinary speed, and that is success that should be celebrated.

Additionally, I have I have heard from Kentucky and many other States that the lack of additional Federal funding for States who distribute vaccine has been the biggest hiccup. We had two vaccines authorized, authorized prior to the latest funding package that was signed into law at the end of December. Let us not forget that this package was stalled for months. Valuable time was lost. When we did move forward, Speaker Pelosi said she moved forward because of a new President and a new vaccine. The money being sent to the States 2 weeks late, when it needed to be weeks if not months before, has cost us valuable time.

From my background in manufacturing, I know it takes time, hard work and detailed planning to get a manufacturing line up and going. Operation Warp Speed's tireless work on supply chains and simultaneous manufacturing during clinical trials meant safe and effective vaccines that were administered to our healthcare heroes and vulnerable populations within a matter of days, rather than months, after receiving FDA authorization.

Each State and some large jurisdictions have been given the opportunity to run their vaccine distribution as they believe is best for their residents.

I am not sure if anyone here is familiar with Utica, Kentucky. It is a rural community in my district that I am proud to represent. I think Frankfurt, our State capital, and Davis County, can do a better job of taking care of Utica than being run out of Washington, DC, which is a person who has probably never stepped foot there. While some States may need to reevaluate their strategy, there are many States that are doing quite well with vaccine distribution.

In addition, I think it is key to remember the work the FDA has done to authorize 320 COVID–19 tests. According to the COVID– 19 tracking project this Monday, we had more than 1.6 million new tests reported in a day. On March 3lst of last year, we had less than 116,000 new tests reported. Over the past year, we have seen the development and authorization of rapid point-of-care diagnostics to reduce instances of delayed results, tests using saliva samples to eliminate the need for swabs in short supply, and even a test that is sold over the counter.

While challenges remain, we have demonstrated that these type of private industry partnerships and the innovative products that are a result are essential to successfully responding to the pandemic.

Lastly, as the Republican leader of the Oversight and Investigations Subcommittee in the last Congress, I believe that oversight is a very important aspect of our response. We have passed around $4 trillion in COVID–19 aid alone. I have supported much-needed relief for American families, workers, and small businesses. We must ensure it is being used effectively and wisely.

And I agree, Madam Chair, that we have an esteemed panel of witnesses. I look forward to hearing their testimony, along with my colleagues, hoping my colleagues will join me in finding solutions and acknowledging how far we have come and work to get even farther as we go forward.

I yield back.

Prepared Statement of Hon. Brett Guthrie

Thank you, Chair Eshoo, for holding this important hearing about the COVID–19 pandemic.Four hundred and forty-three thousand people have died from the COVID–19 pandemic in the United States which is greater than the number of American servicemembers that we lost during World War ll. I believe that all of us who serve on this committee are committed to stopping this horrible virus.

Specifically, I think we must fully evaluate our country's response efforts on what has worked and what lessons we have learned thus far during the COVID–19 pandemic. Our focus needs to be forward looking in order to make continuous improvements that will stop this virus. Each of us have a choice to make—we can stay in our camps and focus on ideological battles or we can sit at the negotiating table and get work done that the American people expect us to do during these challenging times.

We need to examine ways to further expand testing, use of therapeutics, and increase vaccine confidence. We also need to prioritize quickly and efficiently distributing vaccines. Let me be clear: we are not starting from scratch. Without Operation Warp Speed, we would not have two vaccines that are currently being administered to Americans, nor potentially additional vaccines that may be authorized by the FDA in the near future. The Biden administration is taking credit for the pathway to 100 million vaccines in 100 days However, two weeks into Biden's presidency, there have been around fifty million vaccines distributed and thirty-two million vaccines administered, largely thanks to the previous administration's efforts. As we move forward with vaccine distribution, we will find ways to improve, and we should explore those. Let us not forget this is the fastest we have ever had a vaccine move through the development pipeline and come to market. We never cut any safety corners, despite the extraordinary speed, and that is a success that should be celebrated.

Additionally, I have heard from Kentucky and many other States that the lack of additional funding for States to distribute vaccines has been the biggest hiccup. However, let us not forget, Pelosi obstructed additional COVID funding for months. We had two vaccines authorized prior to latest funding package that was signed into law at the end of December.

From my background in manufacturing, I know it takes time, hard work, and detailed planning to get a manufacturing line up and going. Operation Warp Speed's tireless work on supply chains and simultaneous manufacturing during clinical trials meant safe and effective vaccines were being administered to our healthcare heroes and vulnerable populations within a matter of days rather than months after receiving FDA authorization.

Each State and some large jurisdictions have been given the opportunity to run their vaccine distribution as they believe is best for their residents. Is anyone here familiar with Utica? It's a rural community in my district that I'm proud to represent, and I think Frankfort and Daviess County can do a better job taking care of Utica than a bureaucrat in Washington, DC, who has probably never stepped foot there. While some States may need to reevaluate their strategy, there are many States that are doing quite well with vaccine distribution.

In addition, I think it is key to remember the work FDA has done to authorize 320 COVID–19 tests. According to the COVID Tracking Project, this week, we had more than 1.6 million new tests reported. At the end of March last year, we had less than 116,000 new tests reported. Over the past year we have seen the development and authorization of rapid point-of-care diagnostics to reduce instances of delayed results, tests using saliva samples to eliminate the need for swabs in short supply, and even a test that is sold over-the-counter. While challenges remain, we have demonstrated that these types of private industry partnerships and the innovative products that result are essential to successfully responding to this pandemic.

Lastly, as the former Republican Leader of the Oversight and Investigations subcommittee, I believe that oversight is a very important aspect of our response. We have passed around $4 trillion in COVID–19 aid alone. I have supported much-needed relief for American families, workers, and small businesses. We must ensure it is being used effectively and wisely.

I look forward to the testimony from these esteemed witnesses and welcome them to this hearing. I hope my colleagues will join in me in helping find solutions and acknowledging how far we have come from just a year ago. I yield back.

Ms. ESHOO. The gentleman yields back.

The Chair now recognizes the chairman of the full committee, Mr. Pallone, for his 5 minutes for his opening statement.

And, Frank, you need to unmute.

Opening Statement of Hon. Frank Pallone, Jr., a Representative in Congress from the State of New Jersey

Mr. PALLONE. Thank you, Chairwoman Eshoo. And I want to, as you did, welcome everyone back for our first Health Subcommittee hearing of the 117th Congress.

There is no more pressing issue to begin with than the ongoing COVID–19 pandemic and our response so far and our need to increase vaccinations, testing, and mitigation of building a robust supply chain.

This pandemic has taken a devastating toll on communities all around the country. As Members of Congress, we have to do everything we can to ensure that this new administration has all of the tools and resources it needs to crush the virus.

With President Biden in the White House, I am confident that we can move forward with comprehensive actions to stem the tide on the virus. One of the first orders of business will be jump-starting and sustaining a robust vaccination program. After the scientific breakthrough of two safe and effective COVID–19 vaccines, and hopefully more on the way, we must do more to confront the challenge of getting the vaccine into people's arms.

Unfortunately, the Trump administration failed to prepare and provide reasons for a national vaccination campaign, and never developed a comprehensive national vaccine plan. Instead, the administration pushed all responsibility for distributing and administering vaccines to the States, and then they made that job nearly impossible when they opposed providing the States with additional resources to do so. And this failure of leadership led to only 3 million Americans being vaccinated by the end of the year, far short of the 20 million that the Trump administration had promised.

Yesterday, we heard at our O&I Subcommittee, we heard from States on the front lines about these vaccination challenges. While we were pleased to hear about how they have improved vaccination rates in recent weeks, they underscored the need for additional resources and clear, consistent communication as they work to get the vaccines in people's arms. And their insight is critical as we chart a better path forward.

In December, Congress stepped up and provided $8.75 billion for vaccine distribution activities, including $4.5 billion to States in the final omnibus and COVID relief package. And so, vaccination rates are increasing, but if we are to accelerate both production and vaccinations, more resources are needed, especially resources dedicated to the most vulnerable, hard-to-reach Americans.

And the same can be said for ongoing needs related to testing and contact tracing. From the early days of the pandemic, public health experts and House Democrats were calling for a comprehensive national testing strategy that would ensure testing supplies were allocated efficiently, and tests were available to all who needed them. But, unfortunately, just like with vaccines, the Trump administration never created a comprehensive national testing strategy, and turned over virtually all responsibilities to the States, with little support or guidance.

Now, I want to emphasize testing again. Testing reagents and supplies, like pipettes, have continued to face shortages, and as new outbreaks have occurred, new bottlenecks in testing have followed. And while we work to vaccinate all Americans, access to reliable, efficient, and speedy testing, contact tracing, and mitigation support will continue to be critical if we are to reduce transmission and community spread.

And we also need a more robust and reliable medical supply chain. While States are administering more COVID–19 vaccines, they are running up against supply shortages of doses, but also the ancillary medical supplies, such as syringes that are used to extract every available dose, and while some early therapeutics have been authorized by the FDA, their limited availability has also curbed their impact. And so, we also continue to face supply challenges for administering tests, like reagents and swabs, and supply challenges remain for critical personal protective equipment for medical personnel, including in nursing homes, vaccinators, and the public health workforce.

So I am pleased that President Biden has taken swift and decisive action to improve our response to the pandemic, as you mentioned, Madam Chair, but crushing the virus requires more action from Congress.

President Biden has proposed the American Rescue Plan, which includes $20 billion in funds for vaccine distribution administration, public awareness, and additional resources for improving our supply of vaccines. It invests $50 billion for testing and contact tracing, including expanding community-based and mobile testing sites, and it includes $10 billion to help support expansion of medical supply manufacturing capacity.

So, Congress needs to move President Biden's American Rescue Plan as quickly as possible. I know their process is beginning on the floor this afternoon, and I look forward to hearing from our witnesses about their thoughts on the Nation's response to the pandemic so far and how we can improve going forward.

So thank you again, Madam Chair, for this important hearing of the Health Subcommittee.

I yield back.

Prepared Statement of Hon. Frank Pallone, Jr.

I want to welcome everyone back for our first Health Subcommittee hearing of the 117th Congress. There is no more pressing issue to begin with than the ongoing COVID–19 pandemic, our response so far, and our need to increase vaccinations, testing, and mitigation, and building a robust supply chain.

This pandemic is taking a devastating toll on families and communities all around our Nation. More than 440,000 Americans have died from this terrible virus, and the Centers for Disease Control and Prevention has projected that number will grow to more than 500,000 before the end of the month. As Americans, we mourn every loss. As Members of Congress, we must do everything we can to ensure this new administration has all the tools and resources it needs to crush COVID–19.

With President Biden in the White House, I am confident that we can move forward with comprehensive action to stem the tide on this virus, bring relief to struggling families, and rebuild our economy.

One of the first orders of business will be jumpstarting and sustaining a robust vaccination program. After the scientific breakthrough of two safe and effective COVID–19 vaccines, and hopefully more on the way, we must do more to confront the challenge of getting the vaccines into people's arms.

Unfortunately, the Trump administration failed to prepare and provide resources for a national vaccination campaign, and never developed a comprehensive national vaccine plan. Instead, the administration pushed all responsibility for distributing and administering vaccines to the States and then they made that job nearly impossible when they opposed providing the States with additional resources to do it. This failure of leadership led to only 3 million Americans being vaccinated by the end of the year—far short of the 20 million the administration had promised.

Yesterday, we heard from States on the front lines about these vaccination challenges. While we were pleased to hear about how they have improved vaccination rates in recent weeks, they underscored the need for additional resources and clear, consistent communication as they work to get vaccines in arms. Their insight is critical as we chart a better path forward.

In December, Congress stepped up and provided $8.75 billion for vaccine distribution activities, including $4.5 billion to States in the final omnibus and COVID relief package. Vaccination rates are increasing but if we are to accelerate both production and vaccinations, more resources are needed, especially resources dedicated to the most vulnerable, hard-to-reach Americans.

The same can be said for ongoing needs related to testing and contact tracing. From the early days of the pandemic, public health experts and House Democrats were calling for a comprehensive, national testing strategy that would ensure testing supplies were allocated efficiently and tests were available to all who needed them. Unfortunately, just like with vaccines, the Trump administration never created a comprehensive, national strategy and turned over virtually all responsibilities to the States, with little support or guidance.

Testing reagents and supplies like pipettes have continued to face shortages, and as new outbreaks have occurred, new bottlenecks in testing have followed. While we work to vaccinate all Americans, access to reliable, efficient, and speedy testing, contact tracing, and mitigation support will continue to be critical if we are to reduce transmission and community spread.

We also need a more robust and reliable medical supply chain. While States are administering more COVID–19 vaccines, they are running up against supply shortages of vaccine doses, but also the ancillary medical supplies such as syringes that are used to extract every available dose. And while some early therapeutics have been authorized by the FDA, their limited availability has curbed their impact. We also continue to face supply challenges for administering tests, like reagents and swabs. And supply challenges remain for critical personal protective equipment for medical personnel, including in nursing homes, vaccinators, and the public health workforce.

I am pleased that President Biden has taken swift and decisive action to improve our response to the pandemic, but crushing the virus requires more action from Congress, as well. President Biden has proposed the American Rescue Plan, which includes $20 billion in funds for vaccine distribution and administration, public awareness, and additional resources for improving our supply of vaccines, therapeutics, and ancillary supplies. It invests $50 billion for testing and contact tracing, including expanding community-based and mobile testing sites. And it includes $10 billion to help support expansion of medical supply manufacturing capacity.

Congress needs to move President Biden's American Rescue Plan as quickly as possible. I look forward to hearing from our witnesses about their thoughts on the Nation's response to the pandemic so far and how we can improve going forward.

Ms. ESHOO. The gentleman yields back. We thank him for his opening statement.

The Chair now recognizes Representative Cathy McMorris Rodgers, our new ranking member of the full committee, for her 5 minutes for an opening statement.

Opening Statement of Hon. Cathy Mcmorris Rodgers, a Representative in Congress from the State of Washington

Mrs. RODGERS. Good morning, everyone. Thank you, Madam Chair and Republican Leader Guthrie, for holding this important hearing.

Exactly one year ago today, news outlets were reporting that the global death toll from the coronavirus was 362, with all but one of those deaths occurring in mainland China. A year later, this heartbreaking number has surpassed 2 million, with over 425,000 of these tragic deaths occurring in the United States. This pandemic has wreaked havoc on our way of life. The loss of life has been devastating.

Our previous booming economy has been decimated. Our mental health crisis has only worsened, and the long-term impact of our children being kept out of the classroom is incalculable.

Last Congress, we put our political differences aside to make extraordinary investments in the fight against COVID–19 through five separate bipartisan relief packages. These included providing over $30 billion for the States, territories, and Tribes for testing, vaccine distribution, contact tracing, and public health infrastructure improvement; and over $23 billion to the Biomedical Advanced Research and Development Authority for the research, development, and manufacture of novel vaccines, tests, and treatments; and $178 billion for healthcare providers on the front lines of taking care of patients with COVID–19.

This investment and partnership with the private sector has led to unprecedented development of innovative vaccines and treatments coming to market faster than we ever thought possible. Operation Warp Speed is one of the most ambitious and successful undertakings in American history, with two lifesaving vaccines now authorized by FDA and a third hopefully soon to follow. There is light at the end of this dark tunnel.

However, our hard work is not yet complete. Vaccine distribution is ramping up, but we must ensure States have the resources and the flexibility they need to immunize successfully as many people who want it and meet the unique healthcare needs of their individual population.

We heard yesterday in the Oversight and Investigations Subcommittee from West Virginia, which has relied on community pharmacists to get the vaccines to people. Unfortunately, other States, like my own Washington State, have not been as successful. Governor Inslee and others in Olympia have spent a great deal of time pointing fingers at Washington, DC, for the State's slow distribution, instead of figuring out strategies to get people vaccinated.

Clearly, some States were better prepared and used the advice of the CDC career scientists to implement locally targeted strategies more successfully.

While vaccine distribution is critical to safely and responsibly reopening our economy and our schools, we also learned additional challenges during the response to COVID–19. We learned that our medical supply chain is incredibly vulnerable and that we rely too heavily on adversarial countries like China for critically important products, such as protective equipment.

We need to consider policies that will improve our domestic manufacturing without impacting cost and consumer access. Our Strategic National Stockpile and medical supply distribution logistics also need to be strengthened.

While we have met this unprecedented crisis with an equally unprecedented response, our resources are not unlimited. Congress has a responsibility to oversee the money we have spent, understand how it is being distributed and used, and learn what is working and what hasn't.

As Chairman Pallone said during our organizing committee just last week, this committee has a rich history of bipartisan cooperation and hard work, perhaps more than any other committee in Congress.

Between the pandemic, the economic crisis, the social and political unrest, last year was one of the most difficult in our Nation's history. Despite these incredible hurdles, Congress was able to come together on five separate occasions to give the American people the relief they needed. This pandemic and our Government's response is bigger than any single administration or political party. As we discuss these important issues in our path forward with our distinguished witnesses today, I hope our focus will not be about pointing fingers on shortcomings, but the opportunity to learn what bipartisan steps we can take over the next several months to win the fight against COVID–19, restore our way of life, rebuild the greatest economy in our history, and prepare for future pandemics so that a public health emergency of this magnitude never happens again.

I thank the witnesses for joining us today, and I yield back the balance of my time.

Prepared Statement of Hon. Cathy Mcmorris Rodgers

Thank you, Chair Eshoo and Republican Leader Guthrie for holding this important hearing.

Exactly one year ago today, news outlets were reporting that the global death toll from the coronavirus was 362, with all but one of those deaths occurring in mainland China.

A year later, and this heartbreaking number has surpassed 2 million, with over 425,000 of these tragic deaths occurring in the United States.

This pandemic has wreaked havoc on our way of life. The loss of life has been devasting.

Our previously booming economy has been decimated. Our mental health crisis has only worsened.

And the long-term impact on our children being kept out of the classroom is incalculable.

Last Congress, we put our political differences aside to make extraordinary investments in the fight against COVID–19 through five separate bipartisan relief packages.

These included providing over 30 billion dollars for States, territories, and Tribes for testing, vaccine distribution, contact tracing, and public health data infrastructure improvement.

And over 23 billion dollars to the Biomedical Advanced Research and Development Authority for the research, development, and manufacture of novel vaccines, tests, and treatments.

And $178 billion dollars for healthcare providers on the front lines of taking care of patients with COVID–19.

This investment and partnership with the private sector has led to the unprecedented development of innovative vaccines and treatments coming to market faster than we ever thought possible.

Operation Warp Speed is one of the most ambitious and successful undertakings in American history, and with two lifesaving vaccines now authorized by the FDA, and a third hopefully soon to follow, there is light at the end of this dark tunnel.

However, our hard work is not yet complete.

Vaccine distribution is ramping up, but we must ensure States have the resources and flexibility they need to immunize successfully as many people who want it.

And meet the unique health needs of their individual populations.

We heard yesterday in the Oversight and Investigations Subcommittee from West Virginia, which has relied on community pharmacies to get the vaccines to people.

Unfortunately, Washington State has not been as successful. Gov. Inslee and others in Olympia spend a great deal of time pointing fingers at Washington, DC, for the State's slow distribution instead figuring out strategies to get people vaccinated as West Virginia is doing.

Clearly some States were better prepared and used the advice of the CDC career scientists to implement locally targeted strategies more successfully than he has done.

Supply Chain

While vaccine distribution is critical to safely and responsibly reopen our economy and our schools, we also learned additional challenges during the response to COVID–19.

We learned that our medical supply chain is incredibly vulnerable and that we rely too heavily on adversarial countries such as China for critically important products, such as personal protective equipment.

We need to consider policies that will improve our domestic manufacturing without impacting cost and consumer access.

Our strategic national stockpile and medical supply distribution logistics also need to be strengthened.

While we have met this unprecedented crisis with an equally unprecedented response, our resources are not unlimited.

Congress has a responsibility to oversee the money we have spent, understand how it is being distributed and used.

And learn what's working and what hasn't.

As Chairman Pallone said during our organizing meeting last week, this committee has a rich history of bipartisan cooperation and hard work.

Perhaps more so than any other committee in Congress.

Between the pandemic, the economic crisis, and the social and political unrest, last year was one of the most difficult in our Nation's history.

Yet, despite these incredible hurdles, Congress was able to come together on five separate occasions to give the American people the relief they needed.

This pandemic, and our Government's response, is bigger than any single administration or political party.

As we discuss these important issues and our path forward with our distinguished witnesses today, I hope our focus will be not about pointing fingers for our shortcomings.

But an opportunity to learn what bipartisan steps we can take over the next several months to win the fight against COVID–19, restore our way of life, rebuild the greatest economy in history.

And prepare for future pandemics so that a public health emergency of this magnitude never happens again.

Thank you to our witnesses for joining us today and I yield back the balance of my time.

Ms. ESHOO. The gentlelady yields back.

The Chair would like to remind Members that, pursuant to committee rules, all Members' written opening statements are going to be made part of the record.

I now would like to introduce our witnesses, first Dr. Luciana Borio, vice president of In–Q–Tel, an organization that I am very familiar with, former Acting Chief Scientist, FDA, and former Director for Medical and Biodefense Preparedness of the National Security Council.

Dr. Julie Morita, Executive Vice President of the highly distinguished Robert Wood Johnson Foundation. Thank you to you for joining us today.

The Honorable Michael Leavitt, founder and chair of the Leavitt Partners, former Secretary of HHS, and former Governor of Utah. That is really quite extraordinary.

Greg Burel, president and principal consultant of Hamilton Grace and former Director of the United States Strategic National Stockpile. Welcome to you.

And, Dr. Luciana Borio, you are now recognized for 5 minutes. And you need to unmute. So we look forward to your testimony and that of each one of the witnesses. I think we have really extraordinary witnesses today and you are all going to get some good, stiff questions from the brilliant members of this subcommittee.

So welcome. And you can begin.

Statements of Luciana Borio, M.D., Vice President, In-Q-Tel; Julie Morita, M.D., Executive Vice President, Robert Wood Johnson Foundation; Michael O. Leavitt, Founder and Chair, Leavitt Partners; and Greg Burel, President and Principal Consultant, Hamilton Grace

Statement of Luciana Borio, M.D.

Dr. BORIO. Thank you. And good morning, Chairman Pallone, Ranking Member McMorris Rodgers, Chairman Eshoo, and Ranking Member Guthrie, as well as members of the subcommittee. It is my great pleasure to join you today.

As you know, I work at In–Q–Tel, a nonprofit technology investment firm that serves U.S. national security. And before that, I served across four different administrations and most recently as a member of the Biden-Harris transition team in its COVID–19 Advisory Board. I am appearing before you in my personal capacity. The situation is dire, and I fear that our worst days could be ahead, given the variants that emerged recently in the U.K., South Africa, and Brazil, and have spread globally. The South African strain is exceptionally concerning since it invades at least partially the antibody-based therapies and diminishes the protective effect of at least some vaccines.

In my testimony today, I would like to share a few thoughts about the past, present, and future.

I do not wish to dwell too much on the past, other than to say that the Nation learned the consequences of departing from the science-driven response, however imperfect, historically taken during public health emergencies. At the same time, we must recognize that many of the shortcomings of this response are due to factors that preceded the most recent administration, and repairing it will require reckoning with early missteps, a failure of imagination, and a significant complacency that has plagued us for years.

Here are seven priorities for the present:

First, given the variants, CDC must immediately expand its genomic surveillance system in collaboration with public health, private, and academic labs. I am glad to see early steps in this direction.

Second, vaccines. We are quite fortunate. We have two safe and effective vaccines developed in record time, with additional ones on the horizon. This incredible success would not have been possible without decades of investments in U.S. biomedical research, the people of Operation Warp Speed, and the FDA's Office of Vaccines under the leadership of Drs. Marion Gruber and Phil Krause. They guided the rapid development of these innovative vaccines without compromising the highest scientific standards, and ensuring transparency. This is what makes American scientific enterprise so powerful and so hard to replicate elsewhere. Sadly, the chaotic rollout of the vaccines has frustrated millions of Americans. The new administration has taken steps to fix the situation, and you should see more improvements soon.

Third, the virus variants. The threat will not be resolved with travel restrictions. We must take urgent measures to reduce the spread of this virus to lessen the opportunities for the virus to further mutate and become even more dangerous. The virus continues to burn through our country, while many people continue to gather indoors and in large groups and refuse to wear masks or social distance. Small businesses across our country that are lucky enough to have survived thus far simply cannot afford another lockdown. If we care about our jobs, we must mask up and change our behavior urgently.

Fourth, the supply chain. I am encouraged to see vaccine manufacturers taking steps to develop new candidates that may be needed to effectively protect against new variants, but the supply chain for making and distributing vaccinations remains extremely fragile. The Federal Government is using the Defense Production Act to prioritize the allocation of limited critical materials. DPA helps, but it is not a final solution. HHS must urgently expand the industrial base for critical supplies to ensure the U.S. has sufficient supplies for this and future pandemics.

Fifth, we do need better therapies. The quest for cures has been hampered by the lack of a national capability for conducting simple and pragmatic randomized clinical trials. In departure from prior practice and under intense political pressure, the FDA issued a series of EUAs for products that had not been properly evaluated. Patient care needs to be driven not by hope, but by science.

Sixth, diagnostic tests. As the Federal Government worked to increase testing ability, it never developed a strategy to help guide clinical and public health practice. To maximize the impact of testing, I urge the CDC to develop guidance for testing in a variety of settings: travel, workplace, and educational settings, for example. And seventh, the U.S. still lacks an interoperable data infrastructure for public health. This should be one of the principal areas of retention if we are to build a 2lst century public health system.

As for the future, biological threats are not going away. As we continue to battle this pandemic, we must also build a system that can meet future threats, one that integrates the private sector in cutting-edge technology, that values the critical role of public health in our collective well-being, health, and economic security, and realizes that good governance is necessary to bring capabilities to fruition.

A better day will soon come upon us if we let science and the American innovation lead the way.

Thank you.

Testimony of Luciana Borio, M.D., Vice-President, In-Q-Tel, "Road to Recovery: Ramping up COVID-19 Vaccines, Testing, and Medical Supply Chain," February 3, 2021, Subcommittee on Health of the House Committee on Energy and Commerce

Introduction

Good morning, Chairman Eshoo, Ranking Member Guthrie, and members of the Subcommittee. I am Dr. Luciana Borio and have dedicated my career to biodefense. I am grateful for the opportunity to testify before you today. I have had the privilege of serving the American people across four different administrations. Most recently, I had the honor to serve as a member of the Biden-Harris transition team and the transition COVID-19 advisory board.

In 2019, I left government service and joined In-Q-Tel, a non-for-profit strategic investment firm that tailors innovative technology solutions to support the mission of the U.S. national security community. I am appearing before you today in my personal capacity.

The COVID-19 Pandemic

The global situation is dire. We are facing the worst pandemic of respiratory disease in the last 102 years with approximately 103mm cases and 2.23mm deaths globally. The United States has been the worst affected country in the world with more than 26.2mm cases and 441,000 deaths to date. We have experienced several surges since the pandemic started, without ever returning fully to baseline. The most recent surge, which occurred in the aftermath of the winter holidays, was very steep. The numbers of new patients seem to be stabilizing but are pushing hospitals and their staff to their limit.

After several months of the SARS-CoV-2 remaining relatively stable, it is now evolving rapidly, as most RNA viruses do. Several variant strains have emerged in the past few months, notably the B.1.1.7 in the United Kingdom, the B.1.351 in South Africa, and the P.1 in Brazil. These variants have not stayed in the countries where they emerged - they have spread globally. The U.K. variant seems to be highly transmissible and is predicted to become the dominant variant circulating in the United States by March. The South African strain is exceptionally concerning since it evades, at least partially, the antibody-based therapies and diminishes the protective effect of at least some vaccines. The next few months are uncertain; our worst days could be ahead of us.

Past

Today, I do not want to dwell too much on the past. The previous administration, in which I served, made many mistakes and individuals in key positions of trust and responsibility let the American people down. Some officials promoted divisiveness instead of safeguarding our collective health. Some were more interested in protecting their turf than building bridges to summon our collective strength. I do not believe there was a single point of failure – there were many failures.

I believe the prior administration's actions were a significant departure from the imperfect but science-driven response undertaken by the U.S. Government during previous public health emergencies.

However, if we are to do better, we must recognize that many of the Federal biodefense enterprise's shortcomings preceded the most recent administration. Repairing our nation's biodefense enterprise will require reckoning with early missteps and continued deficiencies.

There has been much attention on CDC's diagnostic test kits failures that left us blind to the virus's early spread. This type of technical failure was an accident and could have occurred in any laboratory. However, it was foolish to think that the CDC, in collaboration with public health laboratories, would be able to meet the nation-wide demand for diagnostic tests during a pandemic. The true failing rests with HHS for not establishing a robust national diagnostic capability (similar to what it did for vaccines and other medical countermeasures) prior to this pandemic or in its early days, in cooperation with private laboratories, to respond with the speed and scale that any pandemic requires.

Furthermore, the lack of a robust, large-scale national genomic surveillance system to monitor viral evolution and spread one year after the pandemic began means we are flying blind with respect to detecting the introduction or emergence of new variants or monitoring their geographic spread. That is inexcusable.

Present

Vaccines

Today, we find ourselves amid the most complex and logistically challenging vaccination campaign ever undertaken in America. In many ways, we are fortunate. For the first time in history, two safe and effective vaccines were developed and authorized for use in less than a year. Additional vaccines are on the horizon. This incredible success can be attributed to three main factors: 1) the decades of investment in biomedical research by the U.S. Government that preceded the pandemic alongside a vibrant and innovative U.S. biopharmaceutical sector, 2) the hundreds of career officials at HHS and DoD who worked around the clock under the supervision of Dr. Moncef Slaoui and the leadership of General Gustave Perna to accelerate development and scale up vaccine production, 3) FDA's Office of Vaccines, under the leadership of Drs. Marion Gruber and Phil Krause, who guided the development of these innovative vaccines in an expedited fashion without compromising the highest scientific standards, and ensuring transparency. As a result, we are the only country in the world that has robust, solid, reliable data in tens of thousands of individuals who participated in randomized clinical trials – the gold standard – for evaluating the safety and efficacy of these now authorized vaccines.

Vaccine distribution was initially left to states, which were inadequately prepared to handle the complex logistics. The new administration has taken important steps to improve vaccine distribution within states. It is examining ways to maximize production of FDA-authorized vaccines to make more doses available sooner, provide direct assistance to states that need it, open up vaccination to more priority groups faster, establish more vaccination sites, increase use of pharmacies and mobile units for vaccinations, and make it easier for states to recruit vaccinators. These steps, done in conjunction with a campaign to counter misinformation and vaccine hesitancy, and a focus on improving vaccine access for "hard to reach" populations, will enhance the nation-wide vaccination program.

Even as these challenges are slowly resolved, new ones emerge. The Federal government is relying on the Defense Production Act to prioritize the allocation of limited supplies to vaccine manufacturers (as well as secondary and tertiary suppliers) under contract with the U.S. Government. This helps, but the supply chain remains vulnerable. The interruption of any critical component required for making or distributing vaccine doses (and the list is vast, including, for example, raw materials, consumables, manufacturing and fill/finish equipment, personnel, dry ice and cold storage, and needles and syringes) will disrupt the availability and administration of vaccines.

Variants

The virus variants pose another challenge. Travel restrictions will not solve this because these variants have spread globally and are already here. Travel measures, such as proof of negative testing before entering the U.S. when combined with a period of quarantine upon arrival, may diminish the number of imported cases, but will not stop the spread of variant strains within our borders.

It is essential that we take urgent measures to diminish the spread of this virus because the more spread there is, the greater the opportunity there is for the virus to further mutate and become even more dangerous. If we reduce the number of people getting infected, the chances for virus mutations go down.

To that end, even as we make a push toward a fast and broad vaccination program, we must redouble our efforts to compel the population to mask up and maintain social distancing through a variety of measures, such as restricting social gatherings and encouraging telework where feasible. This virus continues to burn through our country, while many people continue to gather indoors and in large groups and refuse to wear masks or social distance. The fundamental behavioral interventions— masking, social distancing, and avoidance of indoor gatherings— remain the single best tools we possess in the fight against COVID-19, equal in importance to effective vaccines. This requires careful public messaging, so Americans understand the value of both vaccines and behavioral modifications.

Even if not for one's own health, we must do this for our country's economic health. Small businesses across America that are lucky enough to have survived thus far cannot afford another lockdown. If we care about our jobs, we must mask up and heed public health advice.

As an additional measure to reduce the chances that the virus develops more mutations that could evade the immune system, I would encourage the U.S. Food and Drug Administration to rescind the Emergency Use Authorization (EUA) it issued last year for convalescent plasma. We already know that, in aggregate, this therapy does not help patients with COVID-19. But by using it in circumstances where it does not work, we are providing the virus with a roadmap that could help it develop mutations that evade natural and vaccine-induced immune responses even more rapidly.

I am encouraged to see vaccine manufacturers taking steps now to develop novel vaccine candidates that may be needed to effectively protect against the emerging variant strains. Developing and testing candidates is relatively simple when compared to the difficult decisions ahead regarding triggers for large scale manufacturing, given the finite supply of manufacturing materials and capacity, and deployment of newer vaccines on top of an already strained distribution system.

Therapies

Even with authorized vaccines being distributed, we still desperately need better therapies for COVID-19, especially ones that can be manufactured at scale and easily administered. A few therapies, such as remdesivir and dexamethasone, have been shown in randomized clinical trials to improve the clinical outcomes for select patients. Dexamethasone was shown in the RECOVERY trial in the U.K. to reduce deaths in patients requiring oxygen and in those requiring invasive mechanical ventilation.

In the U.S., except for the NIH-led ACTT trials, the system for evaluating new or existing drugs has faltered. Lacking a national capability for conducting simple, pragmatic randomized clinical trials, the U.S. had to repurpose existing clinical trial networks originally designed for other diseases. The process has been slow and inefficient. In the meantime, many industry-driven and independent trials with varying degrees of scientific rigor emerged.

In a departure from prior practice, and under intense political pressure, during this pandemic the FDA has issued a series of EUAs based on a product potentially meeting the EUA statutory bar (which is low and designed to give the Agency maximum flexibility) but with little consideration about the impact of the EUAs on patient outcomes. The EUAs for products that had not been properly evaluated in clinical trials nevertheless provided an "FDA-endorsed" treatment option for patients that could have otherwise enrolled in rigorous yet highly efficient clinical trials, that would have provided definitive answers about a given drug, and allowed patient care to be driven not by hope, but by science.

On 1/30, the New York Times [https://www.nytimes.com/2021/01/30/health/covid-drugs-antivirals.html] reported that despite the wealth of evidence against hydroxychloroquine and chloroquine for COVID-19, there are still 179 clinical trials with 169,370 patients in which at least some are receiving the drugs. Convalescent plasma has been used in more than 150,000 patients despite recommendations by the NIH that its use should be limited to randomized controlled trials, and now the possibility that its indiscriminate use could add more selective pressure on the virus and hasten the day when vaccines become less effective.

Diagnostic Tests

The national diagnostic testing capability remains precarious. To date, the focus has been on managing the supply chain, but the challenges are much broader than that. There is a myriad of diagnostic testing technologies available, but we still lack a national diagnostic testing strategy that can help guide clinical and public health practice.

For example, there is little agreement on the preferred and alternative methods for diagnosing or screening an individual suspected of having COVID-19, and ways to link test results to actionable public health measures (e.g., isolation, quarantine, and contact tracing). We still do not know the optimal strategies for deploying testing programs to workplaces or educational settings, or for screening travelers leaving or coming into the United States.

In addition, there is tremendous confusion about the approach FDA is taking to facilitate access to appropriate tests, while ensuring that tests perform to a minimal standard. In my view, FDA has taken a reasonable and flexible approach to regulating diagnostic and screening tests. At the end of the day, FDA needs some data to allow manufacturers to make certain claims about their tests. These data requirements are not onerous and test developers that want to make their tests available to consumers should embrace the responsibility of properly validating them.

The last administration hurt the American public when it declared that FDA did not have the authority to regulate laboratory-developed tests. Once it became clear that developers of these types of tests wanted to have liability protections available under the EUA framework, HHS directed FDA to review these tests. FDA rightfully resisted since its staff is stretched to the limit and need to focus their work on tests that have the greatest public health impact. HHS then decided to outsource FDA's review to a private company, which may have the expertise but does not have all of the information necessary for an adequate review or the same robust systems to manage conflicts of interest that are in place for federal employees. It is essential for the new administration to undo the prior administration's attempt to privatize the review of diagnostic tests.

Data Infrastructure

The U.S. still lacks an interoperable data infrastructure to capture the results of diagnostic tests conducted by so many disparate entities in so many disparate settings. Our data systems are simply not connected despite the existence of technical standards to do so. Even within states, each county sometimes runs their own program. Federal coordination, and in some cases, mandatory provider participation will be required. I would argue that this should be one of the principal areas of attention if we are to build a 21st century public health system.

Supply Chain

Our supply chain remains vulnerable. I am encouraged by the new administration's initial steps to secure the supply chain of critical materials. However, the path ahead is complex. Using the Defense Production Act will help but will not take us far. Onshoring the production of all critical materials may not be possible, economically viable, or necessary. A secure and resilient supply chain is much like a balanced portfolio of investments. All options, including establishing interdependencies and redundancies, fostering regionalization, and applying novel technological solutions to creating materials de novo when needed, should be explored.

Future

Larry Brilliant, a renowned American physician and epidemiologist, once said "Outbreaks are inevitable. Epidemics are optional." Biological threats are not going away. As we continue to battle this pandemic, we must do so with an eye toward building the system that we need going forward. We must build a system that integrates the private sector and cutting-edge technology; acknowledges and values the critical role of public health in our collective well-being, health and economic security; and realizes that good governance is necessary to bring capabilities to fruition.

The actions that follow are necessary and within reach in the near or mid-term, but many will require support from Congress:

1. To ensure the ability to monitor viral evolution and spread, the CDC must immediately expand its genomic surveillance system and analytic capabilities in collaboration with private and academic laboratories. Currently, approximately 3,000 specimens are sequenced each week, out of 1.4 million positive tests. These efforts are principally led by a patchwork of academic, state and commercial laboratories rather than a formal, centralized, and coordinated national system.

2. To ensure Americans understand the necessity to wear masks, HHS, in collaboration with the Ad Council and others, must launch a national "Mask Up" communication campaign to achieve greater compliance with mask use. At the same time, the CDC should immediately make more specific mask recommendations to the public. Should we "double mask" by donning a fabric mask on top of a surgical mask? Should some people consider wearing a KN95 or N95 masks? Even in the absence of quality data, the CDC is best equipped to make judgements about relative benefits of the different strategies and guide us through these difficult choices. The U.S. Government should also issue a challenge for the development of protective, comfortable, and easy to use masks for the public.
3. To maximize the impact of testing and efficiently use finite testing resources, the CDC, in collaboration with the FDA, should develop a national testing strategy.
4. To save the greatest numbers of lives, mitigate against viral evolution, and help restore our economy, the Federal government must accelerate vaccination campaigns to shorten the time between vaccine production and delivery into people's arms. It must not waver in its commitment to reach hard to reach areas, to counter misinformation, and promote informed decisions by the public and health-care workers.
5. To make sure we are ready to pivot toward second generation vaccines, if needed, in light of new and emerging variants, HHS should develop the triggers that would direct vaccine manufacturers to scale up production of new candidates and plan for a vaccine program that incorporates additional vaccine candidates.
6. To ensure the U.S. has sufficient supplies for this and future pandemics, HHS should expand the industrial base for critical supplies required for medical countermeasures manufacturing and administration.
7. To ensure high quality vaccines are made available in low- and middle-income countries, the Federal government should develop a framework for contributing safe and effective vaccines internationally. America's scientific prowess and stringent regulatory standards have brought Americans high quality vaccines, in contrast to some very low efficacy vaccines produced elsewhere. If we do not act, these low-quality vaccines will dominate the world, which will not help individuals or pandemic containment, and may add selective pressure on the virus.
8. To accelerate development of potential therapies, the NIH should establish a national infrastructure for the conduct of simple, randomized clinical trials for infectious diseases that can be used during a crisis and in the interpandemic period to study infectious diseases and promising therapies quickly and efficiently. In addition, the NIH should immediately notify institutions that receive NIH funding that they must prioritize the nationally-coordinated ACTIV trials over smaller and independent trials at their respective institutions.
9. The Federal government needs to acknowledge the central role of the private sector in achieving national preparedness and engage with it in pandemic planning. Private laboratories should receive priority access to the tools needed to validate their tests at the onset of potential emergencies, on par with public health laboratories. An industrial base for diagnostics and vaccines manufacturing will be required. This base should be built with cutting-edge and flexible technology, adapt to innovations, and be of good value to the taxpayer.

10. The Federal government should reimagine the 21st century public health system. The CDC should not be simply the place where the best public health experts and best laboratories reside, who are called upon to backstop a gap at the State or local level. Rather, CDC should be a coordinating entity that establishes public health standards, interoperable data systems, and a fully integrated national system at every level.

Conclusion

I would like to acknowledge the role of Congress for providing the Federal government many laws that provide the executive branch many vital authorities and critical funding to perform its duties, such as the Project BioShield Act of 2004, the Pandemic and All-Hazards Preparedness Act of 2006, and its subsequent reauthorizations.

Unfortunately, we thought we were better prepared today than we were in 2001, but our systems did not stand up to the challenge of this pandemic. We must do better.

Finally, I would like to recognize the staff at the CDC, NIH, HHS, FEMA, the Department of Defense, and my former colleagues at the FDA, who I know continue to work around the clock to protect Americans from harm and from this epidemic. A better day will soon come upon us if we let science and American innovation lead the way.

Ms. ESHOO. Thank you, Dr. Borio.

I now would like to recognize Dr. Julie Morita. You are recognized for your 5 minutes of testimony. And please remember to unmute.

Statement of Julie Morita, M.D.

Dr. MORITA. Chairman Pallone, Ranking Member McMorris Rodgers, Chairman Eshoo, Ranking Member Guthrie, and members of the subcommittee, thank you for this opportunity to testify. My name is Julie Morita, and I am the executive vice president of the Robert Wood Johnson Foundation, the Nation's largest health philanthropy, and I served on the COVID–19 transition advisory board in my personal capacity. Previously, I served as commissioner and chief medical officer of the Chicago Department of Public Health, an epidemic intelligence service officer at the Centers for Disease Control and Prevention, and a member of the CDC's Advisory Committee on Immunization Practices.

Our foundation believes that everyone deserves a fair and just opportunity to live the healthiest life possible. The pandemic, with more than 26 million Americans infected and 440,000 lives lost, illustrates the critical nature of our mission.

Vaccines offer real hope to eventually end the pandemic, but we must improve distribution by adhering to three fundamental principles: equity, accessibility, and coordination.

We must begin with equity. People and communities of color are disproportionately impacted by COVID–19. These populations historically and currently face discrimination, marginalization, and neglect. As a result, they are more likely to be denied basic necessities, like a living wage, health insurance, and paid leave.

The CDC recommends that frontline and essential workers, predominantly people of color, be among those prioritized for vaccination due to high exposure risk. But today, the country is consumed with total allotments and weekly averages instead of whether shots are getting in the right arms.

We must course correct quickly. Our foundation believes an equitable response to the pandemic starts with collecting and reporting all COVID–19-related data by race, ethnicity, and other socio-economic factors. Yet most States do not publish vaccine data that includes race and ethnicity. Among States that do, the share of vaccinations among Black people lags behind the share of cases and deaths.

We can no longer accept the systemic racism that drives these disparities. Congress and the administration should encourage and enable all States to vaccinate priority populations first and to report vaccine by race, ethnicity, occupation, and neighborhood.

Second, we must increase accessibility. Vaccines are only as effective as people's ability to obtain them and willingness to take them.

Across our Nation, those with means and privilege are increasingly getting vaccinated before those with highest exposure risks. Necessities that some may take for granted—an internet connection to make an appointment online, a car to drive to a large-scale vaccination site, the time that it takes to navigate complex systems—are unaffordable for millions.

A fairer approach simplifies appointment systems and brings vaccines directly to priority populations. In Chicago, during the H1N1 pandemic, we partnered with pharmacies and federally qualified community health centers that provided care to the uninsured in neighborhoods with less access to healthcare providers. More than 700 locations in Chicago ultimately received more than 1 million H1N1 vaccines during a critical 12-week stretch.

We also established meaningful connections with trusted community partners to address vaccine hesitancy, which remains an issue today. More than one-quarter of Americans report they will not or likely will not get a COVID vaccine. Notably, hesitancy rises to 1 in 3 among rural residents, Black adults, and essential workers.

Community groups, faith organizations, and other neighborhood pillars of trust play a pivotal role in helping people make appointments and understanding and addressing their concerns. Our foundation is providing grant support to State and territorial health officials and community organizations to address vaccine hesitancy. As we await additional doses, funding and supporting critical and local efforts will help us move to vaccine confidence and equitable distribution.

Third, the incredible complexity and urgency of this vaccine rollout requires coordination and illustrates the unique role of the Federal Government.

I am proud of how Chicago handled H1N1, but we didn't do it alone. CDC's clear guidance, additional funding, and technical assistance were invaluable. Without that support, our vaccine rollout would not have been as successful.

I am encouraged that the current administration, particularly Dr. Rochelle Walensky, the new CDC Director, is committed to improving coordination at the Federal level. Open lines of communication, increased transparency, such as more specific, accurate, and timely estimates of State allotments of vaccine, and ramping up our public health workforce, will all help State and local health officials perform their heroic work.

In conclusion, the Robert Wood Johnson Foundation is invested in creating a more equitable Nation during this pandemic and beyond. In the short term, America's ability to weather this crisis will require wearing masks, social distancing, washing hands, and additional support from Congress to help those hit hardest. Vaccines will eventually lead us to this pandemic's end, but saving the greatest number of lives will require a recommitment from all of us to equity, accessibility, and coordination in vaccine distribution in all facets of our response.

Thank you. I look forward to your questions.

Hearing Testimony, Julie Morita, MD, Executive Vice President, Robert Wood Johnson Foundation, U.S. House of Representatives, Committee on Energy and Commerce, Subcommittee on Health, "Road to Recovery: Ramping up COVID-19 Vaccines, Testing, and Medical Supply Chain," February 3, 2021

Chairman Pallone, Ranking Member McMorris Rodgers, Chairwoman Eshoo, Ranking Member Guthrie, and Members of the subcommittee:

Thank you for the opportunity to testify. My name is Julie Morita. I am the executive vice president of the Robert Wood Johnson Foundation, the nation's largest health philanthropy, and I served on the COVID-19 Transition Advisory Board in my personal capacity. Previously, I served as: commissioner and chief medical officer of the Chicago Department of Public Health; an Epidemic Intelligence Service officer at the Centers for Disease Control and Prevention; and a member of the CDC's Advisory Committee on Immunization Practices.

Our Foundation believes everyone deserves a fair and just opportunity to live the healthiest lif e possible. The pandemic—with more than 26 million Americans infected and 440,000 lives lost— illustrates the critical nature of our mission.

Vaccines offer real hope to eventually end the pandemic, but we must improve distribution by adhering to three fundamental principles: equity, accessibility, and coordination.

Equity

We must begin with equity. People and communities of color are disproportionately impacted by COVID-19. These populations historically and currently face discrimination, marginalization, and neglect. As a result, they are more likely to be denied basic necessities like a living wage, health insurance, and paid leave.

The CDC recommends that f rontline and essential workers—predominantly people of color—be among those prioritized for vaccination due to high exposure risk. But today the country is consumed with total allotments and weekly averages instead of whether shots are getting in the right arms.

We must course correct quickly. Our Foundation believes an equitable response to the pandemic starts with collecting and reporting all COVID-19-related data by race, ethnicity, and socioeconomic factors. Yet most states do not publish vaccine data that includes race and ethnicity. Among states that do, the share of vaccinations among Black people lags behind their share of cases and deaths.

We can no longer accept the systemic racism that drives these disparities. Congress and the administration should encourage and enable all states to vaccinate priority populations f irst and to report vaccine data by race, ethnicity, occupation, and neighborhood.

Accessibility

Second, we must increase accessibility. Vaccines are only as effective as people's ability to obtain them and willingness to take them.

Across our nation, those with means and privilege are increasingly getting vaccinated before those with the highest exposure risk. Necessities that some may take for granted —an Internet connection to make an appointment online; a car to drive to a large-scale vaccination site; the time it takes to navigate complex systems—are unaffordable for millions.

A fairer approach simplifies appointment systems and brings vaccines directly to priority populations. In Chicago, during the H1N1 pandemic, we partnered with pharmacies and federally qualified community health centers that provided care to the uninsured in neighborhoods with less access to healthcare providers. More than 700 locations in Chicago ultimately received more than one million H1N1 vaccines during a critical 12-week stretch.

We also established meaningful connections with trusted community partners to address v accine hesitancy, which remains an issue today. More than one-quarter of Americans report they will not or likely will not get a COVID-19 vaccine. Notably, hesitancy rises to 1 in 3 among rural residents, Black adults, and essential workers.

Community groups, faith organizations, and other neighborhood pillars of trust play a pivotal role in helping people make appointments and understanding and add ressing their concerns. Our Foundation is providing grant support to state and territorial health officials and community organizations to address vaccine hesitancy. As we await additional doses, funding and supporting critical local efforts will help us move to vaccine confidence and equitable distribution.

Coordination

Third, the incredible complexity and urgency of this vaccine rollout requires coordination and illustrates the unique role of the federal government.

I'm proud of how Chicago handled H1N1, but we did not do it alone. CDC's clear guidance, additional funding, and technical assistance were invaluable. Without that support, our vaccine rollout would not have been as successful.

I'm encouraged that the administration—particularly Dr. Rochelle Walensky, the new CDC director— is committed to improving coordination at the federal level. Open lines of communication, increased transparency—such as more specific, accurate, and timely estimates of state allotments of vaccines—and ramping up our public health workforce will all help state and local health officials perform their heroic work.

Conclusion

The Robert Wood Johnson Foundation is invested in creating a more equitable nation during this pandemic and beyond. In the short-term, America's ability to weather this crisis will require wearing masks, social distancing, washing hands, and additional support from Congress to help those hit hardest. Vaccines will eventually lead us to this pandemic's end, but saving the greatest number of lives will require a recommitment f rom all us to equity, accessibility, and coordination in vaccine distribution and all facets of our response.

Thank you. I look forward to your questions.

Testimony Addendum, Julie Morita, MD, Executive Vice President, Robert Wood Johnson Foundation, U.S. House of Representatives, Committee on Energy and Commerce, Subcommittee on Health, "Road to Recovery: Ramping up COVID-19 Vaccines, Testing, and Medical Supply Chain," February 3, 2021

I respectfully request the following resources be submitted for the hearing record. These resources are either directly funded or supported by the Robert Wood Johnson Foundation or partners working in the public health and health equity space. A description of each resource and a link to the source follows.

Research

Anticipating COVID-19 Vaccination Challenges through Flu Vaccination Patterns
The State Health Access Data Assistance Center released a brief examining flu vaccination rates as the closest possible analog to understanding how the implementation of a widespread coronavirus vaccination campaign will unfold. Key findings f rom the brief indicate that current flu vaccination rates fall far short of the needed targets to reach COVID-19 herd immunity goals not only among the overall population, but also across all subgroups, even those with the highest reported vaccinations (adults age 65 and older), and that vaccinating a sufficient share of the uninsured may pose serious challenges.

COVID-19 and the Experiences of Populations at Greater Risk
The COVID-19 and the Experiences of Populations at Greater Risk survey is a national poll measuring attitudes, views, and values toward health, equity, civic engagement, and systemic racism during COVID-19. Funded by the Robert Wood Johnson Foundation and conducted by the non-profit RAND Corporation, the survey found that less than half (42%) of respondents believe that systemic racism is one of the main reasons people of color have poorer health outcomes, despite well-documented racial health disparities. Black respondents are much more likely than white respondents to believe that systemic racism affects the health of people of color.

Ensuring Access to the COVID-19 Vaccine for Adult Medicaid Enrollees: A Roadmap for States
The State Health Access Data Assistance Center released a roadmap for states to assess their vaccine coverage policies in Medicaid, and, if necessary, to close any coverage gaps that might otherwise inhibit vaccine uptake during a crucial period of mass immunization.

Ensuring Equity: State Strategies for Monitoring COVID-19 Vaccination Rates by Race and Other Priority Populations

The State Health Access Data Assistance Center released an interactive map examining which states publicly report vaccine distribution by age, gender, race/ethnicity, provider type, and location (state vs. county). This data will help states break down and address inequities to ensure that those populations most affected by COVID-19 are able to receive equitable access to vaccines. The State Health Access Data Assistance Center also includes recommendations for states on collecting information about future COVID -19 vaccine administrations via survey data.

For Most Workers, the Latest COVID-19 Vaccine Developments Won't Mean Protection Just Yet

New research f rom the Urban Institute reveals that 57 million essential workers and workers in nonessential industries, many of whom must work in close proximity to others, will not receive the COVID-19 vaccine until production increases. Researchers at the Urban Institute detailed three steps communities and states can take now to protect these workers and reduce community transmission rates.

How Risk of Exposure to the Coronavirus at Work Varies by Race and Ethnicity and How to Protect the Health and Well-Being of Workers and Their Families

Researchers from the Urban Institute found that Black, Native American, and Hispanic/Latinx workers were more likely than white workers to have jobs that placed them at greater risk of exposure to and transmission of the coronavirus. They also found that Black, Native American, and Hispanic/Latinx workers who must work in person and close to others have lower incomes than white workers in these jobs and are less likely to have health insurance.

The Impact of Coronavirus on Households across America

"The Impact of Coronavirus" poll series offers a national look at the problems emerging f rom the pandemic relating to household finances, jobs, health care, housing, transportation, caregiving, and well-being. Researchers interviewed 3,454 adults aged 18 or older across the United States. The series includes five reports examining: the impact nationwide, in four major cities, by race and ethnicity, in households with children, and in households in rural America. Some key f indings include: at least 4 in 10 Latino, Black, and Native American households report using up all or most of their household savings during this time; more than 1 in 3 (36%) households with children face serious problems keeping their children's education going; and, 43 percent of rural households report any adult household members have lost their jobs, been furloughed, or had wages or hours reduced since the start of the outbreak.

Pandemics and Health Equity: Lessons Learned from the H1N1 Response in Los Angeles County

An article in the journal of Public Health Management Practice, authored by Alonzo Plough, chief science officer, Robert Wood Johnson Foundation, focuses on the low demand and uptake of the H1N1 vaccine among African Americans in Los Angeles and makes the case that this was not unique to that city. The f indings suggest that a national race/ethnicity reporting requirement may enhance early identification of health inequities in public health emergency response.

Preemption, Public Health, and Equity in the Time of COVID-19
As governments seek to address the myriad health, social, and economic consequences of COVID -19, an effective response requires coordination between state and local governments. This paper highlights how local leaders need f lexibility and authority to respond to COVID-19 in ways that ref lect local conditions—whether regarding stay-at-home orders, limits on gatherings, or the use of masks. However, there is a concerted effort to pass state laws that limit the ability of local leaders to protect their communities.

Resources

Advancing Equity in the Nation's COVID-19 Public Health Response and Recovery: Options for a New Administration
The George Washington University and the Georgia Health Policy Center released a paper which identifies the services that are essential to an equity -centric approach to the COVID-19 pandemic, as well as the infrastructure and workforce needed to ensure these services are available and have an equity focus. It reviews a set of administrative and legislative steps that the new presidential administration can take to strengthen the immediate response to the pandemic and address the long-term health and social needs the pandemic has exacerbated.

Finally, it offers a strategy for "building back better" in the long term.

ASTHO Bounce Forward
The Bounce Forward initiative helps state public health leadership to advance equity by applying the lessons learned f rom the COVID-19 pandemic, specifically leveraging investments made during COVID-19 to support communities and address equity within the following areas: housing and the built environment; food systems and nutrition; children, families, and social supports; employment and economic security; education (K-12); and health care access.

Center for Strategic and International Studies Panel on Vaccine Confidence and Misinformation
CSIS released a series of recommendations to build trust and confidence in COVID-19 vaccines including the rapid launch of an independent panel on vaccines and misinformation; innovations in reaching diverse and underserved populations with vaccines and other health and social services support; pledges and actions by mainstream media to improve the information climate related to vaccines; great activism by key social and economic sectors; and federal reform.

COVID-19 Equitable Testing Strategy
This strategy, created by Harris County Public Health in partnership with NACCHO, describes equitable testing approaches that are necessary to ensure quality testing services are available, accessible, and utilized by people and places at highest risk for severe health outcomes f rom

COVID-19. For COVID-19's holistic equity solutions, HCPH created the T3 REO equity strategy (Testing, Contact Tracing; Vaccines and other Treatment; Health Supportive Resources; and Community Engagement and Outreach).

Diversity Data Kids & The Child Opportunity Index

The Childhood Opportunity Index measures and maps the quality of resources and conditions that matter for children to develop in a healthy way in the neighborhoods where they live. Dolores Acevedo -Garcia, PhD, project director, has highlighted the impact of the COVID-19 pandemic on children and neighborhoods. Acevedo-Garcia notes that while children are less likely than adults to become ill with COVID -19, the impacts of the pandemic on children will be deep and long lasting. As it has with adults, COVID -19 will disproportionately hurt minority children, because we went into this crisis with very serious, long-standing inequities and higher vulnerability among Black, Hispanic, and Native American children.

Both the health and the economic implications of COVID-19 are affecting and will continue to affect minority children disproportionately.

Language of Vaccine Acceptance Poll and Vaccine Communication Tips

The de Beaumont Foundation and Frank Luntz—in partnership with the American Public Health Association, the National Collaborative for Health Equity, and Resolve to Save Lives—conducted a nationwide poll in December 2020 which found that rural Americans, young Republicans, young Black Americans, and young women are among the least likely to get vaccinated. The poll revealed the urgent need for political and health leaders to adjust their messaging to improve confidence in COVID -19 vaccines.

National Immigration Law Center's Resources Related to the COVID-19 Crisis and Consequences

The National Immigration Law Center has released a series of resources to help immigrant communities understand their rights, the assistance they qualify for, access to testing and treatment, and other resources to keep immigrant families safe and healthy.

US COVID Atlas

The US COVID Atlas is an interactive, open-source data visualization tool connecting near real-time COVID-19 case, testing, and vaccination data with community indicators across U.S. counties and states. Updated daily, the Atlas shows how the virus has spread since the start of the pandemic including historical, persistent, and emerging statistical hotspots. It now also includes state-level vaccination data, as well as customizable features highlighting the impact of the pandemic on vulnerable communities.

Opinion Pieces

America's Last Line of Defense for a Safe Vaccine

Co-authored by Julie Morita and Edward Belongia, this piece highlighted the importance of independent, expert advisory committees the FDA and the CDC rely on to ensure the approval and distribution of vaccines that are safe and effective. "If, in the days ahead, either of these independent bodies are sidelined, ignored or in any way circumvented, a red line will have been crossed, and the safety and/or efficacy of a coronavirus vaccine can reasonably be questioned" *(Scientific American, 10/19/20).*

Pressure Won't Build Vaccine Trust

Richard Besser, president & CEO, Robert Wood Johnson Foundation, asserted that in order to move from vaccine hesitancy to vaccine acceptance the country must patiently and deliberately engage with tens of millions of Americans who have real questions and concerns about the coronavirus vaccine *(ABCNews.com, 12/13/20).*

We Need a Vaccine Distribution Plan—Right Now

Julie Morita asserted that "the federal government must enable the CDC to take the lead in coordinating the nation's COVID -19 vaccine planning. Without swift action and federal funding, existing health inequities will play out again in the distribution and uptake of a potential vaccine" *(CNN, 8/16/20).*

Ms. ESHOO. Thank you, Dr. Morita.

Next, I would like to recognize Governor Michael Leavitt. You are recognized for your 5 minutes, and we thank you for your willingness to be a witness today. Welcome to our subcommittee. And please unmute. We want to hear every word you have to say.

Statement of Michael Leavitt

Mr. LEAVITT. Well, thank you to all of the committee.

This hearing is about looking ahead. The summation of the submitted testimony that I provided can be expressed in a simple phrase: "Scout the next valley." Explorers and others that navigated new territories always sent scouts ahead to help them anticipate the problems. In a pandemic, surprises are just an inherent condition, but we should not be surprised by the fact that, in every phase of this pandemic, there are new challenges.

So today I would like to talk a bit not about the next pandemic, I think we need to focus now on what we should be doing next in this pandemic. What should we be prepared for 3 to 6 months from now? What problems will we likely face 6 to 9 months from now? My submitted testimony lists 11 categories that we need to be planning today for predictable near-term problems. In the 5 minutes I am allocated today, I would like to focus on just one: the need to develop an open source vendor-agnostic digital vaccination and testing credential.

Here is the problem: Of course, we have vaccines and we celebrate that. We are moving with increasing haste to distribute them, and it is happening at an increasing velocity. There is great anticipation this is going to bring down transmission rates and the disease prevalence will fall. But vaccines are, of course, voluntary. Many people are still reluctant. There are still risks even after vaccination.

Inevitably, to open up the economy and to get back to what we consider to be normal, we are going to need to have many parts of our economy adopt a strategy of requiring some form of proof of vaccination as an entrance requirement. Now, dozens of efforts are underway right now by large companies and small enterprises that are building the killer app that would allow people to authenticate their status as a person who has been vaccinated. All of them assume that there is a trusted source of truth on who has been vaccinated, and who has not.

Today, my message is that it does not exist. Let me repeat that: It does not exist. Unless action is taken very quickly, this is going to be a mess. This is a valley we need to scout now, or it is going to present substantial delay in the fulfillment of the need and the promise of vaccines.

Now, we have made this mistake before. While I was Secretary of Health, I was dealing with electronic medical records, the fact that there were 200 different standards, and we couldn't connect up and talk—the computers could not talk to each other. We have seen it in banking. I remember the day when you would walk into an airport and there would be nine ATM machines, and you had to take your card and match up which one would fit into that system. We can't make that mistake again. Consumers need an easy means of voluntarily demonstrating their vaccination status.

Now, to be clear, I am not arguing here about mandatory vaccination. I am saying that consumers are going to need access to their own vaccination records. Yes, they have a card, and they will find that useful. But they are going to need access to their records digitally and on paper. Let's be candid: Paper records are simply not going to be adequate.

Every State has an immunization information system, and that is good, but every vaccination is not being reported, and they need to be.

More importantly, every State should be participating in the CDC/APHL IZ Gateway. Let me explain. HHS developed a technology called the IZ Gateway, which allows State jurisdictions to share vaccination information. This enables individuals and provides access to vaccination information from any jurisdiction in the country. Here is the problem: Unfortunately, only about half the jurisdictions—there are 64 in total, but about half of them are participating in the IZ Gateway. Without that data, such a system of being able to get our economy going based on the existence of validated, trusted records of who is vaccinated will not exist.

If the committee wants a way to scout the next valley, you should include in the next stimulus bill a requirement for States that give Federal vaccine to participate in the IZ Gateway and to ensure that every vaccine that is administered gets reported to the States through their IIS system and allows consumers the ability to access their own vaccination records.

In my remaining time, I will just list a couple of the other areas that have been—that I will add emphasis to. Others have mentioned them, that is, the increased worry of supply chains on syringes and vials and drug ingredients, and so forth.

Madam Chairman, I think my time is up. I will stop. I look forward to the questions.

U.S. House Energy and Commerce Health Subcommittee Hearing, "Road to Recovery: Ramping up COVID-19 Vaccines, Testing, and Medical Supply Chain," February 3, 2021, Governor Michael O. Leavitt, Former U.S. Secretary of Health and Human Services, Salt Lake City, Utah, "Scouting the Next Valley: Preparing for the Next Phase of the COVID-19 Pandemic"

Good Morning, Chairwoman Eshoo, Ranking Member Guthrie, and Members of the Health Subcommittee.

Thank you for the invitation to appear before the Health Subcommittee. The topic of this hearing is of great importance to me personally and to the nation.

As I begin, I want to acknowledge the sobering milestones we recently marked: more than a year into our COVID-19 public health emergency and more than 400,000 Americans lost to this novel virus.

- To the families who have lost loved ones, I convey my greatest sympathies to you.
- To my fellow Americans who have suffered loss of income or job, I empathize with you and hope you are able to use your time and talents professionally again soon.
- To all the heroes in the public and private sectors who have helped us respond to this health emergency, combat the virus, and keep essential businesses open to serve our communities, thank you for your work. We are indebted to you.

This pandemic has affected each one of us in profound and different ways. As the pandemic grinds on, we acknowledge the accumulating toll it places on our friends, families, neighbors, and communities.

That is why the committee is holding this hearing today, even as we seek to assess where we are and to plan for the months and yearsahead. Already, this committee has shown bipartisan leadership in enacting legislation to provide authorities and resources to address the health and economic challenges faced by our country. But we know more needs to be done. We know the months ahead are full of both promise and peril; they hold both hope and hardship.

As we look at the road ahead and what the future of the pandemic holds, I want to share with the committee a leadership framework I call "scouting the next valley." After explaining this framework, I will provide specific recommendations on how we can apply this framework to the current COVID-19 pandemic.

Pandemic Response Requires Strategically "Scouting the Next Valley"

Let me begin by sharing a useful framing concept for how to approach the activities needed for a more adequate pandemic response: the idea is *scouting the next valley*. In exploring new challenging terrain, an essential task for leaders seeking to lead people safely along a journey is to look ahead – not merely to seek the flattest or smoothest terrain, but to assess the potential threats and environmental conditions along the way that can impede progress.

The charge of federal policymakers in pandemic response is to *scout the next valley* – anticipating dangers, developing contingencies, and adopting strategies to mitigate potential threats. While the committee is not tasked with the operational response to the pandemic, you have a critical role to play. Members can help us all learn from past errors or missed opportunities, to understand all the current developments, and to help prepare for the challenges ahead. Members occupy a vitally important role by providing resources and authorities, asking questions, and helping hold accountable the agencies leading the response. Members have the opportunity and the obligation to hear from stakeholders and the private sector as the response is ongoing.

One perspective to emphasize with you is that the road to recovery is a winding one and will likely take much longer than any of us anticipated. From studying the history of pandemics, it is important to say that we should view our response as not just a "this-year" effort but along a multiple-year horizon. Even once we as a country achieve widespread vaccination for COVID-19, we must anticipate that the virus will continue to circulate and evolve. Thus, the pattern of changing course in our response needs to be "par for the course," as we seek to also evolve our response and stay ahead of developments.

To help inform your efforts, I offer you my current assessment of issues I see in the next three to six months or six to nine months that are important for planning. As you would expect, there is more granularity in the near term while the broad outlines of looming challenges further out on the horizon are also included.

Scouting the Next Valley for COVID-19 – Issues and Recommendations

Developing an Open-Source Vendor-Agnostic Digital Vaccination and Testing Credential

Many workers, contractors, small businesses, and large business have been hit very hard by the economic fallout related to the pandemic. As more Americans get vaccinated and testing becomes a built-in expectation in certain sectors of the economy, one way to foster our recovery is to enable individuals to voluntarily, digitally have secure and trusted access to their testing and vaccination information. Giving consumers an easy means of voluntarily demonstrating their vaccination status could help encourage vaccination at a popular level, especially to the extent business leaders in the future require some verification of vaccination and testing to enable sites like football stadiums and theaters to have larger numbers of in-person patrons once again. To help foster the ability for private sector business and consumer interests to make this attractive, we need to remove the barriers to making digital access to an individual's vaccination information a reality. To advance this idea, we need to prioritize supporting efforts that are open-source and vendor-agnostic. We have all seen the challenges in how proprietary approaches in electronic health records slowed the progress of interoperable medical records. It literally took an act of Congress that originated in this committee to prevent information blocking.

- *All vaccinations should be reported to the state Immunization Information Systems.* Vaccinations are being administered both by traditional health care entities and by nontraditional ones. Currently, there is no national vaccination registry that includes personally identifiable information, nor should there be. Public health is administered at a state and local level and that should continue. The challenge is, depending on the state, not every vaccine administration is necessarily reported to the state's vaccination database, which is called the Immunization Information System or IIS. In fact, there are several states that do not require everyone who administers a vaccine to report that information to a state Immunization Information System. Federal policy can incentivize and encourage a future state where individuals administering a vaccine report such information through the proper channels to their state IIS so there is a single, statewide trusted source that houses this information for consumers and others who voluntarily need to access it.

- *Consumers should have access to their immunization information from their state Immunization Information System.* Numerous states do not provide digital access to consumers so they can access their vaccination history from a state Immunization Information System. To ensure we can restart the economy and put more people back to work, Congress should encourage states to provide consumers with digital and paper-based access to this information through the state immunization information system. Federal funding associated with modernizing public health could be tied to enhancing state immunization information systems to allow consumers access to their vaccination history.
- *All states should participate in the CDC/APHL IZ Gateway.* Working in conjunction with the CDC and the Association of Public Health Laboratories, HHS developed a technology called an IZ Gateway, which allows cross-state jurisdictions to share vaccination information. This enables individuals and providers to access vaccination information from any jurisdiction in the country. Unfortunately, only about half of the jurisdictions (there are 64 total) are participating in the IZ Gateway today. I believe that to ensure individuals have dependable access to their complete vaccination history, all states and jurisdictions should be participating in the IZ Gateway. Congress can help encourage and incentivize that reality.

Strengthening Domestic Capacity to Rapidly Manufacture Vaccines after the Emergence of a Virus

Today, there are two COVID-19 vaccines authorized for emergency use by the FDA, with more promising vaccine candidates in the development pipeline. In addition to recognizing the countless efforts that have brought us this far, we should also recognize how fortunate we are to benefit from the unprecedented efficacy of the two approved vaccines. Reflecting on my time at HHS as the H5N1 avian flu emerged as a serious pandemic threat, I continue to be amazed at what seemed unthinkable just 15 years ago. Today, we have seen the development and manufacture, distribution and administration, and ongoing monitoring of a safe and effective, novel vaccine, all under the close and expert regulatory and scientific review of the federal government. The accomplishment is not without its challenges and imperfections, but it is worth remarking on. However, the ongoing scouting challenge for our country is to ensure that we maintain ample supply of the vaccine through the entire course of what may be a multi-year pandemic. Essential to that scouting will be open communication with manufacturers and stakeholders about their needs, to ensure that COVID vaccines and therapeutics remain available. That open communication must also apply, frankly, to non-COVID products. Each product category uses similar manufacturing, supply chains, and even components (such as caps, high-quality glass for syringes and vials, and drug ingredients). That communication should also be collaborative, looking to innovative and non-compulsory procurement tools, especially as we seek to ensure domestic production where feasible.

Pandemics evolve in part because viruses evolve. We are seeing that now as new strains of the virus appear to be more transmissible and thus more deadly. We urgently need to prioritize the development of resourced capacities at scale to analyze the genome of variants of the virus that causes COVID -19, so we can more quickly understand the ramifications of such variants and work to develop interventions to help mitigate the threat.

Anticipating the Potential Needs of Patients with "Long-COVID"

As Dr. Fauci explained last year in testimony before the Senate, "a number of individuals who virologically have recovered from [their COVID-19] infection, [who] in fact have persistence measured in weeks to months of symptomatology that does not appear to be due to persistence of the virus. They're referred to as long haulers." He explained that "they have fatigue, myalgia, fever, and involvement of the neurological system, as well as cognitive abnormalities, such as the inability to concentrate."[2] The CDC said, "persistent symptoms are being reported among COVID-19 survivors, including individuals who initially experience a mild acute illness," and cautioned that "these persistent symptoms pose new challenges to patients, healthcare providers, and public health practitioners."[3]

A few weeks ago, NIH Director Dr. Francis Collins wrote about these patients with "long-COVID." As Dr. Collins explained, "thousands of [people] who've gotten sick and survived COVID-19 are finding that a full recovery can be surprisingly elusive. Weeks and months after seemingly recovering from even mild cases of COVID-19, many battle a wide range of health problems."[4] Dr. Collins highlighted one study in which nearly half of respondents with ongoing symptoms from COVID-19 reported they "had to reduce their hours at work due to the severity of their symptoms," and "another 22 percent weren't working at all due to their Long COVID." Dr. Collins concluded, "while the number of people affected isn't yet known, if even a small proportion of the vast numbers of people infected with COVID-19 develop Long COVID syndrome, it represents a significant public health concern."[5]

Dr. Collins noted that in the appropriations health extenders bill enacted several weeks ago, Congress included funding "for NIH to support continued study of these prolonged health consequences." While research on long-COVID funded by NIH and others is ongoing, the committee should be aware of this growing cohort of patients. With jurisdiction over the ACA Marketplaces, Medicaid, the state Children's Health Insurance Program, and Medicare, the committee has a unique view of understanding to what extent these federal and state programs may be helping meet the needs of patients with "long-COVID."

Anticipating and Addressing the Barriers of Social Determinants of Health and Inequity

In a matter of months, we expect a greater supply of vaccine. Yet a crucial step toward recovery is not merely manufacturing vaccines but achieving widespread vaccination of the American people. As part of pandemic response, states and health systems will have a significant amount of work to do to ensure that minority communities, low-income individuals, rural residents, non-native English speakers, and others who face adverse social determinants of health (SDOH) are not left behind in this process.

While there is a long road ahead toward fundamentally tackling SDOH, for pandemic response today we should recognize that there will be people whose circumstances – such as not having a car, poor broadband access, or language barriers – may prevent them from signing up for a vaccine appointment or reaching a health care provider to receive their shot. There also may be people who are hesitant to take a vaccine. State public health officials, health care providers, and the federal government can all be planning now for how to educate,

[2] https://www.help.senate.gov/hearings/covid-19-an-update-on-the-federal-response.
[3] https://www.cdc.gov/coronavirus/2019-ncov/hcp/clinical-care/late-sequelae.html.
[4] https://directorsblog.nih.gov/2021/01/19/trying-to-make-sense-of-long-covid-syndrome/.
[5] https://directorsblog.nih.gov/2021/01/19/trying-to-make-sense-of-long-covid-syndrome/.

communicate with, and creatively provide access to these harder-to-reach populations to ensure they have the chance to be vaccinated.

While also taking longer to fully address, as part of the pandemic response, we must acknowledge the stubborn persistence of inequities in our health care systems and consider how these can be barriers to receiving care for many of our friends and neighbors. At a state and local level, leaders should look for partnerships and collaboration with community leaders and health care leaders to design and deploy strategies that seek to overcome inequities. We certainly will not get it right every time, but a recognition of the presence of these challenges is the necessary predicate for working to address them.

Resourcing and Sustaining Our Public Health Infrastructure

Public health is often a forgotten function of government, working quietly behind the scenes and not drawing attention to the part it plays when things are going well. But the COVID-19 pandemic has thrust public health into the spotlight, and it is now getting the attention it warrants since we are not likely to see full economic recovery until we have public health risks fully mitigated. We should seek this opportunity to invest in public health. In many cases, targeted upfront investments in public health modernization at the state and local levels can save the federal government money over time. For example, if state and local public health agencies had steady funding to maintain their capacity to trace contacts for emerging infectious diseases, well-trained personnel, IT infrastructure, and surge capacity, it would not be as great of a strain to respond to a pandemic or any other health emergency.

Resourcing and Sustaining Medical and Scientific Innovation

We are fortunate that because of scientific advancements, dedicated leadership, intense collaboration, and private and public sector investments in American innovation before and during the current health emergency, we now have multiple COVID vaccines available. We need to maintain investment in innovation – not only for vaccines against new strains that emerge, but investments in the kind of medical research that will help us better understand the virus that causes COVID-19. Beyond COVID-19, we should consider areas where scientific and medical limitations could metastasize into public health threats. One area in desperate need of fresh investment is antimicrobial resistance. The CDC has reported that more than 2.8 million antimicrobial resistant infections occur in the U.S. each year, and an estimated 35,000 Americans die as a result.[6] Unfortunately, as antimicrobial resistance accelerates, the problem could grow much worse because the pipeline of drugs to fight these infections is very thin. If an antimicrobial-resistant superbug were to cause the next pandemic, the U.S. would not have the ability to fight it like we did COVID-19.

Strengthening Our Commitment to Mental Health

As the COVID-19 pandemic continues into its second year, the mental health consequences caused by the pandemic have become painfully clear. Unfortunately, as the public health emergency continues, mental health needs will worsen.[7] There is much the federal government

[6] https://www.cdc.gov/drugresistance/biggest-threats.html#:~:text=According%20to%20the%20report%2C%20more,at%20least%2012%2C800%20people%20died.

[7] We see Americans' mental health needs growing in several ways. First, the public health emergency has disrupted and stressed the care delivery system of patients who, even before COVID-19, had mental health needs or mental illness. Second, as the CDC has noted, "public health actions, such as social distancing, are necessary to reduce

can do directly to help through existing health programs and authorities, as well as indirectly in its role as a collaborator and partner with states, grantees, the medical and mental health community, and the private sector. Clearly, reviewing federal tools and authorities to help to respond to these unprecedented demands in mental health needs is within the purview of the committee, and should be a priority area of focus.

In recent years, this committee has helped develop and enact important legislation to combat the opioid epidemic and ongoing substance abuse.[8] Given the growing scope of mental health needs this committee may have a key opportunity to reprise its policy leadership role and advance new bipartisan policy that could make targeted improvements in the federal government's response to widespread mental health needs. Some promising policy directions for your consideration might include:

- Improving the oversight of existing mental health parity requirements to ensure that the commitment made to patients under current law occurs in practice. Where workforce limitations make it challenging to effectuate parity, efforts to improve and strengthen the mental health community workforce could help ensure a sustainable supply for increased demand.
- Leveraging workforce funding such as loan forgiveness and repayment to help increase the availability of behavioral health experts, especially in settings of care for at-risk populations.
- Collecting and disseminating through a learning collaborative a wide array of evidence-based practices that providers, plans, patient advocates, and community-based organizations identify to link patients to care, ensure successful care coordination, leverage telehealth services, and improve access to quality peer supports.

Responding to the Challenges that Pandemic Presents to Medicare's Financing

The economic disruption resulting from the COVID-19 pandemic has further eroded Medicare's financing. That is because the pandemic resulted in depressed payroll tax collections compared to previous projections. These payroll tax collections comprise roughly 90 cents of every dollar in the Medicare Hospital Insurance (HI) Trust Fund – and this Fund in turn pays for items and services provided to Medicare beneficiaries in inpatient hospitals. In September, the Congressional Budget Office reported that "[t]he HI trust fund is projected to become exhausted in 2024, two years sooner than CBO estimated this past March. After the date of exhaustion, the Centers for Medicare & Medicaid Services (CMS) could not make payments in excess of the available receipts."[9] CBO explained that "the projections for deficits were revised upward in part because of the economic disruption stemming from the 2020 coronavirus pandemic, which reduced CBO's estimates of payroll tax revenues."

As we anticipate the challenges beyond the current COVID-19 public health crisis, there is an urgent need to focus on Medicare. Medicare beneficiaries are currently among the country's most vulnerable to the virus due to their age and health conditions. At the same time, thousands

---

the spread of COVID-19, but they can make us feel isolated and lonely and can increase stress and anxiety." Third, many Americans have lost income or job, lost a loved one or friend, lost their sense of security and safety, and they worry for the future.

[8] https://www.congress.gov/bill/114th-congress/senate-bill/524/text and https://www.congress.gov/bill/115th-congress/house-bill/6.

[9] https://www.cbo.gov/publication/56541.

of Medicare providers are serving tirelessly on the frontlines of health care delivery, battling the virus in order to save them. Given the committee's jurisdiction over Medicare and your interest in sustainable and strong access for beneficiaries during the pandemic and beyond, I believe this issue merits your thoughtful attention now. I believe remedying them is an important opportunity – not only for keeping our commitment to Medicare beneficiaries, but also for advancing value-based care and the role that value plays in our health care system.[10]

While 2024 may feel like a long way from now, we must acknowledge that we do not know how long this pandemic will persist, the precise course it will run, and the degree to which Medicare's financial outlook could even worsen. Adopting reasonable policies to address the financing gaps early on is a more prudent path than waiting for a more ideal time.[11] While this task requires collaboration and hard work, it is eminently doable. It was not that many years ago that this same committee achieved what was then thought unachievable by leading the Congressional effort to enact MACRA. I believe bipartisan collaboration and cooperation from this committee can again set the tone and pace for needed improvements.

Prioritizing Pandemic Preparedness on an Ongoing Basis

A frequent observation I have shared with many during the past year is that actions taken by federal and state policymakers before a pandemic often appear or sound alarmist, while much they do after a pandemic is already here may feel inadequate. Such is the nature of pandemic planning and response. We must acknowledge that pandemics are a fact of biology and human history. The very goal of preparedness is to recognize this fact and identify potential threats and responses before they happen.

While we cannot take our eye off the pandemic we are in, we must acknowledge the hard reality that additional pandemics will come, whether we are ready, and they will arrive on their own timeframe. Future pandemics could be more contagious or deadly than even this COVID-19 pandemic. Federal and state officials have a unique responsibility to prepare for pandemics, but they are not the only leaders who need to be prepared. Preparedness exercises must be done regularly at the federal, state, and local government levels, as well as by the private sector, communities, and families. In many places, these exercises are a standard practice already, and I think that they should become more widespread, more frequent, and should focus on known and unknown threats.

Assisting the Nation's Governors in Strengthening Medicaid's Response to the Pandemic

The collective footprint of the states' Medicaid programs will provide coverage and care to nearly 100 million Americans this year. Yet the economic effects of the pandemic have reduced the ability of states to resource their own programs, even as enrollment has increased due to the pandemic. Several Medicaid policy areas merit thoughtful review by engaging with governors and Medicaid stakeholders.

---

[10] https://leavittpartners.com/press/leavitt-partners-releases-medicare-drifting-toward-disaster-white-paper/.

[11] To get a sense of the growing gap between incoming revenue and projected outlays, consider what the Congressional Budget Office outlined in its report several months ago. In a hypothetical scenario without interventions in which the HI trust fund was allowed to reach insolvency and the fund's outlays were limited to its income, expenditures in 2025 would be 17 percent below the amounts scheduled under current law.

- *Giving State Medicaid Programs More Tools to Better Integrate Care for Dually Eligible Beneficiaries.* Of the more than 12 million individuals dually eligible for and enrolled in Medicare and Medicaid, many face challenges due to comorbidities, mental health conditions, or the social determinants of health.[12] The Medicaid and CHIP Payment and Access Commission has reported that "dually eligible beneficiaries are at particular risk during the COVID-19 pandemic due to their age and underlying medical conditions." Data released from CMS shows that dually eligible beneficiaries are at greater risk of hospitalization or mortality due to COVID-19 compared to other patient populations.[13] Yet, as MACPAC noted, "covering individuals under two programs can result in fragmented care and promote cost shifting instead of ensuring that beneficiaries receive services that best meet their needs." To help, the Committee should advance MACPAC's recommendation that Congress "provide additional federal funds to enhance state capacity to develop expertise in Medicare and to implement integrated care models." Modest federal investments in state Medicaid programs in this moment can help ensure states maintain the expert staff, information technology, and data capacity to enact needed reforms. Beyond this, the committee should consider the benefit of creating a new option for states that lets them leverage Medicare dollars under a shared savings model to offer a single integrated product to dually eligible beneficiaries while maintaining current benefits and protections.
- *Strengthening Home- and Community-Based Services.* There was bipartisan interest in increasing access to HBCS before the pandemic. Now, with a significant portion of fatalities from COVID-19 connected to institutional care settings during the pandemic, this topic feels even more timely. Going forward, exploring opportunities to increase the provision of HCBS by identifying and addressing complex and interconnected dynamics is an area of great potential.

Learning Continually by Scouting Valleys Beyond

As we have learned firsthand during the past year, pandemics are unpredictable. The thing about scouting the next valley is that, as the journey continues, there are valleys beyond the next valley. While the more distant future may feel abstract at times, blazing trails through new territory always requires looking ahead. This mean there will always be valleys to scout, so we must scout the next valley not just today, but on an ongoing basis. The lessons we learn now will provide important insights for how to fight both COVID and future pandemics. They will also offer insights on how we can address important health care issues outside of pandemics. One way to elicit these insights is to use the following framework of categories, which can help as we conduct our analysis now and as the pandemic continues:

- What we have learned during the last year that should inform how we handle the rest of this pandemic.
- What we are learning that should inform future pandemic preparedness.
- What we are learning that should inform how we do non-pandemic things (e.g., we have learned how to develop vaccines faster – consider how could we apply those learnings to antimicrobial resistance or possibly to brain diseases).

---

[12] https://www.macpac.gov/topics/dually-eligible-beneficiaries/.

[13] https://www.cms.gov/files/document/medicare-covid-19-data-snapshot-fact-sheet.pdf.

Applying this framework will help us capture important insights and employ them appropriately.

Conclusion

Scouting the next valley is a responsibility of leaders. As members of Congress and members of this committee, you have both a special opportunity and unique obligation in this moment of our national public health crisis to work together in this effort. I appreciate that this is not an easy task. Not only is the work of scouting usually unglamorous, but it is also often complex and sobering work.

But this work of looking ahead tobe prepared is as honorable as it is essential. As you undertake this work, you have my support and appreciation for your service to our country. Thank you for the opportunity to address this committee. I look forward to answering any questions you may have.

Ms. ESHOO. Thank you, Governor, very much. And we will follow up on the last point that you made with our questions.

Next, I would like to recognize Mr. Greg Burel for 5 minutes for his opening statement. And thank you again for being with us today.

Statement of Greg Burel

Mr. BUREL. Thank you.

Chairman Pallone, Ranking Member McMorris Rodgers, Chairwoman Eshoo, and Ranking Member Guthrie, members of the committee, thank you for the opportunity to testify today.

It was my privilege to serve as Director of the Strategic National Stockpile for almost 13 years until my retirement in January of 2020. I am now president of Hamilton Grace and am an elected fellow of the National Academy of Public Administration.

COVID–19 has exposed the fragility of our Nation's medical supply chain. It brought to the fore the vital need to consistently and properly resource our preparedness for health security threats. The most glaring supply chain problem was the inability to provide PPE due to political and geographic vulnerabilities. We must channel what we have learned into better policies to prevent this from ever happening again. We must simultaneously address today's response by preparing to meet future health security needs.

To address the fragile supply chain, we must invest in sustained domestic critical healthcare manufacturing. Without regular investment post-COVID–19, domestic manufacturing will wane again as the crisis abates and demand recedes while competition from lowcost foreign sources undercuts new domestic manufacturers. Continued domestic manufacturing is a national security imperative.

We find ourselves trying to successfully vaccinate our whole population. Rapid, mass delivery of medicine will always present challenges, but advanced preparedness investment, planning, and use of operating distribution systems will better facilitate the process. A successful government-led response must engage the whole commercial healthcare supply chain.

We must pivot from our long history of inconsistent, inadequate preparedness funding to long-term mandatory sustainable preparedness. How we drive those policy changes today will define our success in the future. We have witnessed the devastating effects of a lack of preparedness on our Nation's health. To respond now and lay the groundwork for future needs, I offer the following recommendations:

First, we must rely on our healthcare system to bring an end to this crisis. We must engage all commercial healthcare distributors and manufacturers. Vaccines are not readily and easily available at expected dispensing sites. Part of this is due to the shortage, but another part is due to the lack of distribution partnering engagement. A sole distributor cannot reach the full breadth of dispensing capability. This is especially a problem for those unable to spend hours online searching for available vaccines and navigating failing websites to register. It is particularly vexing for those without technology resources or abilities. This affects the most vulnerable of our citizens.

Second, we must clearly assign responsibilities to the appropriate entities. The SNS has long been the lead to acquire, manage, and deliver countermeasures to secure the Nation's public health in emergency. But SNS appears somehow to have been sidelined somewhat during this response. Other Federal departments have been assigned responsibilities SNS can lead effectively. As a result, success in buying and delivering the right products has been, at times, inconsistent. Engaging SNS expertise can make sure we get the right thing to the right place at the right time.

SNS needs significant increased appropriations if it is to be our bulwark against failing supplies of vital medical material in crises. Making such appropriations mandatory rather than discretionary would help achieve better preparedness.

Third, we know as a crisis abates, so does the urgency for sustaining their preparedness. We cannot continue to claim we are ready, only to act shocked when we find ourselves unprepared because we couldn't invest to meet the need. We must invest in purchasing domestic capacity or otherwise providing incentives for manufacturers to sustain domestic production and create greater material stocks. We must support and resource regulatory structures friendly to domestic manufacturing while always respecting the science that assures safe and effective products. These actions, along with using the existing distribution infrastructure, will help create flexibility in an otherwise lean supply chain that can cushion surging needs.

As the current crisis subsides, we must incentivize those manufacturers who now boldly enter a domestic market to continue consistent production. They must be incentivized to improve capability, plants, and machinery to achieve better quality and higher output. Establishment of an aggressive government investment platform driven by clear needs for critical products will allow us to use and develop and maintain this domestic base.

Finally, we must improve planning at all levels. At one time, SNS supported State, local, Tribal, and territorial officials with dedicated consultants. A return to linking the medical logistics professionals in SNS directly with these public health officials will assure strong preparedness planning.

Our path forward must incorporate elements of all of these considerations. We must unyieldingly fund health preparedness in the United States.

I look forward to your questions, and I always remain available to assist our Nation in these endeavors.

Opening Statement of Greg Burel, Committee on Energy & Commerce, February 3, 2021

Chairwoman Eshoo, Ranking Member Guthrie and members of the Committee, thank you for the opportunity to testify today. I had the privilege of serving as Director of the Strategic National Stockpile for almost 13 years until my retirement January 2020. I am now President of Hamilton Grace, LLC, and am an elected fellow of the National Academy of Public Administration.

COVID-19 has exposed the fragility of our nation's medical supply chain. It brought to the fore the vital need to consistently and properly resource our preparedness for health security threats. The most glaring supply chain problem was the inability to provide Personal Protective Equipment due to political and geographic vulnerabilities. We must channel what we have learned into better policies to prevent this from happening again. We must simultaneously address today's response while preparing to meet future health security needs.

To address the fragile supply chain, we must invest in sustained domestic critical healthcare manufacturing. Without regular investment post COVID-19 domestic manufacturing will wane again as the crisis abates and demand recedes while competition from low-cost foreign sources will undercut new domestic manufacturers. Continued domestic manufacturing is a national security imperative.

We find ourselves trying to successfully vaccinate our whole population. Rapid, mass delivery of medicine will always present challenges, but advanced preparedness investment, planning and use of operating distribution systems will better facilitate the process. Successful government led medical response must engage the whole commercial healthcare supply chain.

We must pivot from our long history of inconsistent, inadequate preparedness funding to long term mandatory sustainable preparedness. How we drive policy changes today will define our success or failure now and in future response. We have witnessed the devastating effects of lack of preparedness on our nation's health, our population's mortality, our economic status and thus, our overall national security. To respond now and lay the groundwork for future needs, I offer the following recommendations.

First, to rely on our healthcare system to help bring an end this crisis, we must engage all commercial healthcare distributors and manufacturers. Vaccines are not readily and easily available at expected dispensing sites. This is partially due to shortage but is also due to a lack of distribution partner engagement. A sole distributor cannot reach the full breadth of dispensing capability. This is especially a problem for those unable to spend hours online searching for available vaccines and navigating failing websites to register. It is a particularly vexing problem for those without technology resources or abilities, many of whom are our most vulnerable of citizens. Americans have learned to go to their trusted pharmacy or physician for vaccines but current distribution makes this nearly impossible.

Second, we must clearly assign responsibilities to the appropriate entities. The SNS has long been the lead to acquire, manage and deliver countermeasures to secure the civilian population's health in emergency, but SNS appears sidelined during this response. Other federal departments have been assigned responsibilities SNS should lead effectively. As a result, success in buying and delivering the right products has been at times inconsistent. Engaging SNS expertise can make sure we get the right thing to the right place at the right time.

SNS needs significant increased appropriations if it is to be our bulwark against failing supplies of vital medical material in crises. Making these appropriations mandatory rather than discretionary would help to achieve better preparedness.

Third, we know as a crisis abates so does the urgency for sustaining preparedness. We cannot continue to claim we are ready only to act shocked when we find ourselves unprepared because we couldn't afford to meet the need. We must invest in purchasing domestic capacity or otherwise providing incentives for manufacturers to sustain domestic production and create greater material stocks. We must support and resource a regulatory structure that is friendly to domestic manufacturing while respecting the science that assures safe and effective products. Emerging domestic manufacturers cannot bear long lead times for approvals while consuming investment funds that cannot offer a return. These actions will help create flexibility in an otherwise lean supply chain that can cushion surging needs.

As the current crisis subsides, we must incentivize those manufacturers who will boldly enter a domestic market to continue consistent production. We must incentivize them to improve capability, plants and machinery to achieve better quality and higher output. Establishment of an aggressive government investment platform driven by clear needs for critical products would allow the us to develop and maintain this domestic base.

Finally, we must improve planning for medical supply delivery and dispensing at all government levels and in the commercial sector. At one time, SNS supported state, local, tribal and territorial officials with dedicated "consultants" to assure plans were in place and staff knew how to manage material. A return to linking the medical logistics professionals in SNS directly with these public health officials will assure strong preparedness planning. The reported losses of precious vaccine doses that may have remained viable with better expert support, for example, in simply managing cold chain requirements is a prime example of needed improvement.

The path forward must incorporate elements of all these considerations, and include a stronger partnership between federal, SLTT and the commercial healthcare manufacturing and distribution sector. We must unyieldingly fund health preparedness in the United States.

I look forward to your questions and I remain available to assist the nation in these endeavors.

Ms. ESHOO. Thank you very much, Mr. Burel.

We now are going to move to Members' questions, and I recognize myself for 5 minutes for questions.

First, to—and, please, to the witnesses, know that each Member only has 5 minutes to ask the questions, get the answers. So let's all try to be as—you know, conserve time so that we can optimize it.

To Dr. Borio, the American Rescue Plan provides the resources needed to vaccinate the 300 million Americans by the end of this summer. How do the new mutant viruses affect the timeline, if they do, for this planned vaccine rollout? And what do we need to be doing today to be ready for that tomorrow and the days following?

Dr. BORIO. So, you know, in that short time, nothing really changes. The response remains, which is to decrease transmission of the virus through public health measures, intervention, and, importantly, vaccinations. So it is urgent that we get vaccine rolled out. Every dose that comes out of the manufacturing line should make it into somebody's arm as soon as possible.

Ms. ESHOO. Good.

Dr. BORIO. In the midterm, we do need to begin to be prepared in case we do need to manufacture on large scale the new candidates if there is a significant erosion in protection and revaccinate the population. We do not know right now if that will be necessary. We hope that it may not be.

And also, I would just add that we do believe that these vaccines will need to be boosted periodically, whether it is the original vaccines, modified vaccines. So we do need to build the industrial base and capacity, just like we do for flu vaccines. That is the current thinking.

Ms. ESHOO. Thank you very much.

To Dr. Morita, thank you again for joining us today. In just the first few weeks of vaccinations, Black Americans are receiving them at dramatically lower rates than White Americans. How do the increased resources from the new administration's plan help bring the vaccine to underserved communities? You spoke to this, to the issue and the problem and the inequities relative to the rates, so can you be instructive to us in terms of what needs to change and how those increased resources are going to change the rates that—the really shameful rates in our country?

Dr. MORITA. So you are right. In addition to the disproportionate impact on our communities of color in terms of disease, who is dying, who is hospitalized, what we are seeing is that there are lower rates of vaccination administration in our communities of color as well.

Things that can be done to improve that situation would be to really make sure that the sites that are vaccinating are located in the communities themselves, that the appointment processes are simplified so that people can use the telephone, they aren't just internet dependent, that there are community workers that are going into communities and actually helping people to register, whether it is online or by phone.

So what we have seen are the processes are challenging for people to actually access the vaccine. I, myself, am trying to get my 91-year-old dad an appointment and struggling through use of the internet. These processes themselves have to be simplified, and additional resources will help. Hire staff to actually do the community work. Simplify the stand-up phone so that people can actually make phone calls instead of just going online——

Ms. ESHOO. I just want to get one more question in, so we can follow up with more questions with you, and all Members can do that.

To Mr. Burel, on our Nation's national stockpile, it ran dry. And, as someone that worked with former Congresswoman Susan Brooks on preparedness and the stockpile, it was absolutely maddening to all of us what we experienced. When you were selecting contracts for the stockpile, did you weigh the country of origin versus the cost?

See, I think we should have an American stockpile. This business of being dependent on other countries—some of them who don't wish us well—I think was a national embarrassment. So what can you share quickly with us about this?

Mr. BUREL. Thank you for the question, Chairwoman Eshoo.

We followed all the appropriate procurement regulations in making our purchases.

Ms. ESHOO. What were they? Did we have Buy American only? Or was it first come, first served? Was it China? Others? I mean, it is——

Mr. BUREL. Sure. I appreciate the question.

Ms. ESHOO. Both sides of the aisle care about this. Mr. BUREL. Yes, ma'am, I understand.

What we did is we procured products under Buy American, where that is appropriate, and that is most products. Where there were products that were not manufactured in the United States, we purchased those from a U.S. vendor.

Ms. ESHOO. What is not manufactured in the United States relative to PPE?

Mr. BUREL. So much of the PPE we find is manufactured overseas, particularly N95 masks.

Ms. ESHOO. That is not true. We have a major American manufacturer for that.

I think I need to stop because I have gone over my time, but we are going to follow up with you with more questions.

Mr. BUREL. Thank you. Ms. ESHOO. Thank you, sir.

So the Chair now recognizes our new ranking member, Mr. Guthrie, for his 5 minutes of questions.

Mr. GUTHRIE. Thank you very much. Thank you, Madam Chair, I appreciate it.

And this is to all the panelists. So my question is—and I am not going to get back into why it was delayed—but we had two vaccines approved mid-December. Then we had $4.5 billion approved December the 27th for States to distribute the vaccines. Some States have been successful, some States haven't.

So looking forward, we are looking at, perhaps, doing it different ways. Do you think now that the States have had the money for a month that they are going to improve, or do you think we really need to restructure how we are distributing these vaccines currently? So we have some States successful, some aren't. The money came late. They now have it. Are we seeing improvements enough, or do we need to overhaul how we are getting these vaccines distributed and in arms of people, which we all want?

So I can start with—I can see Dr. Morita in my screen first, so I will just call on you, if that is OK.

Dr. MORITA. Thank you so much for your question. I really appreciate it.

So the challenges that we have experienced with the distribution are because of a lack of initial resources to support States and locals. As much money that went into Operation Warp Speed, which was an incredible process and incredible results with two vaccine being developed and manufactured so quickly, additional resources in equal amounts were needed to go to States and locals so that they could actually ramp up their systems. But they are playing catchup at this point. What we heard consistently during the transition period was that they didn't have enough resources to hire staff, to open up clinics, to actually do community work to improve understanding of the vaccine, to drive demand, enhance the electronic——

Ms. ESHOO. Excuse me. Dr. Morita, can you either maybe get closer to your microphone, speak a little louder? We don't want to miss a word you are saying.

Dr. MORITA. Sure.

Ms. ESHOO. And whatever time I have taken to say that you won't lose.

Dr. MORITA. Additional resources are necessary, so although things are improving, and I am thrilled to see how much the rate of administration is actually improving, additional resources are necessary so we can actually do this as quickly as possible.

What Dr. Borio mentioned in terms of the variants really gives us urgency in terms of the need to vaccinate as quickly as possible. And we can do it equitably if additional resources are made available so they can get in the community, help people sign up for the vaccines. Make sure those who need the vaccine the most are really able to access it as well.

Mr. GUTHRIE. OK. Thanks.

And to get to all of my questions, I am probably just going to jump next, but it is sort of the same thing for Governor Leavitt to touch on that, but also you mentioned in your testimony about Medicaid and how the—the competition with Medicaid and public health spending.

So as a former Governor, I mean, the money has now moved forward. I know they need additional resources. But could you kind of address my question, please, for Medicaid and public health spending issues as well?

Mr. LEAVITT. Well, we have allowed public health to go to seed over the last 25 or 30 years in this country. There are probably a lot of things that have contributed to that, but one of course has been the tension that States are under to deal with both Medicaid and public health. We can pursue that.

Could I just comment briefly on——

Mr. GUTHRIE. Yes.

Mr. LEAVITT [continuing]. The previous question?

I had the privilege of serving as HHS Secretary when we rolled out Medicare part D to 45 million people. That is not a challenge of doing vaccines to 300 million, but I learned something, I think, important, and that is we are going to get better at this. The first month, I am sure there are always going to be issues. The second month will be better. The third month will be better. If we were trying to give everyone in America a hamburger, we can get that done in 30 days because we have the infrastructure. Everyone knows how to do it, and people could go through the drive through and we would be finished. But the reality is we are standing up something entirely new, and we will get better at it. And it is a good thing, because we are going to likely be doing this for some time, well beyond this year.

Mr. GUTHRIE. Thank you.

And, Dr. Borio, just to kind of nuance that question, if you want to address that, you can. But I also have Kentucky BioProcessing in my district, and they are coming up with a new generation vaccine. They are telling me they are having trouble finding clinical trials because, as more people get vaccinated, there are not going to be the test populations, particularly placebo groups that they need. So could you talk about what HHS and BARDA must do to help development of the next generation vaccines?

Dr. BORIO. That is a really great point, because once you have a product that is authorized broadly and broadly available, it makes it more challenging for new products to come in and evaluate them with the same type of standards that we would have accepted for the first trial. So we do the randomized control trials. You may have heard in the news, for example, that a company, Novavax, are now doing studies in the U.S. Some of the older patients in that study are dropping out of the study to be able to get the authorized vaccines. So that is not an issue that is, you know, just to this company.

I know the FDA is working really hard to then develop, you know, more of the pathway forward for these companies. How can we show scientifically and that these products are indeed safe and effective if they are—you know, how to demonstrate that. And it may be that it will require a different type of trial than the original ones. And I know they are working hard at that.

It is possible that, you know, we be able to rely on immune markers to be able to establish the efficacy of these vaccines. I don't have the answers today, but hopefully soon.

Mr. GUTHRIE. Well, thank you very much. I see my time has expired. And sorry, Mr. Burel, but my time has expired.

I will yield back.

Ms. ESHOO. The gentleman yields back.

It is a pleasure to recognize the chairman of the full committee, Mr. Pallone, for his 5 minutes of questions.

Mr. PALLONE. Thank you. Thank you, Chairwoman Eshoo.

I just wanted to comment, I heard when our Ranking Member Rodgers in her opening statement mentioned how we have too much reliance on China and other countries and we needed to do more domestically, including manufacturing. I just want to say I totally agree with you on that, and that is certainly something that we need to continue to look at: you know, too much reliance on other countries, particularly China, for supplies, ingredients and that. And also that we need to prepare for future epidemics or pandemics. One of the things that was always done in our committee every year, including under Greg Walden and Mr. Upton when they were chairs, was an annual flu hearing. So we would always, like, prepare for the future, and that continues to need to be done.

But I, of course—with Mrs. Rodgers, I don't agree about her analysis of the Trump administration. I don't want to dwell on the past, but I think it is important to understand the message the Trump administration left behind. And one of the areas of concerns that we heard from States yesterday at the hearing was the lack of communications, lack of national preparations, guidance, and resources when it came time to roll out the vaccination program. And States were given a vaccine supply under Trump, but very few resources to carry out distribution.

Now, I know that, Dr. Morita, you talked about this, so I don't went to dwell on it, but give me a little more analysis, if you can quickly, about the lack of resources. And particularly, I don't know if you have seen or want to comment on Biden's American Rescue Plan, which we have put into legislation form, we are going to start the process today. How can we benefit from additional resources moving forward if we are going to meet President Biden's goal of vaccinating these 300 million people by summer or fall? I am only going to give you 30 seconds or a minute because I have to move on to testing.

Dr. MORITA. Sure thing. Thank you so much for your question.

In my past experience, whether it was H1N1, Zika, or Ebola, the best responses were those that were really coordinated at the Federal level, because the Federal agencies work so closely with State and local health officials. That kind of coordination is reflected in the American Rescue Plan, and we heard about it during the transition period as well as the planning was being developed. There is a strong commitment for there to be this coordination so that supplies are arriving appropriately, places that are doing well or recognized places that are struggling get the support and resources they actually need.

So this level of coordination that CDC and other Federal agencies can do is really, really critical. That and this clear and consistent communication regarding the science. So the science-based recommendations and guidance usually flow from CDC to State and locals were incredibly valuable. And that kind of issue, those guidances are already starting to flow, and the communication is much more consistent and regular. So we are really seeing signs that this can be a more coordinated and robust response moving forward. So those approaches are clear in the American Rescue Plan, but also in the strategy that was released the day after inauguration.

Mr. PALLONE. Well, thank you.

Now let met get to Dr. Borio. I want to emphasize the importance of our vigilance in testing and contact tracing in doing other mitigation activities. I don't think that vaccines alone are going to be enough to protect people as we continue to have outbreaks. So, Dr. Borio, as you noted in your testimony, the Federal Government never developed a comprehensive national testing strategy, despite the fact that we know one of the keys to controlling outbreaks relies on access to reliable diagnostic tests. And, of course, I was critical of the lack of a national strategy under President Trump.

So can you talk about the importance of national coordination in a testing strategy and the importance of providing resources to carry out mitigation such as contact tracing? Do you think—you know, tell us about additional national investments to increase testing. And if you want to comment on Biden's American Rescue Plan in that regard, I would appreciate it as well. You have only got 45 seconds.

Dr. BORIO. So, yes, just like a clinician, you know, has usually a menu of options to care for patients and which tests to use, public health practitioners also need the menu of options to be able to optimize the use of these finite supplies of testing. It is not an infinite supply, and there are strategies that are more effective than others. And we need Federal guidance for that.

With respect to contact tracing, it is very critical. We cannot do it without technology, I will say that. And to be able to have, you know, people—it is important, it is a critical aspect, but we are also going to have to need technology to be able to do it with a speed of which a pandemic requires. We need Federal coordination for that to develop the standard, the privacy standards, and to evaluate the effectiveness of these technologies that are just emerging. Other countries have deployed it. We need do it too.

Mr. PALLONE. Thank you so much.

And I yield back, Madam Chair. Thank you.

Ms. ESHOO. The gentleman yields back.

It is a pleasure to recognize the ranking member of the full committee, Congresswoman Cathy McMorris Rodgers.

Mrs. RODGERS. Thank you, Madam Chair. It is great to be with you.

And, Mr. Pallone, chairman of the committee, I just want you to know that the Republicans stand ready to go to work, to identify the gaps, and to work together to continue to address the needs around the pandemic. And we really appreciate the chance to talk with our witnesses today. Thank you all for taking the time to be with us.

I wanted just to start by asking each one of you: At the start of this pandemic, did any of you anticipate that we would have a safe and effective COVID–19 vaccine to distribute and administer only 10 months later? And if you would just answer yes or no, maybe beginning with Dr. Borio.

Dr. BORIO. Well, I'm an optimist, and I did. I did have deep hope. I wasn't 100 percent sure, but I have great confidence in, you know, the type of science that underpins the current technologies and also in our ability to be able to move fast, given the tools that we have today at our disposal. And thanks to the FDA for helping with that.

Mrs. RODGERS. Thank you.

Dr. MORITA. So I too was not certain, was hopeful, and have been so appreciative of the work that Congress had for supporting Operation Warp Speed, because the amount of resource and attention that was provided guaranteed that this effort was actually going to be successful. So it is the amount of resource and attention that will be supported.

Mrs. RODGERS. Very good.

Mr. LEAVITT. I will just say, based on past history and what I know about historic process, there was not a lot of reason to be optimistic. It was truly a remarkable feat.

Mrs. RODGERS. Thank you.

Mr. BUREL. I was hopeful as well, but I was not convinced. I do think we have made a lot of progress in being able to do these sort of things in public health emergencies. We need to continue to invest to be able to do this in the future.

Mrs. RODGERS. Yes.

Has vaccine distribution of this magnitude and complexity ever been attempted in the United States before? And, again, I would just like to ask each one of you to answer yes or no.

Dr. BORIO. Not even close.

Mrs. RODGERS. OK. Thanks.

Dr. MORITA. This is the largest I have seen in my lifetime.

Mrs. RODGERS. Great.

Mr. LEAVITT. I think it is clear it is unparalleled.

Mr. BUREL. No, we have never done anything at this level before.

Mrs. RODGERS. Great.

Governor Leavitt, given your experience serving in government and your tremendous service both at the State and the Federal level, I just wanted you to speak, and I know you did some in your opening testimony, but a little bit more about the appropriate role of the Federal Government when it comes to vaccines. If you would just talk a little bit more about that. And what flexibilities you believe need to be preserved to the State or local authorities to best respond to the unique needs facing their individual constituencies.

Mr. LEAVITT. Well, I will start by saying there is a role for both, and both need to do their job and work together to make this work. The point that has not been made that needs to be: Both of the vaccines that we have in the market today are based on new technologies that were actually developed under Federal procurement and/or other Federal investment beginning in 2006, 2007, and 2008, when we were dealing with the H5N1 and Congress responded by appropriating at nearly $8 billion.

The point here is, if you want to have this kind of result, it doesn't just happen in 11 months. It requires perpetual investment and perpetual vigilance to be ready.

Mrs. RODGERS. Thank you. Good point.

To Dr. Borio, you mentioned in your testimony the complexities of the vaccine supply chain and how the disruption of any critical component will disrupt the availability and the administration of the vaccines. I just wanted to ask you, are there any immediate additional actions that you believe that we need to be taking right now to ensure a stable supply chain for COVID vaccines?

Dr. BORIO. Thank you. I really do believe that Operation Warp Speed has done everything to maximize the process, to optimize it, and to basically rely as much as they could have already on DPA, the Defense Production Act.

I think to be able to—the next step really is about expanding the industrial base, domestic base, to manufacture some of the critical supplies here. We are talking about filters and columns and syringes and needles and bags that are required for the biomanufacturing. We are talking about filling finish lines to be able to bottle the vaccines. Every little single component, no matter how small it seems, can really bring the whole process to a halt if we don't have access to it.

Mrs. RODGERS. Very good. Well, I ran out of time. Again, thanks all. I will save my questions for later.

Ms. ESHOO. We thank the ranking member.

And just to remind everyone that we leave the record open so that questions can be submitted to our witnesses. And I will do another reminder of that at the end of the hearing.

It is a pleasure now to recognize the gentleman from North Carolina, Mr. Butterfield, for his 5 minutes of questions.

Mr. BUTTERFIELD. Thank you, Madam Chair. Good morning, good afternoon to all of you. And thank you, Madam Chair, for you leadership, and thank you for the direction in which you are taking this subcommittee.

And let me just say in the outset to our new ranking member, Mr. Guthrie, I look forward, sir, to working with you as we worked together in previous Congresses. I look forward to not only working with you, but also to all of you on the other side of the aisle.

Let me just take a moment to thank the witnesses. I have listened very carefully to your testimonies. Your testimony is very much appreciated today. And thank you for all the work that you do in the space in which you operate.

But I am going to concentrate my three questions, if I have enough time, on Dr. Morita.

Dr. Morita, thank you for your willingness to give the Nation the benefit of your expertise.

Since the very beginning, it has been clear that, while COVID– 19 affects us all, it does not affect us all equally. And I think some of the witnesses made reference to that in their testimonies. African-American and Latino, Asian, Native Americans, all of these individuals are more likely than White Americans to be infected. That is a fact. More likely to be hospitalized. More likely to die from COVID. This reality is why health equity must be at the center of any plan for distributing the vaccines. Unfortunately, the trends from the first several weeks are headed in the wrong direction.

The previous administration failed our country in so many ways. And the chairman of the full committee is right: We are not going to dwell unnecessarily on the past, but the previous administration did fail, including not putting forth a clear plan for vaccine distribution. Because of this failure, we now have a lack of reporting and incomplete data.

According to the CDC, we only have race and ethnicity data for about half of those receiving the vaccines. And where do we have data, only 5.4 percent of individuals getting the vaccines are African-American, 11 percent are Latino, 6 percent are Asian, 2 percent Native American, despite the fact that these groups bear a higher share of the COVID burden and often serving on the front lines of our healthcare workforce. And we have got to fix this now. I think we can all agree on that.

Dr. Morita, with such limited data, the situation might be worse than we know. How can we improve data collection and vaccine distribution?

Dr. MORITA. Thank you for your question. The equity issue is critical. In order to respond appropriately, we need to really improve the data systems that are being used currently. And there need to be additional resources made to make the systems better but also to support the manpower necessary to enter the information. It takes time to enter additional fields like race, ethnicity, gender, geography, occupation. And so it is manpower and it is also data systems.

What can be done? While we already acknowledge that there are some discrepancies in terms of who is getting vaccines, improve the systems by making it more accessible to people. So making sure the sites are located in geographies where people can easily access them without cars if they don't have them. Make sure they can make appointments by telephone, to make sure that there are community workers going into the communities to actually help people register and make appointments. All these kinds of things are necessary to make sure that we are reaching the people who are most likely to die and be hospitalized because of COVID, and those things often require additional resources.

Mr. BUTTERFIELD. Let me share this with you, if I can: Ninety percent of Americans live within 5 miles of a community pharmacy. Retail pharmacies are accessible. They are convenient. They are based on recent modeling. They have the capacity to administer 100 million vaccine doses in 30 days.

From your experience as the chief medical officer in Chicago, what more can be done to utilize retail community pharmacies?

Dr. MORITA. Retail community pharmacies played a major role in our response during H1N1. They do have reach into communities. And so, just yesterday, the Biden administration announced that they will be making more vaccine available through pharmacies throughout the Nation, particularly focusing on communities of color. They are one mechanism for getting vaccine to these communities.

Federally qualified health centers or community health centers and rural health centers are also places that are located in these communities and have trust within the communities to actually help address some of the concerns that people have about the safety or the efficacy of the vaccines. So a full-court press really needs to happen right now with healthcare providers, health centers, pharmacies, mass vaccination clinics, all those things need to be happening right now so we can get these vaccines out quickly and equitably.

Mr. BUTTERFIELD. Thank you very much, Dr. Morita.

And I yield back the 5 seconds that I have, Madam Chair.

Ms. ESHOO. We thank the gentleman. And thank you for your continuing focus on this issue. I don't really know whether our public health departments across the country are even equipped to gather the information that is needed in a very efficient and effective way, and I think that we need to do a little deeper dive on that.

The Chair now recognizes the former chairman of the full committee, someone that is always—he is really, I think, one of the most popular guys on the committee. Everyone loves Fred Upton.

So, Fred, you have 5 minutes for your questions.

Mr. UPTON. Well, thank you for your generous words. I am delighted to participate in this most important hearing.

I just have to say we all have to work so hard together. I mean, we are just hearing all these frustrating stories, not only from our constituents, but you see the news at night and the long lines of people in folding chairs in other places all around the country just waiting. The serious concerns about folks of color not having access. I mean, all these things just tear at our heartstrings, and we need to work together to do the very best that we can to improve the infrastructure.

Ms. ESHOO. Excuse me, can you speak up? I don't know if it is my computer or what.

Mr. UPTON. Is that OK? Is that better?

Ms. ESHOO. A little bit.

Mr. UPTON. All right.

The question that I have, I guess, for Greg Burel, what are your thoughts on the steps that we need to make sure that domestic manufacturing is, in fact, doing the right job being prepared as we look at the Defense Production Act? Where are we actually short in providing PPE for our communities that really need it? Is it masks, is it gowns, is it gloves, is it testing supplies? What products can you identify that we really need to step up, particularly as we have looked at the private sector, at least in my district, a whole number of different entities are producing that, which is a really good thing, but where do we need to go from here?

Mr. BUREL. Thank you, sir. I think that we are short in almost every area of PPE, both in the medical field and for the public who might want access to those kind of, say, N95 masks.

I think what we have got to do is find a way to invest better in onshoring or nearshoring some of that work. Most of that is not manufactured in the United States anymore. And there are a lot of manufacturers that want to get into this business and stay in this business, not just to respond to a DPA. So I think that we need to continue to invest. We need to encourage those manufacturers after this event ends to increase their capability, to make better quality products, to make products faster.

Mr. UPTON. Thank you.

Governor Leavitt, as you well know, our committee and most of the Members here, you will remember that we worked in such a bipartisan way to get 21st Century Cures done, which really led to Operation Warp Speed so that we could actually get a vaccine approved within the 10 months. For me, it was obviously very personal, not only with the legislation that Diana DeGette and I worked on together, every member of the this committee, but even more so in my own district. Pfizer's largest production facility is in Portage, Michigan, and it was so exhilarating to see the trucks roll out on that December Sunday morning to distribute with UPS and with FedEx all around the country. But now we are hearing obviously troubling reports, at least in Michigan, a number of counties having to cancel or reschedule second doses of that Pfizer or Moderna vaccine because they are getting differing amounts than what were expected from the State.

FDA's data indicates that the second dose needs to be given about 21 days after the first one; in the case of Pfizer about 28 days, in the case of those two companies in order to have the proper efficacy. So timing is critical. What steps do we need to take within the supply chain to ensure that the second doses are not foregone, especially in light of the recent decision not to reserve them, knowing that there is a line at virtually every entity of people ready to roll up their sleeve and get vaccinated?

Mr. LEAVITT. Well, Mr. Upton, let's remember first of all supply. We have to have a steady supply. Second, could I say coordination and communication between every level of government. This is a coordination and collaboration exercise. And finally, may I say that we have to be persistent in improving continually our process. And that will include our data systems.

I recently had the privilege of getting my first vaccine. I was scheduled for an appointment to go back for my second. I thought that was a very important step. I know when I am going, and assuming that the supply is there, I will get it. I think we will get better at this as we go, and we need to. This needs to be an iteratively improved process with lots of communication between Federal, State, and local governments.

Mr. UPTON. The last thing, and I wonder if you can—knowing that my time is quickly expiring, can you provide us a list of the States that are complying with the IZ, the form that you talked about in your testimony? It is so easy—you know, I have seen the little cards that people have. Obviously, it is so easy to counterfeit or whatever. I mean, we need a standard form. Whether getting on an airplane or going to a stadium, you would think that there ought to be some device that you can show on your iPhone or some program showing that you were vaccinated, to assure the folks around you and to your family members and others that, in fact, you have had that vaccination.

Mr. LEAVITT. Thank you for highlighting that. Yes, we can. I will submit it to you and for the record.

Mr. UPTON. Great.

And with that, my time has expired. Thank you, Madam Chair.

Ms. ESHOO. Thank you, Mr. Upton.

It is a pleasure to recognize the gentlewoman from California, my friend, everyone's friend, Ms. Matsui.

Are you unmuted?

Ms. MATSUI. I am unmuted now.

Ms. ESHOO. There you are. Five minutes. Thank you.

Ms. MATSUI. Thank you very much, Madam Chair, for really calling this important hearing.

And I want to thank all the witnesses. We are learning a lot with you and from you, so it is very important. Yet the sad thing is we are about to hit 450,000 COVID–19 deaths in this country. And nearly 300,000 Americans over the age of 65 have died from the virus. And that we probably can estimate, by the time we look back on this pandemic, some 250,000 older adults will have died from COVID–19 while living in a nursing home, assisted-living facility, or a group home.

You know, these are people who have died and will continue to die until we improve our response to managing the pandemic for vulnerable older adults and the frontline staff who care for them. And that is really why, as cochair of the House Democratic Caucus Task Force on Aging and Families along with Jan Schakowsky, I have called on the Biden administration to involve a geriatrician or expert in aging services on the COVID–19 response team. An aging expert, someone with a deep understanding of a long-term care system, will help ensure that moving forward we are really addressing the unique needs of older Americans as we take critical steps to get the virus under control and safely and equitably distribute vaccines, therapies, PPE, and tests.

Now, while the Trump administration left the delivery of most vaccines to the States, officials at Operation Warp Speed pursued a Federal public/private partnership with chain pharmacies to supply and administer vaccines to long-term care residents and staff. Now, the former HHS Secretary Azar said in mid-December that we could have every nursing home patient vaccinated in the United States by Christmas. The only State that met this mark was West Virginia, which opted out of the Federal program and instead used local pharmacies to administer vaccines.

Now, like many aspects of the vaccine rollout, leveraging the existing network of chain pharmacies like CVS really has worked in some places but not in others.

While I am encouraged by the centralized leadership being taken at the Federal level, it seems like the one-size-fits-all approach to vaccinating long-term care residents may cause further delays.

Now, Dr. Borio, in your view, what are some of the challenges with one-size-fits-all distribution and that leadership model? And what needs to be done to make the vaccination process more efficient?

Dr. BORIO. You know, I think you really—first of all, I would like to acknowledge that the pharmacy programs have done a tremendous job in preparing for one of the most challenging vaccination components of this challenging program. And, you know, this is not an easy task.

I think that nobody was prepared, for example, for the amount of hesitancy associated with vaccinating the workers in those facilities. The receptivity to the vaccine has been extraordinarily low, given the high-risk population that they serve. There were also issues with informed consent, and I think that they really wanted to make sure that patients, for example, were—that the vaccinees or their families were comfortable. There is still an investigation of vaccine authorized by the FDA. Investigation is important to make sure that people are comfortable receiving those vaccines.

So these are things that—I mean, you know, the other member said, you know, we are always going to have a lot of challenges when we launch a new program, and we have picked the most challenging component of this program as the step one of this.

But to answer your question directly, I think it is true, there needs to be a coordination and communication, as Secretary Leavitt says, because there is no such thing as one size fits all. You do need to be able to have Federal leadership and standards, but also tailor it to the needs of the community at the local level.

Ms. MATSUI. Absolutely. When you brought up vaccine hesitancy, you know, there is no question that staff are a primary source of transmitting the virus in long-term care facilities. Now I am deeply concerned about the large percentage of long-term care workers nationwide who are declining to take the COVID–19 vaccine.

Dr. Morita, what needs to be done to better support higher uptake of the vaccine by staff members of nursing homes and assisted-living facilities and group homes? And I think I only gave you 25 seconds.

Dr. MORITA. I will speak fast. Thank you so much for your question.

Vaccine hesitancy needs to be addressed across the board, and the way that we do that is really—it is not easy work. It is hard work. It means talking with those who are actually hesitant, understanding what their concerns are, what information do they need, who do they want to hear from to have their questions addressed, because it is not one size fits all for that either. And so really getting into these communities and understanding what are their concerns, and that requires resources.

There are many States and locals who are actually doing that kind of work right now, but they need the dollars to pay the community workers, the trusted voices to engage with the people to address their concerns so that demand increases.

Ms. MATSUI. OK. We have run out of time, and I appreciate it. And I yield back. And I have got further questions I will submit. Thank you.

Ms. ESHOO. The gentlewoman yields back.

The Chair now recognizes the gentleman from Texas, Mr. Burgess, for his 5 minutes of questions.

Mr. BURGESS. Thank you.

Secretary Leavitt, it is so good to see you in our committee again. You know, in this committee a year ago, we received a number of briefings from the top people in public health, and one of the things that, of course, people have brought up this morning, it still stands out in my mind, was Dr. Fauci telling us that, under the best of circumstances, if absolutely nothing goes wrong, that it would take 18 months to deliver a vaccine. And he also emphasized that it almost never goes perfectly. But here we are now a year later with not one but two highly effective vaccines, perhaps two more waiting in the wings to rapidly come forward, and really we should celebrate [inaudible] former Chairman Upton that [inaudible] watching my local news show about the trucks leaving. Fred, I thought it was from Kalamazoo. Maybe I was mistaken. But just the emotional response to seeing those trucks leaving the factory with the vaccines on board, I wasn't prepared to be as affected as I was, but the enormous sense of relief and joy at having those vaccines now on the road to get into the arms of people who would now be protected from this terrible virus. It really was a significant moment.

And, you know, I think some credit does go to the previous administration. They made it a priority. The 18 months was perfectly reasonable in January, February of 2020. Now we know that that timeline can be significantly condensed.

And, Secretary Leavitt, I also—your reference of your earlier work, and you are right, another thing short of stunning to get the rollout of part D done in the timeframe that you did. And I would remind members of the committee, that was on top of a public health emergency when Hurricane Katrina came ashore Labor Day weekend in 2005. And, in fact, I remember questioning you and Administrator McClellan at the time if it was even possible to go through the rollout of part D while this public health emergency was tearing across the country. And you assured me that it was, and I certainly became a big fan of your administrative capabilities at that time because, clearly, you were correct.

And one of the things I also remember from back then, 2005, I think the Defense Appropriations Bill where you got money for Sanofi to begin manufacturing vaccine in this country. Apparently, vaccines were no longer manufactured in this country, but in the advent of the bird flu, you thought it was important and got those dollars in that appropriations bill to start that. And the reason that is significant, I mentioned yesterday in our hearing, Sanofi is one of those companies that was in development of its own vaccine. Things didn't go perhaps as they wanted, but they are now partnering with a rival, with Pfizer, to manufacture more vaccine, more of the Pfizer vaccine that has gotten through the FDA approval and shown to be so effective.

So that really brings up the point, one of things that is hindering our getting vaccine into people is the amount of vaccine that is available. So this type of partnering between private companies seems something that could be enormously effective. So I just wondered, Secretary Leavitt, if you had any thoughts on that.

Mr. LEAVITT. You properly point out the fact that there has been investment in the vaccine infrastructure for some time now. And may I say that is a very important component. I would point to three other things that have added to this.

One is that we did enter into partnerships, as you have said, and that kind of collaboration is essential in this kind of emergency. The second thing I will mention is that we planted many seeds, knowing that not everything would turn out. And lastly, I will point out that the Federal Government did accept a lot of risk here. That kind of risk could not have been taken by the private sector or any State. Only the Federal Government could do that. And because there was a relentless concentration on delivering those four and many other ingredients, this has been a great success, one that we will have to perpetuate, because I have a feeling that, over the course of not just this year but probably 2 or 3 years, COVID is going to be with us. We are going to see variants. We are going to have to respond with different vaccines. And we have got to get better at this.

Mr. BURGESS. Certainly, again, thank you for your long service to our country. And I have a number of other questions. I will submit those for the record.

And I will yield back my time.

Ms. ESHOO. It is a pleasure to recognize the gentlewoman from Florida, Ms. Castor, for your 5 minutes of questions. Unmute.

Ms. CASTOR. There we are. Thank you, Chairwoman Eshoo and Chairman Pallone, for calling this very important hearing. And congratulations to my good friend Brett Guthrie for serving as ranking member. I look forward to our continued work together. And thanks to the witnesses for your excellent testimony.

It is clear that we must act with urgency on vaccines, on the next generation of diagnostic tests and more, because we have got to get kids back into school safely and folks back to work. And Americans just want to live their lives again.

So my takeaway from the witnesses and your great testimony is you believe Congress must act with urgency and with greater specificity in support for our partners all across the country. I think that means that we must ramp up the equitable vaccine distribution. And thank goodness President Biden now has a robust plan in the American Rescue Plan. And then we have got to improve our public health infrastructure. It needs modernization, especially accurate and timely reporting of data. That transparent information allows our scientists and community leaders, everyone, to make the right decisions and ensure we are acting in an equitable way.

This has been a real problem. I mean, just in my home State of Florida, it has been very difficult at times to get transparent information simply on mortality rates, on what is happening in our skilled nursing centers, what is happening with testing.

So, Dr. Morita, you have a very unique perspective on this as the former chief medical officer in Chicago and your work at CDC. In your testimony, you say that an equitable response to the pandemic starts with collecting and reporting all COVID–19-related data by race, ethnicity, and socioeconomic factors. Yet most States don't do this, and especially with vaccine data, they are not publishing and collecting the data that way. How can we improve our reporting and make sure that States are following through with what they need to do?

Dr. MORITA. Thank you for the question. The Robert Wood Johnson Foundation issued some health equity principles early in the pandemic because we recognized that there were disproportionate impacts on communities of color. And the top recommendation that we have is really to have data [inaudible] by race, by age, by ethnicities, by socioeconomic factors, geography, all those things. That work, though, requires dedicated resources and higher education. And so the problem that we have had with past response is that the same people that were doing testing, contact tracing, arranging the—investigating the outbreaks, were also asked to ramp up the vaccination systems. And some of the systems weren't equipped. They actually lacked this kind of information. So there are resources needed to support enhancement of our systems and also manpower to actually collect that information and then analyze the information, because it is not enough just to have the information. There have to be people to actually analyze the data, to generate reports, develop the systems to reporting consistently.

So all these things are critical. They need to be prioritized so that actually the work that is being done can be guided by what we find. When we see there are populations or communities that are underserved, we can actually get the resources to them, meet their needs, provide the services needed so they can actually have access to the vaccines just as much as everybody else.

Ms. CASTOR. And, Dr. Borio, you have made similar recommendations. And, Governor Leavitt, I heard you loud and clear as well on your specific recommendations.

I introduced the Ensuring Transparent Honest Information on COVID Act, or the ETHIC Act, last Congress with Reps Underwood and Haaland. We are going to be updating that and introducing it soon to make sure that we are providing that specific direction to States in the next emergency aid package.

And, Dr. Borio, it is hard to believe that here we are a year later, and we do not have a true national testing strategy. I would have thought by now that our diagnostic testing capacity with public and private labs would be state of the art, but the prior administration just did not prioritize this. What else needs to happen in the next emergency aid package to ensure that we have the most robust diagnostic testing system?

Dr. BORIO. So, as I recommended in my written testimony, I would like to see the CDC working alongside sister agencies—the FDA, HHS and others—to be able to provide much more clear guidance for testing in the different types of settings.

What are the options, for example, for an employer? What are the options for workplace? What are the options for travelers? What are the options for higher education? Right now, there are so many different types of strategies being deployed in a very ad hoc manner. We don't have that much data about, you know, which strategy is the most efficient. And, again, the supply of testing is just not something that can grow infinitely. We have a finite supply, we need to be able to optimize what we have through a really public-health-oriented guidance.

Ms. ESHOO. The gentlewoman's time has expired.

The Chair now recognizes the gentleman from Virginia, Mr. Griffith, for your 5 minutes of questions.

Mr. GRIFFITH. Thank you very much, Madam Chair. And I am going to——

Ms. ESHOO. Good to see you. Speak up.

Mr. GRIFFITH. OK. I will try to speak up a little bit. I have this mask on. There you go.

I am going to tag team with your questions earlier, Madam Chair, and, Mr. Burel, if you will help me out here. I agree with Ms. Eshoo that, you know, there were some suppliers in the country for PPE and that we need to have more domestic production. That being said, I need help and the committee needs help. We need to figure out, assuming that we can't bring all the production necessary for the United States back to the United States, what percentage—and you may not have an answer today, but I want us to work on this going forward—what percentage of our Nation's needs when it comes to, whether it be PPE or, as Dr. Borio mentioned, filters dealing with the manufacturing of vaccinations, et cetera, what percentage of that needs to be in the United States? And then, as a sidebar to that, we were having the discussion here that, you know, we had that problem when Puerto Rico got hit by the storms, and what percentage of that then needs to be split up so that we are not being hit by various storms? I mean, different parts of the country have different issues, but it would seem to me we need to make sure that we have a diversity of geographic locations. But I do think on these important matters we need to have production in the United States.

Knowing that we probably could have done better before, what can we do better going forward? And what percentage is necessary to be on our home territory, whether it be one of our territories, like Puerto Rico or Micronesia, or wherever it is, where we can get our hands on it when we need it?

Mr. BUREL. Sir, I appreciate the question. I am going to have to come back to you with some thoughts on percentages or possibly other measures we might consider about what should be manufactured here. But I think it is absolutely vital. We have made efforts to invest in the vaccine infrastructure, as Governor Leavitt discussed. I think we have got to make investments at the Federal level in the PPE infrastructure, because regardless of what pandemic event hits us again in the future—and I am sure there will be another—we have got to be better prepared.

So we need to encourage people to enter the PPE market that are not currently in it. We need to encourage those that currently manufacture PPE to do that. And I agree with your discussion of, for example, the small saline bags that were manufactured only in Puerto Rico. We cannot limit ourselves to a single manufacturer or a single location geographically. We must have diversity.

Mr. GRIFFITH. Well, I appreciate that.

And let me say that, in relationship to the PPE infrastructure, earlier this year we had a hearing where we had some of those people in. In fact, it must have been pretty early because I think we were live here in the room. And they said, if the Federal Government would just issue contracts to purchase it, we don't necessarily need to buy the equipment. But if we said we were going to buy a certain amount of PPE, they felt like they could ramp up much easier. And in my district, several folks came forward. I know one is going to continue long term, I don't know if the others are, to make masks and to make other PPE, and they are ready to go. But if the market were to suddenly drop out, we would be back in the same boat we were in before. So I think that that is important.

Do you agree with that, Mr. Burel?

Mr. BUREL. Sir, I do agree with that. I think that, once we create more market, more manufacturing capability for these things in the United States, we have got to continue to support that market or the bottom will drop out again and we will have wasted investment. So my concern here is that we have a diversity of suppliers, we bring other people into the pipeline.

And one thing I would encourage your thoughts about are, it is difficult to hold this PPE because it is large. It occupies a lot of space. Maybe we need to hold bridge stocks and then have capability to turn directly, immediately to domestic manufacturers to bring in rapid surge directly to where the government would direct or directly to fill behind government needs.

Mr. GRIFFITH. And, Dr. Borio, I want to get one more question to Mr. Burel, but if you could think about it and we might ask you to answer that question after this hearing, because my time is almost up.

Mr. Burel, you specifically mentioned in your testimony the need to engage all commercial healthcare distributors and manufacturers. You reference the single vaccine distributor. Are you aware of other situations in which additional parties stand ready to partner with Federal, State and local governments?

Mr. BUREL. Sir, I believe that most parties involved in the typical day-to-day healthcare supply chain are very much prepared to partner with the Federal Government. We have a system that operates every day. And, if we make ourselves take advantage of all aspects of that everyday operating planning and distribution system, I think we will have a better, stronger result going forward. As we see vaccines increase——

Mr. GRIFFITH. I have to cut you off, because I do want to say one last thing and my time is just out.

Dr. Borio, you always are so good to give us testimony in this committee, and I always appreciate it. So I apologize I didn't get to you live today, but I would love to see some of your thoughts after this meeting is over. Thank you so much.

And, Madam Chair, I yield back.

Ms. ESHOO. I thank the gentleman. And I just want to say I look forward to working with you on the supply chain. In my book, it should be all American. This business of maybe we should do this and then be dependent on so-and-so, I just—excuse the expression, I just don't buy that.

Mr. GRIFFITH. We certainly need to have a big percentage of it here.

Ms. ESHOO. Exactly, exactly. We guaranteed a market for the pharmaceutical companies to buy vaccines. So, if we can do that, we can certainly promise a market for American manufacturers of American products to be used by the American people in their hour of need. So thank you very much.

I now recognize the gentleman from Vermont, Mr. Welch, for his 5 minutes of questions.

Mr. WELCH. Thank you, Madam Chair. And I agree with all your comments. And, Mr. Guthrie, congratulations to you as well. I really look forward to working together to get some things done here.

You know, the last administration, I think, could be credited with doing a good job in public/private partnerships to create the vaccines. The challenge, however, is how do you get them injected into the arms of all Americans? And there really wasn't a plan.

Vermont is doing pretty well, but it is very rural and there are lots of folks who are homebound. And in the original package, the Federal Government passed legislation to work with our pharmacies. And we have got like 40,000 pharmacies that are well situated to provide help to rural Americans.

And the question I wanted to ask Mr. Burel and Dr. Morita is, how could we make that plan work better? The two things that our Department of Health director has said is there has to be predictability on the delivery of the vaccine. And, number two, there has to be better Federal and State coordination.

Mr. Burel, do you have any comments about that?

Mr. BUREL. Thank you for the opportunity, sir. I believe that we can rely on our everyday outlets for healthcare delivery that our American citizens are accustomed to seeing. But I think one of the important things is we must engage the entire supply chain, all distributors who are accustomed to dealing with specific clientele across the country who are specifically ready to deliver to their normal clients. I think that we need to, as vaccine supplies increase, make sure that all the distribution capability we have in healthcare in the U.S. is engaged with assuring products are available at all of the outlets that people expect them to be.

Mr. WELCH. Well, Dr. Borio, maybe you could follow up on that. And just, you know, this is operational now. We are not talking just general and abstract. This is like the really hard work of systems that are repetitive, reliable, and sustainable.

Dr. Morita?

Dr. MORITA. Thank you for your question. I completely agree with your health director in that having a predictable awareness or knowledge of how much vaccine the health directors can actually anticipate on a regular basis really helps to do the kind of planning and operational work that you are talking about. That was part of the challenge with some of the cancellations that people were experiencing early on, is because the health directors weren't actually hearing about the supply of vaccines, except for a couple of days before the vaccine actually arrived.

So what we are hearing now is the health directors are actually getting 3 weeks' notice. So they actually can predict and plan how to schedule their clinics, how to hire people, where to locate their clinics, how much vaccine can they give to their healthcare providers. So this predictability is really critical.

The other thing is this level of coordination, because, as Mr. Burel mentioned, we have a strong infrastructure for delivering healthcare services, vaccines included. But there really does need to be a coordination to understand where does one system work and where does one system not work, because it is not a one size fits all. And so having this Federal coordination which CDC is overseeing what is working, where is it working well, how do you share those best practices among various jurisdictions is really, really critical to having a successful ramped up system that optimizes all the different ways of delivery of vaccines.

Mr. WELCH. Thank you very much.

Madam Chair, I yield back. I appreciate the time of the panel.

Ms. ESHOO. The gentleman yields back.

It is a pleasure to recognize a great Greek American from Florida, Mr. Bilirakis.

Mr. BILIRAKIS. Thank you very much.

Ms. ESHOO. How are you feeling, Gus?

Mr. BILIRAKIS. I am doing good. I appreciate it.

Ms. ESHOO. Do you feel better?

Mr. BILIRAKIS. I am feeling much better. Thank you.

Ms. ESHOO. Good.

Mr. BILIRAKIS. Thank you for the letter too. I appreciate it very much.

It is great to serve on this committee again in this term. It is a wonderful committee. And I want to congratulate my good friend Brett Guthrie as well for being the ranking member.

I have a couple of questions. The first is for Mr. Burel. I want to follow up on Mr. Griffith's question. Were States and localities properly set up to order and receive shipments from the Strategic National Stockpile? If not, how did that impact the effectiveness of the response for those particular States?

Mr. BUREL. Sir, I think one of the things that we need to make sure of going forward is that the Strategic National Stockpile has direct communication with State public health officials. We used to have a strong connection to those so we all understood what to expect from each other. That kind of got lost somewhere a few years back as priorities changed, money moved away from the Public Health Emergency Preparedness Cooperative Agreements.

We talked to them in the past around flu about allocations per capita, but some of those conversations I think have been broken and we need to reenter those between the SNS and those States so everybody really understands each other well.

Mr. BILIRAKIS. Absolutely.

Governor Leavitt, I have a question. Tell me a little bit about the availability of therapeutics. You know, I am all for the vaccines, don't get me wrong, but tell me the availability of therapeutics. Where are the challenges that we are facing in administering therapeutics?

Mr. LEAVITT. Yes, we have failed to make the robust progress on therapeutics that we have on vaccines. And I think we can learn from that and realize that it requires perpetual investment, that we have got to enter into the same kind of partnerships, and we have got to plant a lot of seeds to make this happen. And as COVID elongates—and I think it is going to; we will I hope go back toward normal, but we are all going to be managing this for a long time—we need more tools. Even vaccines are not such that it guarantees our success. So those would be my suggestions.

Mr. BILIRAKIS. Thank you, Governor.

Mr. Burel, today's leading manufacturing supply chains often operate just in time instead of the just in case to reduce costs and maximize efficiency. However, this is a dual edge that can present challenges, obviously, in the midst of a pandemic response. As we saw with personal protective equipment, how can supply chains balance resiliency with value moving forward? Again, this is for Mr. Burel.

Mr. BUREL. Sure. I like your words of "just in case." And I think that what we can do is, one, we can build stock in the Strategic National Stockpile. We can build stock at State and local levels with Federal assistance to do that. We can encourage manufacturers and distributors to hold some flexible stock for that really bad day that we just went through that we hoped we never would. I think that there are ways to incentivize that, and I would love to think about that and come back to you with further answers.

Mr. BILIRAKIS. Please do. I would appreciate that very much.

Again for Governor Leavitt, as policymakers consult the data to direct response efforts, where should the goal post be erected—talking about the—you know, we have the Super Bowl coming up. Go Bucs. In other words, where should the bulk of our attention and the resources be directed as States reopen? Is it about total confirmed cases, hospitalizations, or deaths? And, again, this is for Governor Leavitt.

Mr. LEAVITT. Look, it is a combination of those things, every one of them. Everyone has their own metric they like to watch. But the reality is we have got to take a holistic view of this. But I would like to underscore the point that Julie Morita and others have made today, and that is the need for data systems, because we won't get the data if we don't begin to invest in the system.

And might I add, this has been a challenge. And I might suggest also a priority for multiple administrations, and that part of the dilemma isn't that they have not been asking, it is that they haven't been funded. And so I think we need all of those metrics available in readily assessable ways in an integrated, open source fashion that give us the tools we need.

Mr. BILIRAKIS. Very good.

Thank you, Madam Chair, I appreciate it very much. Take care. And, again, go Bucs, everyone. Kathy agrees with me on that one.

Ms. ESHOO. Well, we are all relieved that you are feeling 100 percent better.

Mr. BILIRAKIS. Thank you.

Ms. ESHOO. And, Governor Leavitt, I couldn't agree with you more about funding of the public health agencies. They are not in good shape across the country. Some of them have systems. I mean, there are all kinds of levels, and I think the grades that we would attach to them, many of them are not where they should be in the second decade of the 21st century. So I think that is a point that Members need to—that we all need to take seriously, because we are not going to get beyond this lack of reporting of the kind of data that we need unless we have agencies that have the systems that are necessary to collect them. So thank you.

I now call on the gentleman from Oregon, a wonderful member of our subcommittee, Mr. Schrader, for your 5 minutes of questions. You need to unmute.

Mr. SCHRADER. All right. It takes a while.

I agree with you on the public health piece, Madam Chair, 100 percent. It is time for us to start to incentivize public health at the State and local level, certain—we should have some base funding that we put out there and then, frankly, use the database collection as an incentive to have local governments and States report good data on vaccines and other critical and public health pieces of information, and they get more money. I mean, that is the way the system should work.

I will add my voice a little bit to the whole PPE situation. I am not sure I think it all has to be made in America to start with, but we have to have at least a base level made in America to make it worthwhile for American manufactures to be online and have that capacity.

And to Congressman Griffith's point, I think we need to put a panel together, a board, if you will, of manufacturers, public health officials, and other certified smart folks, to come up with what is a plan for ongoing manufacturing in this country. We have had testimony that it is mostly just a lack of having the ability to keep manufacturing going. So we should invest in that, I think.

And I am curious, Mr. Burel, you know, very specifically, what can we do to encourage, in this capitalist system of ours, the manufacturers to set up and continue to manufacture? I assume it has to do with churning over the stockpiles at a certain rate that it makes sense for manufacturers, making sure there is a percentage that providers of their gear, of their PPE gear that has to be coming from America. What specific recommendations would you have for us going forward?

Mr. BUREL. So I think there are several things. I would like to come back with you for a longer list, but a couple of things immediately come to mind.

The first is we know there are people who want to enter this market. There are people who have already taken risks to enter this market. We need to support them, whether that be through some sort of subsidy program, possibly investing in a joint venture of certain lines with them, guarantees of certain sales into the Federal Government, so that they can continue to manufacture, but not only manufacture, improve their ability to manufacture.

What we have found is the use of machinery made to do this are made offshore as well. So we need to invest in how to make our own machines.

I would like to come back with you with a more fulsome list, if that would be possible.

Mr. SCHRADER. That is great. That is very, very helpful and totally on point.

Dr. Borio——

Mr. LEAVITT. Mr. Schrader, would you be open to me commenting on this?

Mr. SCHRADER. Please.

Mr. LEAVITT. This points, I think, to a very important principle, and it is that there are certain expenditures that are just a cost of doing business for a country to be safe, and we make those expenditures in the area of defense every year. But we now find that there are enemies that are substantially more debilitating than anything we face as far as hostile opponents. And we need to invest not just in PPE and vaccines, but in readiness every year as a matter of national security.

Mr. SCHRADER. I would totally agree. And as the chair and the committee knows, active ingredients are largely manufactured in China and India for pharmaceuticals, and we need to bring some of that back as another discussion.

Dr. Borio, what about treatment? I mean, there are a lot of different treatment options hawked out there, some more realistic and successful than others. I think a lot of folks are facing difficulties accessing treatment and knowing what treatments are peer-reviewed and actually going to be successful.

What can we do to make sure that folks are getting the right information regarding effective treatments?

Dr. BORIO. Thank you for the question. It is indeed the wild west out there.

I have to say that in 2014, the U.S., the U.S. Government, led the way in the conduct of very rigorous clinical trials that were very effective and very fast in West Africa during the outbreak, when the rest of the world did not think it was possible. We did the same thing in 2017 in the Democratic Republic of the Congo in the middle of conflict. We actually did clinical studies of vaccines and therapeutics. And here in the U.S., we had a proliferation of trials being conducted that did not meet standards, that did not have any hope for giving us really interpretable data that we need to be able to inform patient care.

We do need to establish a national infrastructure that can be used in peacetime for studying infectious diseases, but also that can rapidly be able to evaluate products quickly, but in a scientifically valid manner, similar to what the U.K. has done with recovery. And it is not too late to start. We need to do this today, because there are so many promising therapies out there, and we just do not want to waste more time in tiny little studies that are not going to help us get information we need to confidently use these products and ramp up supplies and really go the extra mile to make sure that that we can deliver them. We need data to make decisions in those investments.

Mr. SCHRADER. Very good. Thank you so much.

And I yield back, Madam Chair.

Ms. ESHOO. I thank the gentleman.

It is a pleasure to recognize the gentleman from Indiana, Dr. Bucshon, for his 5 minutes of questions.

Mr. BUCSHON. Thank you, Madam Chairwoman.

And, Dr. Morita, I just want to touch on something. In your testimony, you talked about the equitable distribution of vaccines, and I represent a rural America area, which is 98 percent White. But we have a lot of the same challenges in my rural counties that we do in inner cities, which, in certain areas of the cities, are mostly African-American.

It is a complicated process to register a vaccine, and what I want to talk about is, do you have data to back up the premise that currently there are people out there in our States that are purposely not distributing vaccines equitably to communities of color? Because if that is true, I was a physician with—that is an appalling and unacceptable situation. Or is it because of the difficulty that I have in rural America, in actually accessing the vaccines that have been distributed? I know that is a distinction, but it is very important that we understand that.

Can you comment on that?

Dr. MORITA. Thank you, Dr. Bucshon.

That is a critical distinction to make. I did not mean to suggest that there are people that are withholding actively the vaccine from communities of color. My concern is——

Mr. BUCSHON. Yes, I didn't think that you meant that, but I wanted to clarify that because, as a physician, it would just be an appalling and shocking thing if people were doing that.

Dr. MORITA. What you described, though, in terms of the challenges of rural communities in terms of accessing the vaccine, are still the same in some of our inner cities, challenges they have in terms of making appointments, making it on time to the places as well. So it is really—the challenges are very similar, so the systems in both rural communities as well as in urban areas really need to be overcome.

Mr. BUCSHON. Yes, and we need to do better, no doubt about that. Thank you for that.

And, Dr. Borio, in your testimony, you speak at length on testing and warning that we are still not meeting the capacity and rapid response that we need in order to limit the spread of COVID–19 most effectively. I know some of this has been touched upon, but increasing our testing capacity is something I have been working on since the onset of the pandemic. When I heard from my constituents, they are unable to access the test, and even then—even when they are symptomatic—and then once they were able to find a test, they had to wait 7 to 12 days. And let me tell you, in certain areas that has not changed.

And while our testing has come leaps and bounds since March, we still are not where we need to be. Turnaround times have improved for some, but in rural parts of the country, which I represent, I continue to hear from my constituents that the turnaround times are long. And, in fact, nearly 20 percent of U.S. counties lack a single testing site that administers for COVID–19.

And as of last fall, nearly 40 percent of our public health labs still lacked access to a single high throughput testing platform.

If we can increase our capacity and have more rapid test results, it will continue—if we can't do that, it will continue to make it difficult for us to limit the spread. That is why today, my colleague and I, Diana DeGette, will be reintroducing the Access for Test Act, which would aid our public health labs in acquiring high throughput platforms and hospitals and doctors and pharmacists in also acquiring these tests. I think we have already touched on our lack of funding for public health.

Dr. Borio, could you speak more again to the need our country still has for greater testing capacity and more rapid results, and how arming our public health labs with more rapid high throughput testing platforms and supplying our doctors and hospitals with more point-of-care tests might achieve that goal, and better prepare us for the days ahead with variants now making their way across our borders?

Dr. BORIO. Sure. So, you know, clearly, testing is critical for us to be able to know what are we dealing with and to provide the appropriate patient care and public health interventions.

But let me go and make a link that may not be so evident. You know, we have these monoclonal antibodies that have been authorized by the FDA based on very limited data. Initially they were designed, or hoped that they would be very effective in treating patients who were sick with COVID. It turns out they don't work very well then. We have to give them very early.

Now, if patients cannot access testing when they are sick, the delay in the results, they will miss the opportunity to be able to access the therapeutics that need to begin very early on. So you see how really difficult it is to break this into very discrete systems, because it is really about the patient, and the patient needs all of this to work——

Mr. BUCSHON. Yes.

Dr. BORIO [continuing]. They can have some good outcomes.

Mr. BUCSHON. Yes. I mean, long turnaround times just are not acceptable. I mean, you need to be able to get a result the same day, especially, like you said, if you have early symptoms, and it takes you out of the window of getting these therapeutics, these antibody therapeutics, if you can't get your test results for 4 or 5 days, and then you get really sick, and then you are out of the window where maybe you could have been helped and prevented hospitalization.

So thanks for that answer. And, Madam Chairwoman, my time has expired. I yield back.

Ms. ESHOO. Thank you, Doctor.

I would just add that there is $50 billion in this plan of the administration that will be coming before us, $50 billion, with a B, and $3 billion relative to the therapeutics that you were just asking about, which are really so important, because time has gone by, but we have not really developed what needs to be developed there. So I just wanted to add that to—add that layer of money on the issues that we are talking about.

It is a pleasure to recognize a good friend, a wonderful member of our subcommittee, the gentleman from California, Mr. Ca´rdenas, for his 5 minutes of questions.

Mr. CÁRDENAS. Thank you very much, Madam Chair Eshoo. And also, I am looking forward to working with you, Mr. Ranking Member Guthrie, and all the members of the committee.

Four hundred thousand lives have been taken by COVID–19 in America. Tens of millions of Americans have been affected. I personally believe it didn't have to come to this. The numbers are too high. We are the greatest country on the planet, and when it comes to research, when it comes to development, when it comes to being able to step up when the country or the world is faced with, whether it be a pandemic or something that threatens the lives of human beings across the planet.

One of the things that I would like to report, put on the record, is President Biden met with some of us this morning, and this morning he, once again, reassured us that, as the President, he is committed to provide every resource that our country can provide to save American lives and to reignite our economy.

And one of our presenters today, I quote, said "a trusted source of truth," that is what people are looking for. And I believe, in this current Biden administration, we are going to get that.

I also want to point out that vaccinations need to be recorded and reported, as some of our witnesses have mentioned, and also when it comes to details as to who is getting the vaccination and some of the background information, because everybody knows, especially if you are a scientist, if you believe in science and you believe in progress, information is critical, and accurate information is important. And, again, I believe that we are going to have more of that going forward.

Also, I would like to point out that it is not enough, in my opinion, to just make sure that we got a vaccination to the market and available in record time. That is a feat, and it is phenomenal, and I am sure everybody applauds that. But I think about it when I grew up in a family where my mother and father had 11 children, and my mother used to serve 13 of us every single day. She didn't just put the food on the stove and leave it there and say, "Come get it and find your own plate or find your own utensils and figure out how you are going to put it in your mouths."

No, no. She went the whole way. She went ahead and served it. She went ahead and provided everything that we needed to make sure that we got that nourishment every single day for decades.

And yet, at the same time, I personally am disappointed that the greatest Federal Government on the planet just decided to focus on a few things, and really allowed everybody to be to their own devices without the critical support that our Federal Government has proven that we are amazing at.

So with that, I would like to ask Dr. Morita, do you think there is a risk in the United States investing too little today in going forward, or should we invest as much as the science requires us to?

Dr. MORITA. Thank you for sharing your story with us.

This is the biggest public health emergency we have experienced in our lifetimes. And the resources that are needed to respond to this public health emergency are large. And so, as much money that went into creating and supporting development and manufacturing a vaccine, also there needs to be a similar amount of resource and support given to assure the delivery of the vaccine into all Americans throughout the United States. And we recognize that some of the systems that are in place aren't meant——

[Audio malfunction.]

Mr. CÁRDENAS. I am sorry, I think you cut off a bit.

I would also like to ask Dr. Borio the same question, but I would also like to insert that my father stayed married to my mother for 48 years. So that partnership, it wasn't just my mother. It was also somebody going to work every single day, 6 days a week, for decades to make sure that that partnership could provide that food on the table.

Dr. Borio, a similar question to you as far as—let me get a little bit more specific. If we don't include good and robust appropriate funding for State and local governments and our local providers, would we be able to address this pandemic properly if we don't include that component in the next tranche of support legislation?

Dr. BORIO. Clearly, funding it underpins a lot of the activities. So I can't say that we can respond adequately without the resources. As Governor Leavitt just mentioned, you know, there is a cost of doing business to be able to keep our citizens safe and—but, I think I would go beyond that, which is there is a need at this point to provide more direct technical assistance as well because of the chronic underfunding that has existed over the years.

So each locality has different needs. Some funding is all they need. Others will require a lot more of a hands-on approach to be able to get us to the other side of this crisis.

Mr. CÁRDENAS. And when we don't do that, the people who suffer the most are the people who had lacked before the pandemic hit. So thank you very much. My time has expired, and I yield back.

Thank you, Madam Chair.

Ms. ESHOO. Thank you, Mr. Ca´rdenas.

I would say God bless your mother. Imagine the work that woman did.

You didn't mention who cleaned up. Maybe—hopefully most of the kids did after all the work she did.

Mr. CÁRDENAS. Yes. Yes, we all had chores. Thank you very much, Madam Chairwoman.

Ms. ESHOO. God love her. God bless the mothers.

It is a pleasure to recognize the gentleman from North Carolina, Mr. Hudson, for your 5 minutes of questions.

Mr. HUDSON. Thank you, Madam Chair. Thank you for holding this very important hearing. I also want to congratulate my colleague, Mr. Guthrie, on taking over as ranking member here in this first hearing. I look forward to working with both of you as we move forward.

It is no secret Washington is sharply divided, but this committee must focus on the areas where we can work together. Today, I have seen a lot of finger pointing, so I must remind my colleagues that finger pointing and assigning blame gets us nowhere. We need to focus on solutions.

From what I hear back home, our immediate priorities must be increasing our manufacturing capacity for vaccines and creating better systems of coordination for vaccine distribution.

If we had held this hearing a year ago and an expert witness told us we would not have one but two vaccines and over 20 million Americans vaccinated at this time, they would have been laughed out of the room. Thanks to President Donald Trump's Operation Warp Speed, we have two vaccines approved, hundreds of millions of doses manufactured, and more promising candidates in the pipeline.

In fact, despite all of the partisan sniping today, President Biden inherited from President Trump a million vaccines per day. President Biden came into office saying he had a better plan to end the COVID–19 pandemic and promising better vaccine distribution. I am pleased this has been a priority for the President, but we are eagerly waiting to see what he will do differently than the Trump plan. I am eager to work with President Biden to get vaccines in the arms of my constituents.

And there is much room for improvement. We need every entity, from the Federal Government to the States down to the individual facilities that are administering these tests, talking to each other and coordinating vaccine supply. As an example, my Governor told me he finds out how many vaccines he is going to get less than a week before. I learned this morning that a new system is being stood up to allow 3-week windows in the coming doses, which is good but I fear may not be good enough.

Another example is a facility in my district declined to receive the vaccine they were offered this week, while another facility in the same large suburban county has a 7,000-person waiting list for the vaccine. This same county did not receive any doses of vaccine for the 2 weeks prior. There is simply not enough coordination to this effort yet, but I have faith we can get there.

Governor Leavitt, given your extraordinary experience as a Governor and Secretary of Health and Human Services, how do you recommend increasing coordination among the many entities responsible for vaccine distribution: the facilities, the counties, the States, and the Federal Government?

Mr. LEAVITT. Mr. Hudson, earlier I spoke of my experience rolling out Medicare part D, where we had a much lesser challenge, but it was 45 million people in a very short time. In the weeks prior to that, I spent a lot of time as Secretary going from community to community, drawing them together, Federal, State, local, civil society, and other aspects, churches, schools, and saying to them, "We have to collaboratively work together to make this happen." And that is what it is going to take to make this happen, collaborative action among all levels. And if we do, we can do better, and over time we will get better.

Mr. HUDSON. I am sorry I muted myself, but I think you are exactly right, Mr. Secretary.

And I would just say, Madam Chair, I think this committee could look at ways that we can promote better coordination in the communities like that. We, as individual Members of Congress, could play a role in this. In my State, I have got a Democratic Governor, I am a Republican Member of Congress, but we have worked very closely together. You know, we have had issues, but we have tried to resolve them together, not in the media. You know, I think that is the model.

I think that is what we as a committee ought to be looking at, is how we can help with this coordination problem, because there are people out there who desperately want this vaccine, and there is plenty—I wouldn't say plenty, but there is a lot of vaccine out there. We need to make sure it is getting to the right places.

So I appreciate the testimony from you, Mr. Secretary. And, Madam Chair, I hope this will be a good starting point for us to work together on this.

With that, I will yield back to you.

Ms. ESHOO. I very much appreciate the comments of the gentleman, and let's put our heads together about how best to do that. Sometimes—my grandmother used to say the most uncommon of the senses is common sense. So I think that we can make some real headway together. And I sincerely appreciate what you said.

It is a pleasure now to recognize the doctor from California, Dr. Ruiz, for 5 minutes for your questions. How are you feeling, number one?

Mr. RUIZ. I am feeling much better. Thank you for asking. I am——

Ms. ESHOO. But you are not all better yet? You still have a ways?

Mr. RUIZ. Not all better. I am still at home. I still have some of those long lingering symptoms, but I am much better.

Ms. ESHOO. Well, get all better fast. We need you.

Mr. RUIZ. Thank you, thank you. Thank you, Madam Chair. Ms. ESHOO. Get your shots. Listen to your elder.

You are recognized.

Mr. RUIZ. Thank you, Madam Chair. Thank you for holding this very important hearing.

Large vaccination centers serve an important purpose, and they are good for getting large numbers of people vaccinated in a short period of time. And sites like that work for someone who has a computer to sign up for an appointment, a car to get there, and a job with flexibility that allows them to wait hours to receive the vaccine.

But those are not useful for everyone, like high-risk farm workers and other essential workers who are working for and also high risk of getting infected from COVID.

I know this from personal experience as a physician. Very early on in this pandemic, I have been coordinating and organizing testing outreach for the homeless as well as farm workers, in trailer parks, churches, school areas, and so, I have had a really up close and personal interaction and have heard their stories, their concerns, their difficulties.

And many don't have internet to make an appointment. They don't have hours to spend on a phone trying to reserve their slot. They don't have transportation to get to the vaccination site, let alone spending hours waiting to receive the vaccine. And they don't have information in their own language to help them navigate the system.

So what we are doing now is just not working, and it is disproportionately harming underserved populations and communities of color.

A recent Kaiser Family Foundation analysis found that, in Mississippi, Black people account for 15 percent of the vaccinations while accounting for 42 percent of the deaths. In Nebraska, 4 percent of vaccinations are to Hispanic individuals, even though they make up 23 percent of the cases. So this is not only a moral failure, this is prolonging the pandemic.

We need a science-based public health approach that serves the hard-to-reach communities, and we can't simply rely on our broken healthcare system that has produced the disparities in infections and deaths due to COVID to begin with to address equity. This means making better use of local physician offices and FQHCs. By and large, physician offices, outside of large group practices, have been left out of the effort to vaccinate patients that have heightened challenges, particularly in communities of color where vaccine hesitancy remains high. People trust their doctor, and they must play a critical role in addressing issues of access and hesitancy. According to a recent Harris Poll, the majority of Americans would prefer to get their shot in their family's doctor's office, and less than a quarter Americans want to be vaccinated at special sites built to administer the vaccine.

Activating primary care and vaccination efforts will open up thousands of access points providing broader reach and better accessibility. And FQHCs, the sites that are there to serve the very communities we are trying to reach, have been massively underutilized during this vaccination process. And they are ready. They just don't have the vaccines and resources to activate their plans.

We need to provide our FQHCs with vaccines and the resources to administer them both in their clinics and out in the community. We need to provide funding for mobile clinics. We need to provide funding for promotoras and the community health workers, or for providers to take vaccines directly to the people, like this past Monday where I joined a collaborative of growers, nonprofits, and public health officials to literally go into the fields to talk to the farm workers about the safety and efficacy of the vaccine, and then inoculate them on the spot. If we don't give them the resources to carry out a vaccination plan, it won't work, and we are seeing that play out now.

The Trump administration told States and counties to develop their own distribution plans but left them no resources to do it. States, county, and travel budgets are already strapped from this pandemic. They need more resources if we expect them to do this right.

So I urge this committee as we move forward in this reconciliation process to make this a priority.

Dr. Morita, let's talk about FQHCs as a source of access point for vaccinating our hard-to-reach areas, rather—and how could FQHCs play an important role? And do you foresee any barriers for them that we need to address?

Dr. MORITA. Thank you so much, Congressman.

The federally qualified health centers played a major role in Chicago's H1N1 response because they are so well connected to our hard-to-reach communities. They are used to providing the social services, as well as they are the trusted messengers in sources of information for those communities. I think that can play a critical role as we are trying to develop a more equitable distribution system.

Mr. RUIZ. What were the barriers that you had to address with FQHCs, so we can learn from those?

Dr. MORITA. The barriers were really resources and adequate staffing, adequate vaccine, adequate—just compensation for the work that was actually being done. So, in order for those FQHCs to be able to provide the services, they really need the resources and support to get the work done. They are fully capable of doing it. They just need resources to ramp up the services they actually provide.

Mr. RUIZ. Thank you very much.

Ms. ESHOO. Does the gentleman yield back?

Mr. RUIZ. Yes.

Mr. LEAVITT. Madam Chair, this is Mike Leavitt. Would you allow me 20 seconds to say and echo the community health center comment?

Ms. ESHOO. I would be glad to with the, I think, graciousness of the Members. Go ahead, Governor.

Mr. LEAVITT. As a former Secretary of Health, and, I might add, Governor, I experienced directly and firsthand the importance of community health centers, and it is evident to me that they have to be a part of being able to solve the equity issues here. And I could break into song longer, but you have been gracious to allow what I have.

Thank you.

Ms. ESHOO. Governor, on that, there is full support—first of all, full understanding and full support from both sides of the aisle in community health centers, and Congress has increased funding for community health centers, I think really quite exponentially, so they are—you are absolutely right, we agree with you. But we want you to know where we all are and that, as they say, it is preaching to the choir because, thank God, all of the Members have a deep appreciation of them.

It is now a pleasure to recognize Mr. Dunn from Florida, and it is great to have you on our committee.

Mr. DUNN. Thank you very much, Chairwoman Eshoo. It is an honor to join you on this committee, and I certainly look forward to the many hard tasks that we have ahead of us.

I appreciate the opportunity today to discuss ideas relating to ramping up vaccine distribution testing and ensuring America has a robust medical response to this and to future pandemics.

As we pass one year from the date that the Trump administration declared a public health emergency, I would like to extend my sincere condolences to those who have lost loved ones to the virus. I also extend my thanks to all of the healthcare heroes who have risked everything to help us all through this emergency.

As COVID–19 began to spread in America last year, the Trump administration got to work implementing timely travel restrictions, launching the active partnership and Operation Warp Speed initiative to enhance agency coordination and, more importantly, to bring private industry ideas and capabilities to the Federal response. The pace at which Pfizer and Moderna, J&J and others, who have developed their vaccines, is truly unprecedented, and I commend the administration's actions for the fastest vaccine development in history.

As States ramp up their vaccine distribution capabilities, they must also continue to employ robust diagnostics, and, importantly, we have to continue to evaluate available therapeutics, that is to say treatments, for COVID–19. We also have to turn the lessons we have learned into action when it comes to supply chain challenges, all the way from production to distribution.

Dr. Borio, we are hearing about the different variants of COVID– 19 and the challenges that they may present us with. Do you agree that the efforts to identify new and existing therapeutics are an important piece of our arsenal to combat COVID and epidemics in general?

Dr. BORIO. I do. Dr. Dunn, I mentioned in my——

Mr. DUNN. You did.

Mr. BORIO. Yes, I think it is a very critical component. I mean, I think we know that vaccines—in public health measures, vaccines are the most important tools to deal with pandemics, the contagious disease we are facing today, but we also need treatments to be able to take care of patients who are ill.

Mr. DUNN. So I like the vaccines for the specific, but I was thinking here more broad, about the broad-spectrum therapeutics, which should enjoy activity against many of the mutations as well as the original virus that we are combating. If you will forgive me, I am going to move on simply because the time is so short.

Governor Leavitt, in your testimony, you stress the importance of preparing what lies ahead, especially as it relates to ensuring the manufacture of vaccines and other epidemic-specific products can be sustained.

In December in a supplemental appropriations bill, Congress authorized $500 billion for domestic manufacturing capabilities. How, briefly, would you spend that money?

Mr. LEAVITT. Briefly, that is a hard question to answer.

Mr. DUNN. Five hundred billion dollars, just blow through it like that, right?

Mr. LEAVITT. Well, I think we need to acknowledge what got us here in such a short time. We planted multiple seeds. We need to keep doing that.

The second is that we entered into partnerships. This was not just about the government, it was about the government and private sector, and we brought people in the private sector together. We need to continue to do it in this setting in the supply chain matters. And we invested in new technologies along the way, and I commented at various times through this hearing about the need for that to be an ongoing process, not simply when we are in the midst of a pandemic or another public health emergency.

Mr. DUNN. I could not agree with you more.

I had—was party to doing that when I worked in the Army with USAMRIID, the Institute of Infectious Diseases, so I am on your side on that. You are going to get more—or hear more from me about this after today.

And, Mr. Burel, you are too. I am going to be reaching out to you on some ideas of what we should be spending that $500 billion on. I have my own ideas. I want to hear yours.

In the short time left, Governor Leavitt, you also recommended communication—you know what, I am going to skip to my last question, because I care about that more. What advice do you offer the Federal Government to facilitate the use of future and currently available therapies for COVID–19? For example, monoclonal antibodies, you know, they are available. They are out there. They are approved. There are many providers who would have the—do have the ability and willingness to set up outpatient infusion sites. What can we do to get this out to the people and other therapies?

Mr. LEAVITT. Well, it happened with vaccines because we put the emphasis on it, because we put the dollars behind it, and because we operated in parallel—we operated rather in parallel on certain parts of the process as opposed to requiring it at every case that it be sequential. That same formula will work in producing and enhancing our supply there.

Mr. DUNN. Our time has expired. I do think that we could use monoclonal antibodies more, in more cases effectively.

And thank you very much, Madam Chair. Certainly a pleasure to join your committee.

I yield back.

Ms. ESHOO. It is wonderful to have you with us, Mr. Dunn. I agree with you on the concern that you raised, and I think it is worth repeating again that in this recovery act that there is—as the Governor said, we put money behind the development of vaccines. There is $3 billion to develop exactly what you reference.

So thank you, and welcome again to the committee.

Pleasure to recognize the gentlewoman from Michigan, Mrs. Dingell.

Mrs. DINGELL. Thank you, Madam Chair, and to Ranking Member Guthrie, it is great to be here for the first hearing of this year to talk about a subject that means so much to all of us and our constituents.

And I think, before I dig into what I really want to talk about, I want to associate myself with many of the comments of my colleagues. But what Dr. Ruiz was saying, I have spent the last—last Thursday night I had a town hall that, if anybody could believe, it was worse than the John Dingell one on affordable care, with people desperate that can't get answers. They feel like they are being deliberately discriminated against. They don't know where to call.

And, you know, we don't have—we have a national strategy—we are trying to get one, to give it to the States. The States are giving it to State and local governments, and there is simply not enough vaccine right now. And there is not a central number to call, and people are—if you call the hospital, the hospital says, "Well, they are now giving it to the public health departments more," and the public health department is sending you someplace else. I was on phone calls with public health departments and hospitals not being on the same page yesterday.

And, quite frankly, members of the African-American community, communities of color, are feeling very isolated.

So I want to talk about that today. This—you talked about today defining the public health challenges, that we ensure equitable vaccine access for disadvantaged communities addressing vaccine hesitancy and clearly communicating availability for all Americans. And I think we have got to be realistic about what that really means, because we can't get them all in everybody's arms right now.

Dr. Morita, in your testimony you highlight the need for an equitable response to the COVID–19 pandemic as one of the fundamental principles required to improve distribution. I agree, couldn't agree more.

Yesterday, Dr. Khaldun, who is our chief medical executive in the State of Michigan and has been working this really hard, reiterated that my home State's commitment before—she said it before the committee—is that no disparity exists in vaccination rates across racial and ethnic groups or by social vulnerability index. However, despite these extensive efforts, we continue to face challenges in Michigan and across the country with meeting this commitment.

What additional steps should States be taking to address the racial disparities in vaccination rates? Michigan is partnering with local health departments and school-based health centers. Should we be looking at leveraging additional nontraditional spaces? Is there other outreach that you are seeing that is effective here? We talk about community health centers, but they are not being given the vaccine to even be a place for it to be used. I would welcome your wisdom.

Dr. MORITA. Thank you for your questions.

The accessibility of the vaccine is dependent on having the vaccine broadly available in multiple locations. When the vaccine supply is limited, it is really hard to do that, and so there has to be a closer hold on the vaccine. As supply improves, more and more locations will actually be able to get it.

Currently, what needs to happen, since there is a limited supply, is that the locations need to be strategic, so they are equally accessible to all communities. And, in addition to that, there is effort that is being made to simplify the registration process for people who don't have access to internet, who don't have a car, who have to work during the day and have to access the vaccine later in the night or on weekends.

So, the systems have to be developed in a way that actually helps people that are most difficult to reach or most likely to get sick to access the vaccines themselves.

Simultaneously, what needs to be happening as well is work needs to be done within communities to understand what their issues are in terms of concern or hesitancy, because there is an element of hesitancy that exists. And the way to overcome that is really to understand from the community what is happening. What are their questions? What are the concerns? Who do they want to hear from?

There are activities going on right now to support those efforts, but they are just ramping up. To use get out the count, get out the vote in rural America type of approaches, with community members going into their communities because they are trusted voices to really reassure the communities about how to access the vaccine and why they should get the vaccination.

So it is going to have to be a stepwise approach, because we don't have sufficient vaccine for everyone to be vaccinated. But, while we have limited supplies, we also have to simultaneously make it available to the communities who are at greatest risk of getting seriously ill and dying.

Mrs. DINGELL. And you said it is a real challenge, and there isn't one—the problem is that no State, no local has one simple process of figuring out who to call. And I think it would be useful if we could figure that out nationwide.

I am out of time.

Dr. BORIO. If I may add? I was going to add an observation that may be helpful to keep in mind. Because of the temperature control requirements of these vaccines, the early vaccines, as well as the presentation in multidose vials, it does present an additional hurdle to making them available at all of the sites that we would have liked, in addition to the supply constraints, of course. Hopefully this will get better with other vaccines being authorized that are less stringent.

Mrs. DINGELL. You know, I think that is true, but in Michigan we have had fire departments and community health centers actually buy the freezer wanting to be able to do it. They have got— it is the supply right now. But then those that are able to access the system aren't necessarily some of those that need it the most. It is a real challenge.

Thank you.

Ms. ESHOO. The gentlewoman yields back.

Mrs. DINGELL. I do yield back.

Ms. ESHOO. Thank you, Debbie.

It is a pleasure to welcome Mr. Curtis as a new member to our committee, and for his debut of asking his questions.

So welcome, and you are recognized.

Mr. CURTIS. Thank you, Madam Chair, Ranking Member Guthrie.

Yes, this is my first Energy and Commerce meeting, and I want you all to know you pass what I call the elevator test, which is if I were to get stuck in an elevator, I would love to be with all of you. I am just really pleased to be on the committee.

I would like to jump in and discuss an issue. At lot of my colleagues, and rightly so—and, Congresswoman Dingell, I think you did a really good job of emphasizing some of the inequities in our minority communities. Julie Morita talked about inequities in urban neighborhoods.

Governor Leavitt, hello. It is great to have one of my fellow members from Utah on the panel. As you well know, my district in Utah and many of the districts in the country represent vast areas of rural areas. And, if not careful, these areas too are underserved. They bear the burden of poor medical care in many cases, long distances, and also have the problem, I think, of being underserved in this.

What is the right way to think about distributing doses in rural areas? You brought up community health centers, and they are helpful, but they are still far and few between in rural places.

And, Julie Morita, if you would jump in after Governor Leavitt and maybe share your perspective on this as well.

Mr. LEAVITT. Congressman, let me say I resonate strongly with many of the things that have been said about the need for us to get vaccines to these areas that are hard to reach, and, like you, I have become very familiar with the dilemmas that happen in rural areas. And I think the first thing to remember is that the infrastructures in urban areas are not available in rural areas, and so you have to deal with them in unique ways and customize the approach to each one. Without that, we will never be successful.

Dr. MORITA. So thank you for your question. I would add into that as well.

The approach that—I understand the challenges associated with rural communities as well, and mobile units can be used more regularly [audio malfunction] vaccines that are available that don't require the ultra-cold storage or freezer, freezer storage. So I think there is potential for increased access through mobile-unit type of approaches in the future.

I think it is really, again, as Governor Leavitt mentioned, really working with the communities to understand what are the challenges they are actually experiencing so they can inform the solution-making as well because, from an equity perspective, whether it is rural, whether it is urban communities, the communities know their needs best, and hearing from them and listening to them to understand what the solutions are will help to inform a more equitable response overall.

Mr. CURTIS. Thank you.

I would love to give the State of Utah a little shout-out here. We are in the top 5 percent in the United States in our distribution, and my congratulations to our new Governor and so many that are doing a great job.

Governor Leavitt, you are unique in that you had experience on the State level and on the Federal level. There seems to be a little clash from time to time about who best handles certain parts of the responsibilities. Some have advocated the Federal Government should have taken over all distribution.

Can you kind of share, from your perspective, what the right marriage is here between Federal and State government, and how can we maximize each of these two subsets?

Mr. LEAVITT. As you pointed out, I served as the chief executive for the State, and I also served as the chief executive at HHS. And I can tell you from that experience, that both have unique jobs and both have limitations. One limitation the Federal Government has is that it does not execute the capacity—it doesn't have arms and legs to move around communities. It depends on the States, and it depends on the local communities. And so, to some, that somehow the Federal Government will execute on this at the local level simply is not acknowledging the reality.

On the other hand, there are many things that States could never do. States could, on their own, never have developed a vaccine. States need the resources that the Federal Government can apply at a point like this. States require the kind of international coordination that this kind of thing takes place. States cannot provide situational awareness. You have to have data from 50 States to be able to know what is happening and what can be done.

There is a role, a critical role, literally, a role that simply cannot be done without at both the State and the Federal level. This requires a collaborative attitude as much as it does any degree of statute or any degree of regulation. It requires us all to sort of put down—lay down our swords, sit around the table, and solve a problem.

Mr. CURTIS. Thank you, Governor. I regret that I am out of time.

I yield my time, Madam Chair.

Ms. ESHOO. I thank the gentleman for his questions.

And it is a pleasure to recognize the gentlewoman from New Hampshire, Ms. Kuster, better known as Annie.

Ms. KUSTER. Great. Thank you very much, Chairwoman Eshoo. And thank you, Governor. I think you said it exactly right, we need a coordinated approach between the Federal

Government and the States. And I think the title of this hearing, "Road to Recovery," is exactly intended for that.

Last spring, after dozens of conversations with our public health officials and business leaders in New Hampshire, my staff and I wrote a comprehensive outline of steps that Congress should take to mitigate this pandemic and support our economic recovery. And we titled that document "Road Map to Recovery" because there is so much work to do. And while many of these proposals were included in COVID legislation last year, we have more work ahead of us specifically related to the vaccine and improving our health data systems.

While some public health departments have access to the latest and greatest public health infrastructure, others are literally collecting case reports with pen and paper and can only transmit data via telephone and fax. In other cases, COVID vaccination appointments are made and canceled and remade and canceled again, while older Americans sit at home frustrated that they are locked out of the website that thinks they already received the immunization. So I am glad that Congress has put resources towards modernizing our public health infrastructure.

I want to ask you, Dr. Borio, you said in your testimony, "Improved data infrastructure needs to be one of our principal areas of attention." And I couldn't agree more. Can you give us a sense of what that data infrastructure will look like for a 2lst century health data system?

Dr. BORIO. Sure, and I will be happy to elaborate in writing for you. But fundamentally, the way I see this is that, you know, a company like Uber did not disrupt transportation business by hiring the best drivers. They did so with technology, to provide a capability at the hands of every driver. And we need to do this—think about public health data similarly. We need to have an integrated interoperable and, at the Federal level, tremendous analytic capability and link those to actual actions to information to the public.

And I just want to say that hearing Secretary Leavitt speak today, too, makes me miss his leadership when I was young in my career at HHS. So thank you for that.

Ms. KUSTER. Thank you, thank you. I appreciate that.

I just want to share with the entire committee, Congressman Bucshon and I have introduced bipartisan legislation to improve our data infrastructure by expanding the enrollment and training of vaccine providers, modernizing public health information technology, and communicating with patients and providers in real time.

Dr. Morita, can you tell us some of the current challenges that healthcare providers and public health departments are having on the ground due to inadequate immunization information systems? And how can we strengthen these systems?

Dr. MORITA. So, as you pointed out, there are huge needs. What Dr. Borio mentioned was this critical need for interoperability, and I would say that is a major challenge for immunization information systems right now, because each of the 50 States have different systems that they are using. They have all been created separately and distinctly, and so they aren't necessarily interoperable.

But, in addition to not relating to each other, they don't necessarily relate to all of the vaccinators within the jurisdictions. So hospitals, pharmacies, healthcare providers, mass immunization clinics—there is not one system where all of the information comes together.

So, as we look forward to the future, having an interoperable robust system for information to be shared within a State and then also between States is really, really essential. What I would say we have seen play out this year has been a consistent lack of support. It is a boom or bust in terms of public health infrastructure, and the data infrastructure is where you see it play out most statistically.

In order for us to really be prepared for the next pandemic, or even to do better during peacetime, we really need sustained levels of support so we can actually maintain these systems in a way that keeps up with the times.

Ms. KUSTER. Well, I love your analogy to Uber.

What steps can be taken to give confidence to the American people that the information shared in these data systems will be protected and only used to further public health response efforts? I know in my district, people are very concerned about privacy of their healthcare data. And can you mention the precautions and protections that would be in place?

Dr. MORITA. So the public health data, when we access public health data at the health departments in the State or local levels, or at the Federal level as well, those data are protected by HIPAA. And so the only way that we can use that information is to really guide or inform public health intervention.

So when we see there is a community that is not being reached or we see a population that isn't getting vaccinated, we can actually target and direct our resources to them.

When information is shared, it is shared in aggregate so that individuals can't be identified. And, if there are too few people that have similar characteristics, that information is not shared, out of respect for the privacy of these individuals. So because of HIPAA being in place——

Ms. KUSTER. Thank you. I have to apologize. I have run over my time. I need to yield back, but that was very helpful. Thank you so much.

And I yield back.

Ms. ESHOO. The gentlewoman yields back.

I do have legislation on privacy relative to these systems, so we can talk more about that later.

It is a pleasure to welcome to the committee and recognize Mr. Joyce from the great State of Pennsylvania. We are thrilled that you are part of the committee. And your debut, 5 minutes.

Mr. JOYCE. Well, first of all, thank you, Chair Eshoo and Ranking Member Guthrie. I am truly honored to be part of the Health committee on Energy and Commerce, and specifically, I want to thank the witnesses for appearing today at this incredibly important time.

President Trump's Operation Warp Speed has been successful at delivering multiple FDA-authorized COVID–19 vaccines in less than a year. This truly is an unparalleled achievement. However, we are now facing new strains originating from the United Kingdom, Brazil, and South Africa. Now is not the time to let up on innovation in face of this additional health challenge.

Many experts believe the coronavirus might continue to be a public threat into the future. And while these first-generation vaccines are nothing short of incredible and significant achievements, I believe that it is imperative that we as a Nation begin thinking about the United States' approach to how we fight this virus in the years to come.

It is also critical that we not lose sight of the development of new therapeutics to treat the virus, in addition to second-generation vaccines that will speed the public's access to the latest therapies and the latest therapeutics.

My questions first are for Governor Leavitt. In your testimony, you said that the role of Federal policymakers in a pandemic's response is to scout the next valley, anticipating dangers, developing contingencies, and adopting strategies to mitigate potential threats.

Given the emergence of more COVID–19 variants that may be resistant to the limited treatments that we currently have, how can we in Congress do what you said, plant the multiple seeds? As the grandson of an Irish immigrant who planted beautiful gardens, and I know the importance of planting multiple seeds, how can we best prepare to face these variants?

Mr. LEAVITT. First, we acknowledge that this is likely to be a much longer process than just the time it takes to get people vaccinated one time throughout the country. It is very possible that over time we will need to have booster shots or we may have to have vaccinations, much like we do the annual flu, that this is going to be mutating, that we have to be prepared.

And there are supply chain issues. This is an ongoing issue. And there will be infrastructure issues that need to become more permanent, not just temporary.

That is what I think we have to be thinking about in terms of scouting the next valley. We have to anticipate that we need to get better.

I said earlier in the hearing that, if we were talking about distributing 330 million hamburgers, we could do that in our sleep because there is something on every corner that can disperse a hamburger, and we all know how to get it.

We need to become good at distributing and receiving vaccines, and over time our capacity to do this will improve.

Mr. JOYCE. Governor Leavitt, what can we do now to equip agencies like BARDA to ensure that we have access to vaccines that can provide broad immunity so we aren't crippled by a new mutation in 2 or 4 or 10 years?

Mr. LEAVITT. You start with funding them, make certain that they have the relationships that they need and the money that is needed to deploy it. You have to connect them with the regulatory agencies who are going to need to be partners. One thing I believe this committee could do that would move this, move our capacity forward, it has been referenced that we have learned a lot of lessons. We need to harvest those lessons and incorporate them in the normal process, not just the emergency process, because this may be an ongoing need.

Mr. JOYCE. My next question is for Dr. Borio. In your testimony, you mentioned vaccine manufacturers who are taking steps now to develop and test vaccine candidates that may be needed to protect against existing and emerging variants that we certainly will face in the future.

How do you recommend Federal officials lead large-scale vaccine manufacturing efforts and approach these challenges?

Dr. BORIO. Sure. So, at this point, as they develop the candidate, if they were to make a decision to go to full-scale production for the new candidate, they are taking away from what is already being produced for the strain that is also circulating. So the most direct way to answer your question is that we do have to expand the industrial base for manufacturing these vaccines so that we can make more than we are making today, so that we have more flexibility and not make these very difficult choices.

Mr. JOYCE. Thank you very much.

Madam Chair, my time has expired. It is great to be with you on this road to recovery.

Ms. ESHOO. Thank you, Congressman Joyce, and we are delighted that you are with us and part of the team. We love this subcommittee, and for good reason. It is so important, and Members take the work very seriously and have been highly productive. So it is an honor for each one of us to be on the committee and to be together.

With that, the Chair recognizes the gentlewoman from California, Ms. Barraga´n, for her 5 minutes of questions.

Ms. BARRAGÁN. Thank you, Madam Chair. Thank you to our speakers, and for this hearing.

Let me start first by responding to one of my colleagues who asked, what is this administration doing differently than the last one? We will also remind people that we inherited over 400,000 deaths from this pandemic, partially for inaction that was taken.

The first thing that was done is the mask mandate. It is making sure that we are putting science first and making sure people understand the best thing we have against this virus right now is wearing a mask, social distancing, and doing those things that are necessary until people can get a vaccine.

This administration is calling for more dollars from Congress, which is why it is important that we invest, so that we can make sure we are getting money to local, State and local governments to be able to give more of this vaccine. The new administration has also ordered more vaccines when the prior administration wouldn't do so and turned it away. So there is a lot being done now. But our job in this committee is to say what can we do to help with what is going on right now. And I want to thank all the conversations we have had about the inequitable distribution of vaccines.

I represent a district that is almost 90 percent Latino, African-American, low-income, poor. And we have seen firsthand the inequities that are happening. We are having some constituents having to take three buses just to get to a vaccination site. We just learned the other day that the pharmacies were no longer going to get vaccines. They were going to be pulled away and be given to mega PODs, which is harder for constituents like mine to get to. And so I appreciate [inaudible] about the creative solutions.

And let me take a moment to say thank you to Governor Leavitt for your testimony. You had an entire section about anticipating and addressing the barriers of the social determinants of health and equity in your testimony and spoke very specifically about not leaving those behind in low-income communities, rural communities, and minority communities. And you talked about the concerns that we have about transportation and people's situations.

The one common theme I am hearing today is long-term investment, and so making sure we are investing in things like social determinants of health and making sure we are addressing that long term, not just when the pandemic comes out. So it is something I hope that we will also look into one of my bills on social determinants of health.

But I want to start the questioning with you, Dr. Morita. You have spoken about one of the things that needs to be done is to use federally qualified health centers and community clinics. When I was a kid, I relied upon them quite a bit. And so I have heard that, number one, many of them, the majority of them, are not getting the vaccine. There are shortages on gloves, shortages on the needles to be used.

Is there anything that you want to either elaborate again on or tell us as Congress on what we should be focusing on to making sure that the community health centers are getting what they need, whether it is staffing or supplies, to be able to reach target communities and those that are underserved?

Dr. MORITA. I reviewed the Biden administration COVID strategy that was released the day after inauguration. Within that strategy is a commitment to providing additional resources to federally qualified health centers, recognizing the important role that they play in reaching some of our harder-to-reach communities who have been so devastated by this pandemic. And so I think that there is what is necessary. The equities are committed. They want to do this work. What they need is the resources to actually ramp up and scale up their ability to deliver the vaccine and to deliver the healthcare that is necessary.

I appreciate also your point about the social determinants of health. What the pandemic has done has made a clear connection between the systemic barriers to people having good health. So it is access to insurance, access to good pay, a good-paying job, access to paid leave. All of these factors contributed to why certain populations actually are at higher risk for having hospitalizations and dying. And so these underlying conditions really need to be addressed for the long term so that we are not in the same state with the next pandemic.

Ms. BARRAGÁN. Thank you.

I think this is a good opportunity to emphasize the need for us to invest in community health centers and clinics long term. Oftentimes we are not funding them long term. We are going year by year. And guess what? We are not giving them the increases that they need yearly to invest in our community health centers.

So I want to thank the panelists. There is a lot to cover, but I am out of time.

And with that, I yield back.

Ms. ESHOO. The gentlewoman yields back.

It is a pleasure to recognize the only pharmacist, I think, in the entire House of Representatives, Mr. Carter, for his for 5 minutes.

Mr. CARTER. Thank you, Madam Chair. I have to correct you, though, we have another pharmacist now.

Ms. ESHOO. Oh, good.

Mr. CARTER. We have two pharmacists in Congress now.

Ms. ESHOO. Well, that is great.

Mr. CARTER. My colleagues are giving me——

Ms. ESHOO. [Inaudible] some of the distribution.

Mr. CARTER. Yes, yes. But I am the oldest pharmacist in Congress, if it matters.

Ms. ESHOO. OK.

Mr. CARTER. So, nevertheless, I thank all of the panelists for being here and discussing this extremely important subject, obviously.

Governor Leavitt, I wanted to start with you and just talk about the distribution process. It is so vitally important. And one of the critical aspects is to pharmacies and to pharmacists, making sure that we are utilizing retail pharmacists. Whether it be independent or chain pharmacists, it is extremely important. As has been mentioned during this hearing, 95 percent of all Americans live within 5 miles of a pharmacy. Pharmacists are the most accessible healthcare professional in America. We need to utilize that. And I think we would all agree with that.

HHS has made some changes to authorize pharmacists to be able to administer the vaccine. In fact, early on, they, during this pandemic or during the administration distribution of the vaccine, the administration of the vaccine, they passed a rule where the people—that pharmacists could give it to anybody 3 years or older, and that was very important. And just yesterday, they also passed a rule to say that the vaccines can be shipped directly to pharmacies, and that is very important during this pandemic as well.

I wanted to ask you, Governor Leavitt, you have served at the State level, you have served at the Federal level, as have I. I have served at both levels as well. And is it your belief that all pharmacists should be able to administer the COVID–19 vaccine, if it is approved by the FDA, no matter what the State laws may be, no matter what varying State laws there may be?

Mr. LEAVITT. I have referenced a couple of times in this hearing my experience with Medicare part D, which is another moment in time when millions of people all at one time were seeking some type of new Federal or new government service. The pharmacies were the main—they were the heroes of that whole effort, because people went to the pharmacy, they knew they could get good advice, they knew they could find out the answers, and I became a great supporter of that. And I think they are a great support in the annual flu. Typically, that is [inaudible] I get my flu vaccine is at the [inaudible].

Now, I personally would not go so far as to say that the Federal Government has an interest in being able to override local decisions that are being made on what is best in every community. But I think many communities are and will realize even more how important the [inaudible] to your important statement is in being able to serve [inaudible] those communities, particularly the underserved communities.

Mr. CARTER. And I would agree with that. And thank you, Governor, for that point.

One thing that I wanted to point out—and I would be interested in knowing your opinion on this as well—is that, during this pandemic, we have both relaxed some rules and implemented some new rules. And one thing that I hope that we do at the Federal level is to review this before we just go and put them all back into place. I mean, there are things that pharmacists can do that they need to be doing, not just during this pandemic, but they need to be doing the whole time in order to improve healthcare services here in the United States.

Governor, another thing that I wanted to ask you——

Mr. LEAVITT. I concur with you having pharmacies operating at the top of their license being able to do all of [inaudible].

Mr. CARTER. Absolutely.

I represent an area that has a high minority population as well. And it is very important and very concerning to me about vaccine hesitancy, particularly in the minority community. Just wondering what your experience is. What works? What doesn't work? Just some advice, if you would, on how we can improve that.

Mr. LEAVITT. [Inaudible.]

Dr. MORITA. I think he is having difficulty. I am glad to jump in on this question.

Mr. CARTER. Yes, please, please do. Thank you very much.

Dr. MORITA. Sure. So I think in addition to the challenges with people accessing the vaccine from our [inaudible] to our communities are color, there are also challenges of vaccine hesitancy because of distrust of the vaccine. Because of mistreatment in the past or discrimination in the past, people aren't trusting the vaccine itself. So it is really important for there to be community efforts where there are trusted messengers from within the community, engaging with the communities, to understand what their questions are, what their concerns are, who they want to hear from so we can actually address the concerns. So, when a vaccine becomes more readily available, the communities that are at highest risk actually have more access to it and their concerns are addressed and they can demand the vaccine to do it.

Mr. CARTER. That is so very important. Thank you, Doctor, for mentioning that. And I for one, as a member of the Doctors Caucus and as a Congressman, I went through the clinical trials myself to try to set a good example. And I was fortunate enough to be able. Of course, it was a double blind study, but I did get the vaccine. So I want people to know that it is safe and effective.

Thank you very much, Madam Chair. And I yield back.

Ms. ESHOO. The gentleman yields back.

It is a pleasure to recognize the gentlewoman from Delaware, Ms. Blunt Rochester, for 5 minutes of questioning. Great to see you.

Ms. BLUNT ROCHESTER. Good to see you too. And thank you so much, Madam Chairwoman. Congratulations, Ranking Member Guthrie. And thank you especially to all of the witnesses.

I want to start by associating myself with the comments of my colleague Ms. Barraga´n on illuminating the social determinants of health. It is an area that we have legislation on as well, and it is vital, especially we have seen it illuminated during this pandemic.

And as our Nation marks the 1-year anniversary of declaring the coronavirus outbreak a public health emergency, it is clear that Congress must move swiftly and boldly with a pandemic response that protects the health and the economic well-being of our constituents and solves this public health crisis at last.

I am preparing to introduce or reintroduce my bill, the Coverage for COVID–19 Treatment Act, to guarantee access to COVID–19 treatment with no cost sharing, because no one should have to worry about how they can afford treatment if they contract COVID–19.

Like President Biden, however, I want to make sure that treatment isn't just affordable but that it is widely accessible and effective. This is especially true for people dealing with long-term health impacts of COVID–19 or long COVID syndrome. And I would like to focus my first questions there.

Dr. Borio, in your testimony, you said that we desperately need better therapies for COVID–19. Why do you think we should continue to focus on investing in and support for the development of therapeutics and treatments for COVID–19?

Dr. BORIO. The currently available treatments are very limited. They are limited in benefit, they are limited in on whom they work, when they work. They are difficult to scale up. They are intravenous drugs. So we do need treatments that are more easily administered, more easily scalable to manufacture, more easily accessible. And also, this is not going to be the last biological pandemic. COVID is likely going to become endemic. We need better antivirals to treat COVID going forward.

Ms. BLUNT ROCHESTER. Thank you.

Dr. BORIO. [Inaudible] research program—it is already late. We have to start a research program that comprehensively tackles it as soon as possible.

Ms. BLUNT ROCHESTER. And following up on that, Governor Leavitt, thank you for your testimony. And you mentioned that Congress should be aware of the growing cohorts of patients with long COVID syndrome. What should Congress do to ensure there is better access to effective therapies to treat people with long COVID syndrome?

Mr. LEAVITT. I will simply under—I will first underscore the importance of this. This is a significant challenge. This is one we ought to be looking into the next valley, scouting the next valley and getting ahead of. And I would point to three things.

The first is data. We need more data about this. The second is the need for us to begin to isolate clinical pathways for those who have it, even to the point that we still can't—we don't know how to diagnose it. We don't have a name for it. We don't have billing codes for it. We need to make progress in the context of clinical care. And lastly, payment. We have to begin to think about the impact this is going to have on payment systems.

Ms. BLUNT ROCHESTER. Thank you.

And, Dr. Morita, how can Congress help ensure equitable access to COVID–19 treatments for the growing number of people with long-term care COVID symptoms, many of whom are experiencing economic hardship right now?

Dr. MORITA. I have to agree with Governor Leavitt. Having data and understanding who is actually getting treatment, how is the treatment working, making sure that those things are all in place so that it is that when treatments are available and they have been studied, that we actually can make sure that they are providing the right places.

In addition, though, as trials are being done with experimental medications, making sure that we have adequate representation in communities of color in the trials themselves so they can feel confident that the medications themselves have been tested in appropriate populations in those that look like themselves.

Ms. BLUNT ROCHESTER. Thank you.

And I am shifting gears. In the early months of the pandemic, I joined my colleagues Congressman Pocan and Crist to introduce legislation to harness the full power of the Defense Production Act. And I know invoking the DPA is a priority for President Biden.

Dr. Borio, how will using the Defense Production Act alleviate supply shortages in our country? And I think you also mentioned that we still remain vulnerable. Can you talk about vulnerabilities?

Dr. BORIO. Sure. Thank you. Look, I am not an expert on DPA. It is quite a complex set of authorities we have. All I know is that Operation Warp Speed has leveraged it very heavily to be able to provide priority allocation to limited resources, to the vaccine manufacturers under a U.S. contract. It is not a final solution. You know, it is very important to recognize that sometimes allocating priorities for filling finished lines for vaccine manufacturers is critical right now, has bumped products in those finished lines that were destined to other patients with some very critical diseases. So it is just not a final solution.

Ms. BLUNT ROCHESTER. I am out of time, but I do want to thank Mr. Burel as well, and I am looking forward to his recommendations on supply chain and DPA. We look forward to that.

Thank you so much. And I yield back.

Ms. ESHOO. The gentlewoman yields back.

It is a pleasure, a real pleasure, to welcome a new member to our committee, the gentlewoman from Minnesota, Ms. Angie Craig. So it is just great to have you with us.

I might add, and I don't know how many Members realize this, but all of our new members on the Democratic side are women. We have a whole new team. So watch out, gentlemen. Here we come. We are coming.

Ms. CRAIG. We are here. We are here.

Ms. ESHOO. We are here.

The gentlewoman is recognized.

Ms. CRAIG. Thank you so much, Chairwoman Eshoo. And thank you to our panelists for sharing your expertise with us here today.

It is really an honor to be here for my first Health Subcommittee hearing. I ran for Congress to tackle the very issues under this subcommittee's jurisdiction, particularly expanding healthcare access and affordability. And I look so forward to working with all of you.

I represent the State of Minnesota where, tragically, we have lost more than 6,200 lives to COVID–19. Like the rest of the country, people are struggling to survive both a global pandemic and widespread economic uncertainty.

With the new administration in office, we have an opportunity to provide the American people with the assistance that they desperately need. I am encouraged by the Biden administration's efforts to provide States with more transparency and increase the vaccine supply, both of which will accelerate the number of shots in arms.

While our vaccine and testing capabilities continue to trend in the right direction, it is clear the Federal Government must do more. Our lives and our economies are depending on it.

My first question is for Dr. Morita. As you noted in your testimony, an equitable vaccine allocation and distribution strategy relies on robust data. Last Congress, I introduced the Vaccine Fairness Act, which directed HHS to provide regular updates on their efforts to ensure the COVID–19 vaccine reaches the groups most at risk.

This week, the CDC released demographic data for the vaccines administered between December 14 and January 14, about half of the total vaccines administered to date. These data points support long-held concerns by public health experts about disproportionately low vaccination rates among Black and Hispanic Americans. These trends are reflected in Minnesota, where we are seeing lower vaccination rates in the areas outside the Twin Cities and among long-term care staff.

I am encouraged by the Biden administration's commitment to provide real-time data, and I would further encourage the administration to include racial and ethnic demographics in on the CDC dashboard.

Dr. Morita, my question is, what impact does Federal data collection and reporting have on State and city efforts to implement an equitable vaccine administration program? In other words, why is it so important that we have centralized and transparent data?

Dr. MORITA. So having disaggregated the data by race, by ethnicity, by geography, by occupation is fundamental to the response being coordinated and an equitable response. In order for us to make sure that we are reaching the people that we actually need to reach who are at highest risk, we really have to have the data available.

What the Federal Government can do is really establish the expectation, require that these fields actually be included. So, as the programs are rolling out, they actually are collecting—the vaccinators are actually collecting this information. I talked with Walgreens at the beginning, prior to them actually rolling out their pharmacy vaccination effort in the long-term care facilities. And they said that they were required by Federal law to collect that information, race and ethnicity information, as they were vaccinating.

The challenge is that the systems within the States and local jurisdictions aren't necessarily equipped to handle that information or haven't been updated in time so that they can accept the information in a quick and efficient way. So what has to happen is the standard has to be established and an expectation for these collections of information, and then resources to support the systems so the information can be collected in an efficient way and then used and reported in a consistent way so there is transparency.

Ms. CRAIG. Thank you so much.

My next question quickly is for Mr. Burel. While the Department of Health and Human Services holds the primary responsibility for responding to and preparing for public health emergencies, a crisis as large as this requires assistance from FEMA. In your assessment, what have the contributions from FEMA had on the availability of medical supplies? And I only have about 30 seconds left.

Mr. BUREL. I apologize, I wasn't prepared to answer that question. Let me give it some thought and come back to you. I do think it is important that, when FEMA takes on those roles, it works with the people who are the subject matter experts in that space to make sure we get the right thing to the right place at the right time. And I think sometimes there is a disconnect there. Having worked both for HHS and FEMA, I know it is something that we always have to work on to coordinate better.

Ms. CRAIG. I appreciate that very much.

And, Madam Chairwoman, I yield back.

Ms. ESHOO. The gentlewoman yields back. And, again, I am so thrilled that you are on the committee.

And speaking of being thrilled, it is a pleasure to recognize Dr. Schrier from Washington State, also a new member of the committee, and our fourth doctor, a pediatrician. So I know that she is going to bring a great deal to our deliberations. We will learn from you, and we are really thrilled to have you as part of our subcommittee. It is already enhanced. So you are recognized for your first 5 minutes of the subcommittee.

Ms. SCHRIER. Well, thank you for that welcome, Madam Chair. And thank you to our witnesses.

Like all of us, I am incredibly relieved that we have two highly effective vaccines, and more to come, in less than a year's time. And I cannot overstate how grateful I am to the scientists behind these achievements. With that said, as we all know, it will take months to immunize the country, and the more this virus spreads, the more mutations we will see.

To successfully reopen our communities and especially our schools safely, we just need more tools in our toolbox to contain the virus and prevent its spread. This is really hard when asymptomatic people spread the disease and much of the Nation still does not mask or distance.

So surveillance testing helps pick up evolving outbreaks once a disease is under control. But, right now, rapid at-home antigen tests done on a regular basis could dramatically slow the spread. So, for regular at-home testing to work, the test would have to be cheap enough for people to use every day or two to see if they are shedding the virus and then just take themselves out of circulation. Guess what? Homes tests like this already exist. So we are really close. But the ones that are currently available are way too expensive for daily use, at $25 to $50 per test. Some require a prescription and equipment.

But here is the thing: The components are really cheap. Produced at scale, they could cost less than $1 each. Did you know that the $15 pregnancy test in the store wholesales for 70 cents? And this is the same concept. So why aren't they already in our hands?

Well, there are lots of reasons, but one is that big companies are buying up those components, and their profit margin is higher to making 1,000 $30 tests as opposed to 30,000 $1 tests. So another is that the Trump administration didn't put its weight behind this concept, and meanwhile a year later, 441,000 dead, more than 3,000 dying every day, and daily at-home testing would have been the curve. So I want to ask about that.

Dr. Borio, thank you for your service. In January of last year, you coauthored an excellent article called "Act Now to Prevent an American Epidemic," and you encouraged government agencies to work with private partners to achieve robust testing. And so I want to ask you about antigen tests.

To your knowledge, Dr. Borio, has there been an effort to establish an independent comparative evaluation of different antigen tests, like a head-to-head comparison of test accuracy to find the best ones?

Dr. BORIO. No, I am not aware of a head-to-head effort. I am encouraged that the new administration has established a pandemic testing board which will look comprehensively across all issues around testing.

Ms. SCHRIER. Great. And I understand there is this kind of test at the Frederick National Lab for serology or antibody test. And so it sounds like we could do the same thing for these lateral slow antigen tests.

Dr. BORIO. There is no reason why not to do comparative assessments of the different tests.

Ms. SCHRIER. Great. And then, if we did this comparing apples to apples and found the best test, could we procure the materials at scale to drive down the price for the American people?

Dr. BORIO. That, I do not know.

Ms. SCHRIER. OK. Because we would need millions every day.

And then, to your knowledge and from your prior experience, did the Trump administration dive in and take an active role in the testing, approval, procurement, and manufacturing of these sorts of tests?

Dr. BORIO. So the prior administration did quite a bit to interfere with FDA's independence in regulating these tests in public health emergencies. There has been a lot of confusion as a result of this interference. I think FDA's now poised to be able to regain its mission to make sure that the American public has access to tests that work as intended. And they don't have to be the best test in the world, they just have to work as intended and do we understand their limitations.

Ms. SCHRIER. That is exactly right. We could have an imperfect test, but if you do it every day, if you don't catch it on Monday, you will catch it on Tuesday and you will stay home from work or school. Thank you for that answer, and that explains some of the holdup.

So thank you, Dr. Borio and all of our witnesses. This has really been a pleasure today. I can't wait to get these tests into every home in the country and open up our economy and get our kids back to school safely and kind of layer these layers of Swiss cheese. You know, we can have masks and distancing and cleaning and rapid tests and vaccines, and we will get much farther much sooner.

Thank so much. I yield back.

Ms. ESHOO. Thank you, Dr. Schrier. Wonderful questions, wonderful points. I agree with you. I think in terms of testing, that so far we have missed the boat. Because these tests really should be 79 cents, $1 each. People should be able to buy a packet for a month or 2 weeks, especially essential workers. And I think the money in the recovery plan will go a long ways to making that happen.

We really have to put our pedal to the metal. This is the United States of America, for heaven's sakes. We can do this, and it is a source of embarrassment to me that we have these gaps. But, boy, with this committee pushing, we can close them and then some.

It is now a pleasure to welcome another new member to our subcommittee, the gentlewoman from Massachusetts, Mrs. Trahan. And I know that she has a great deal of biotechnology in her congressional district and that she will be a voice for issues coming out of that particular segment of the healthcare industry.

So welcome, and you are recognized.

Mrs. TRAHAN. Thank you. Thank you, Chairwoman Eshoo and Ranking Member Guthrie, as well as to all the witnesses.

I will start by just saying, as Chairman Eshoo, Chairman Pallone, the Ranking Member Rodgers stated, I too want to emphasize that, in order to build a system to address future threats and protect our national security, we must revitalize America's manufacturing industry. And I won't say much more about it, except that I welcome my colleagues to join the bipartisan Pandemic Preparedness Caucus that I started with Congressman Balderson and Congresswoman Axne.

I will echo the concerns of my colleagues about ensuring equitable and accelerated access to COVID–19 testing, treatment, and vaccination. Now, I recently spoke with healthcare providers at Lawrence General Hospital in Lawrence, Massachusetts, a majority minority gateway city in my district, and they shared that the mortality rate for Hispanic patients rose from below 2 percent pre-COVID to nearly 13 percent—a massive spike, and one we are seeing predominantly in our communities of color across the country. Conversely, the mortality for White Americans climbed just 1 single percent. So we can't allow inequities like this to persist. Rather, equity has to be our central concern.

And I too celebrate the miracle of having two highly effective vaccines. But we must be focused on dramatically accelerating the distribution while also addressing the fact that we have fallen behind in testing innovation, as Congresswoman Schrier mentioned, and capacity building central to opening our schools and businesses. We have fallen behind on genomic research, specifically sequencing surveillance that identifies new variants. And we have fallen behind on developing treatments that mitigate the most severe symptoms.

So today I just want to zero in on one method to help reduce mortality for all Americans, and that is developing new therapies for COVID–19. The development of effective therapeutic agents can greatly decrease the severity of the disease while we are vaccinating Americans and preventing hospitalizations, long-term effects, certainly death.

So, Dr. Borio, you have answered in your testimony and here today why it is important to continue to invest in developing COVID therapies but also mentioned that the U.S. response was hindered by its lack of a clinical trial network that could be utilized quickly during a pandemic. Can you explain how a network like this can be established and adapted to different novel diseases?

Dr. BORIO. Thank you. Absolutely. So, you know, just taking a step back, we had to rely on existing clinical trial networks that existed for other diseases, for oncology, for et cetera, and we had to repurpose them. That took a long time.

NIH did some quicker studies. Actually they brought us remdesivir, for example. But they were limited to certain of number of sites across the U.S. And we really need to be able to leverage technology and leverage advances in how we conduct clinical studies, including around the oversight clinical studies, to really be able to capture patients where they are.

If you do the math and see how many cases we are seeing today across America, only a very, very tiny fraction of those patients are really able to enroll in clinical research. That allows us to have a learning system where we can learn as we go through this and be able to modify our practice according to new knowledge. So we need to be able to, you know, really use all of our healthcare systems, our networks, hospitals, medical centers, VA, et cetera, into a clinical research enterprise.

Mrs. TRAHAN. Great. Thank you for that.

You know, vaccine development for COVID–19 leveraged major biomedical research investments, and it created these public-private industry partnerships to get a vaccine to market in record time. What lessons should we take from our early approaches to testing potential therapeutic agents as well as the success of vaccine development that would help catalyze better treatments for COVID–19 as well as other emerging infectious diseases?

Dr. BORIO. I will say that just trust the importance of the adequately conducted studies, rigorous studies that give us definitive answers about whether a product works or doesn't, so we can go all in into making sure that we have sufficient supplies and ways to administer them.

Vaccines are a great example where we did, you know, the gold standard in a most efficient way, very thoughtful approach, and we have definitive data about their safety and effectiveness. We do not have that same degree of information from most therapeutics. There are very few exceptions. So we can't cut corners in therapeutics if we want to really be able to provide cures that we can send support to our patients.

Mrs. TRAHAN. Understood. Well, thank you. I appreciate your answers.

And I will yield back. Thank you, Madam Chair.

Ms. ESHOO. The gentlewoman yields back.

And, boy, today is filled with a lot of pleasures relative to our subcommittee. Another great new member, the gentlewoman from Texas, Ms. Fletcher. Welcome to the subcommittee. We are thrilled that you are part of it. And it is your debut, your first 5 minutes of questions.

Mrs. FLETCHER. Well, thank you so much, Chairwoman Eshoo. I am just delighted and honored to be here and to serve on this subcommittee. So I thank you and Ranking Member Guthrie for holding this vital hearing today. And I am so glad to be able to do the critical work to combat this public health crisis. And I thank our witnesses today for their time and their excellent insight.

My colleagues have touched on many of the critical issues before us. Focusing on vaccines and vaccination rates are vital issues in my district in Houston as well. But I want to pick up on the line of questioning that my colleague, Dr. Schrier, was asking about just now about testing. Because as we understand it now, that administering the vaccine will take time and that those vaccinated may still be carriers of the virus even if there—you know, the impact of the disease that emerges from it with COVID–19. So that really brings us back to the need to having an effective testing strategy.

And, Dr. Borio, in your testimony, you talked about the need for CDC and FDA to develop still a national testing strategy. Part of any good strategy is ensuring that you have adequate supply to follow demand, and we know that if it is done right, there will be demand for a long time.

We saw last summer, particularly where we had outbreaks in the South, that there was driving demand, some labs had excess capacity and others were having long testing delays. So can you discuss a little bit how we can efficiently get testing supplies to labs where there is need and how we can do this on an ongoing basis?

Dr. BORIO. So part of making sure that we have sufficient supply has to do with having the strategy so that we know where to focus, where to be able to put the dollars behind. And we don't have that today. So it is not sufficient to say let's, you know, increase the supply of every possible available test. We need to know which ones really need the most attention, which ones might be fine, and what is the balance of rapid tests and other high throughput tests. We don't have that information today because we don't have a strategy.

Mrs. FLETCHER. OK. Well, and I guess there is sort of a related strategic issue that I want to touch on with the time I have left for Dr. Morita and then anyone else who wants to weigh in, because I think another important aspect of understanding the supply issues is also ensuring that we have the adequate public health workforce to conduct the testing and the contact tracing while we are still vaccinating individuals. And I was glad to see that the American Rescue Plan includes resources for testing and a greater public health workforce. I also understand there was some testimony just yesterday in another hearing that State and local governments have diverted some of the resources for testing and contact tracing to vaccines.

And so what do you think, starting with Dr. Morita, what do you think can and should be done to ensure that the proper resources and personnel are allocated to testing and tracing?

Dr. MORITA. Your point is well taken. During the transition period of time, we spoke with a number of State and local health officials, and what they reported was they were really struggling in terms of manpower, because it was the same people that were being asked to do the testing, to do the contact tracing, to do the outbreak investigations, and to start planning for the vaccine. This is prior to the vaccine being available. And so there are just insufficient numbers of staff that are actually available.

What has to happen is really ramping up and shoring up that infrastructure with staff right now for the immediate response but in looking at how to sustain that for the long haul, because it is really difficult to hire a bunch of staff within State or local government and to get them mobilized and have them trained up to actually do the kind of work that is necessary, rather than having an existing solid network of workforce that could actually respond when the crisis actually occurs.

I think I agree with Dr. Borio in terms of there needs to be a testing strategy. And in order to have a strategy, there really—it won't all be just public health workforce that is doing the testing. It can rely on healthcare providers that are in the community, in health centers and clinics and hospitals doing some testing as well, just because I don't think that the workforce necessarily has to do the testing on an ongoing basis. It can be a coordinated effort with other providers as well.

Mrs. FLETCHER. Terrific. Thank you for that.

Would anyone else like to weigh in with their thoughts on that question?

Mr. LEAVITT. I will simply remind us all that, during the early part of this pandemic, we were in a big hurry to get tests, and a lot of tests went on to the market. And a lot of damage happens when tests are inaccurate on either side. And so there needs to be a testing strategy. Part of that has to be accuracy and dependability. And a test is not a test that is not a test. They are not all the same.

Mrs. FLETCHER. Thank you for that. And thank you all again for your insights today.

I am just out of time, so I will yield back. Thank you, Chairwoman Eshoo.

Ms. ESHOO. The gentlewoman yields back. Again, welcome to the committee.

And now I would like to recognize the gentlewoman from Illinois, Ms. Kelly, a really valued member of the committee.

Where are you, Robin? I don't see you. There you are. You are recognized.

Ms. KELLY. New glasses. Thank you, Chairwoman Eshoo. And thank you to all of our witnesses. Thank you for your patience. And, again, welcome to all of our new members.

As the chair of the Congressional Black Caucus Health Brain Trust, vaccine equity is very, very important to me, and testing. I mean, there was a story on CNN about a vaccine that was supposed to go to a more Latino neighborhood, but the appointments were taken by Whites coming into the neighborhood and them not getting their vaccines. And also stories around hospitals who are coding the way they give their vaccines out so doctors and nurses and folks like that come first and Black and Brown folks who are janitors are pushed to the background. So those stories are very, very concerning.

And the other thing that I am worried about: What happens with people with disabilities? Like, do you know anything about what is happening with people who are deaf or people that are blind? We don't seem to talk about that that much. And I was just curious, do any of you know anything about that population?

Dr. MORITA. I can jump in on this question. Nice to see you, Congresswoman.

Ms. KELLY. Nice to see you.

Dr. MORITA. In terms of just what is happening with communities of color and the challenges that are being experienced, the systems have to be developed. And whether it is communities of color or it is disabled communities themselves, the systems have to be developed in a way that everyone has easy access to them. So it can't just be a one-size-fits-all, internet-access appointment-making schedule, because that is just not going to work for everybody. And it can't just be vaccines offered in hospitals, large hospitals.

And so what really is happening right now is on the ground, and I have heard this from many jurisdictions, they are making the plans to broaden out how they actually make the vaccine available. They focused on hospitals and healthcare systems because that is who was supposed to get it first, but now as the groups are broadened, they will be broadening out to the locations and places. But they also are working on developing systems to actually have community workers go out into the communities to help people register for the vaccines, making the vaccines available in the appropriate sites, working with federally qualified health centers that actually provide services to those communities themselves. And also that they should be building into the systems and are building for people with disabilities to actually access the systems as well. So it is a comprehensive type of approach.

And you mentioned it earlier and have been saying it pretty consistently, that in order to build the systems out and have the people to actually do this kind of critical work, more research is really needed to flow to the States and locals who are on the ground doing this critical work.

Ms. KELLY. I actually just got a phone call from one of my mayors. In our local supermarket, they are vaccinating 500 people today, and then they will be backs in 3 weeks to vaccinate 500 more. And this is in a suburban town outside of Chicago.

Just also out of curiosity, we can just go down the panel, how do you feel about school opening? It is a big issue in Chicago, as I am sure that you have heard about. And, you know, our Catholic schools have been open, but it is a big issue about public schools. I am just curious how each one of you see that.

Mr. LEAVITT. Well, I will just say, as Governor I learned that those decisions are not well made at State capitals or Washington, DC. They are best made by local school communities, because every school community is different, and it changes from time to time and it needs to be managed in a very direct, individualized way.

Ms. KELLY. Thank you.

Dr. MORITA. There was a recently published article in JAMA by the CDC that described schools that have reopened safely and what assistance needed to be in place to allow them to open safely. So I think it is really important that these kind of publications are coming out. There is a lot of natural experiments that have been happening over the past year where school systems have been open, and understanding how to open them safely is really, really important. We all want our kids to be back in school, because we know learning is optimal in that school setting. And yet we have to make sure that the systems are in place, appropriate social distancing, requirements for mask wearing, or appropriate ventilation. Those kinds of assistance are critical for State schools to be open safely.

Ms. KELLY. Ms. Borio?

Dr. BORIO. I think the data is really critical, and I think we begin to see the data. I agree with Governor Leavitt as well that it is important to make decisions locally. But we do—the Federal Government has a duty to be able to provide schools with information and with guidance and with assistance to be able to reopen safely.

Ms. KELLY. Thank you, Doctor. Mr. Burel, my last few seconds.

Mr. BUREL. Sure. I think that I agree with all of my colleagues. One of the things that I think we have talked about here is the need for availability of testing, the need for availability of personal protective equipment. I think all of these things would go a long way to creating a safer environment for schools and businesses to reopen faster.

Ms. KELLY. Thank you.

And thank you, Madam Chair. I yield back.

Ms. ESHOO. The gentlewoman yields back.

It is a pleasure to recognize the gentleman from Maryland, Mr. Sarbanes. And thank you for your patience.

Mr. SARBANES. Thank you very much, Madam Chair. Can you hear me OK?

Ms. ESHOO. Yes. Just speak up a little louder. I don't know if everyone's systems are as dim as mine, but everyone's voice seems awfully almost muted to me today. So do speak out.

Mr. SARBANES. I will try to speak clearly for the benefit of you, Madam Chair, and other members in the panel.

I want to thank our witnesses today. This has been an exhaustive and long session, but I think you covered really important dimensions of the crisis that we are facing, particularly this vaccine distribution challenge.

Dr. Borio, I am very interested in your thoughts, and perhaps Governor Leavitt as well, when it comes to workforce challenges. We already had a public health infrastructure that lacked the kind of robust workforce component that you would need in normal times. The pressure that has been placed on our public health infrastructure and just broadly on our healthcare system by the pandemic has exposed these workforce shortages and, of course, has aggravated them in many places, because the healthcare workers themselves have come down with the pandemic and they have been knocked out of work, many have lost their lives and so forth.

Could you speak, beginning with Dr. Borio, to what strategies you see for deploying in this moment additional healthcare workers, anyone, for that matter, who would be viewed as qualified to administer vaccines? Because, as we tried to deliver the vaccine more creatively, whether that is having mass vaccination sites or mobile vaccination sites, reaching out to communities that have less access, et cetera, we are going to need the people. And that is often the bottleneck that we face. Along with protective equipment, along with the availability of the vaccine itself, along with the cold chain custody and all the rest of it, speak specifically to the workforce part of this crisis and what we are doing in the moment to try to ramp up that capacity to handle all of these things, but in particular you could talk to the vaccine distribution.

Dr. BORIO. So, briefly, I think that we always know about the four S's: the supply, system, space, and staff. And we sometimes forget that staff is also a supply chain issue. There are efforts to now find a way to create more flexibilities with allowing practitioners to move from State to State as well as rehire retired healthcare professionals to be able to participate in the program. Look at other types of health-related professions to be able to administer, whether it is EMS, dentists, and pharmacists. I think that there are ways to be able to do that in the short term. But in the long run, it is really about expanding public health workforce to be able to tackle the types of threats that we are going to face, continue to face in the future.

I don't want to over—also take this moment to just share that, even in the manufacturing of this vaccine [inaudible] to staff it, because it is about staff. We think about the back, the filters, the columns, the space. But staffing with people that really understand vaccine production has been a challenge as well. So it is all around the whole response program.

Mr. SARBANES. Thank you.

Governor Leavitt?

Mr. LEAVITT. Yes. I am of the view that, in the long term, this has to be an all-hands-on-deck exercise. One of the things that I believe is limiting about a highly centralized distribution process is that it in many ways is not convenient for people, and hence, it will be less accessible. However, what militated against that in the early stages of distribution is that it takes infrastructure to do it. And I believe one of the things that will occur as time goes on, as this becomes an elongated process—that is to say, it has to endure for a long time—there needs to be mobile units, employer-based units, all kinds of different mechanisms. But they not only need to know how to give a shot, they also need to be able to access the records so that, as we begin to deploy what I spoke of earlier, which is a vaccine credentialing process, that people can gain access to their own vaccination records and have them digitally presentable to people. They need to be part of that system.

Mr. SARBANES. Thank you very much. I yield back, Madam Chair.

Ms. ESHOO. The gentleman yields back. And we thank him for his always excellent questions.

So this concludes all members of the subcommittee that were with us today in having their time to question. We also extend a legislative courtesy to members of the full committee that wish to join us. And we have Mr. O'Halleran, the gentleman from Arizona, who is waiving on. And I would like to recognize him for his 5 minutes of questions.

So welcome back, Tom. It is always great to see you.

Mr. O'HALLERAN. Thank you, Madam Chair. Thank you for the panel. This has been an excellent presentation.

The first cases of COVID were detected in the United States a year ago. Early in the pandemic, Congress acted in four bipartisan bills, which is important for the unity that we need in America today.

Secretary Leavitt in testimony noted that we will get better at this. We are a year in, actually more than a year in, because we need to be working 24 hours a day. And so that year is really 3 years of work, hopefully.

Mr. Burel noted that we are short on everything. And Dr. Morita said that, today, we are going to need a full-court press. We needed a full-court press from the beginning.

Over the summer, in one of the hearings, I asked Dr. Fauci, would we be ready in the fall and early winter. He said, "I hope so." Then I asked him again in another meeting, will we be ready in the fall or winter? In fact, he said that, as we were getting into the fall, he said again, "I hope so."

It is obvious from the testimony today that we are nowhere where we need to be in relationship to where we should be. From April until the end of December, Congress was unable to come together to provide additional support to build out a robust national testing contact tracing system. And, in fact, almost every other discussion we have had today.

Despite claims to the contrary, it became overly reliant, the prior administration, on States to implement their own testing strategies. That is clear. They are needed, but it has to be a coordinated process. Test kits, everything else, we are still in short supply.

I am going to try to cut some of this out because it has been talked about. But the national strategy has been talked about time and time and time again, and not just today but the need for it, and here we are sitting, talking about it still a year later. Time is of the most importance.

In my district, I have people in my district, similar to others, mostly rural areas, not being able to get tested. And when they get the first shot, they can't get to a second shot. The computer systems are in a situation where they are mostly, if you are dealing with somebody from the Hispanic community or some other Tribal communities, which I have a lot of, they have problems even having a computer, and it is required in many areas. And I am glad to see that the President has called for $50 billion to build out a national testing program, which we have talked about so many times over the course of this last year.

We have to ask so much from our frontline workers, and we are still where—I can remember when this first started, they still don't have where we need to be.

Dr. Borio, I appreciate the honesty and self-reflection in your testimony. One of your recommendations called for the CDC to immediately expand its genomic surveillance system. Can you expand upon how, in conjunction with President Biden's plan to spend $50 billion in testing, this will help quickly identify new variants of infectious diseases like COVID–19 and how that will impact public health recommendations offered by scientists at the FDA or the CDC, and how it will help in the future?

Dr. BORIO. Thank you. I will elaborate in writing for you afterwards. But, briefly, the fact is that, early on, we knew this was an RNA virus. They mutate, they always mutate, and we didn't really have a system to be able to begin to sequence, to receive viral samples from patients, to locals, to State labs, to the CDC, or under the sequencing labs, sequence them and then do a data analysis so we can really track the evolution of the virus, detect the emergence of variants, and understand where they were spreading. So we took, you know, the alerts in the U.K. and South Africa to get us then to begin to scale up our systems, but it still is very inadequate for what the need is.

Mr. O'HALLERAN. Doctor, I have to interrupt you because my time is almost up. And I would like to ask you, how long has this system been needed and how long have the professionals been asking for it?

Dr. BORIO. The need precedes this pandemic.

Mr. O'HALLERAN. Thank you very much.

And I yield. Thank you, Madam Chair.

Ms. ESHOO. The gentleman yields back. And always know how welcome you are at the subcommittee, Mr. O'Halleran.

Well, that concludes all of the questions for today. I want to thank our witnesses, Dr. Julie Morita, Dr. Luciana Borio, Governor Leavitt. It was really wonderful to have you join us. I think Members—well, Members have learned from each one of you, and, of course, to Greg Burel as well.

I need to request unanimous consent to enter the following into the record, which includes documents submitted by both Democratic and Republican Members. It is a rather long list. I am going to speed read. And if any of my colleagues want to interrupt and ask for unanimous consent before I finish reading it, otherwise bear with me.

A January 31, 2021, Politico article entitled "'It's a mess': Biden's first 10 days dominated by vaccine mysteries"; a statement from the Association of American Medical Colleges; a letter from AARP; a statement from the National Immigration Law Center; a statement from the Asian & Pacific Islander American Health Forum; a letter from the American Academy of Family Physicians; testimony from Dr. Arthur C. Evans, CEO and executive vice president of the American Psychological Association; a statement from the American Society for Microbiology; a statement from Steven C.——

Mrs. FLETCHER. Madam Chairwoman?

Ms. ESHOO. Yes.

Mrs. FLETCHER. Madam Chairwoman, I rise to request unanimous consent that all of the items be included in the record.

Ms. ESHOO. Is there a second to the motion?

Ms. SCHRIER. I second. I second.

Ms. ESHOO. Wonderful. Thank you, Dr. Kim.

Mr. GUTHRIE. Madam Chair? Can we just make sure the list— can we read—I don't want you to have to read. That is fine. Is there a procedure that we can verify that if we had something that was left off for some reason that we submitted, gets admitted?

Ms. ESHOO. Absolutely.

Mr. GUTHRIE. Just make the motion that if something we agreed to as admitted can be included in the record? That is all. I am fine with you not reading them. I just want to make sure we double-check.

Ms. ESHOO. Absolutely. And as I said, this includes documents submitted by Democratic and Republican Members.

Mr. GUTHRIE. OK. All right. Thank you.

Ms. ESHOO. So, if there are any Members that have something, please submit it and we will gladly add it to the list.

I hear no objections to the motion. So ordered.1A[14]

And, let's see, it is 3 o'clock, so 4 hours on the dot. And this has been quite an extensive hearing, but I think every moment, every comment, every question, and all of the information gleaned from our witnesses are absolutely essential to this national effort to crush COVID. So thank you, everyone.

Again, it is really a joy to welcome the new members from both sides of the aisle.

And I don't think we have any other business before us. So the Health Subcommittee hearing of today has now ended. Thank you. Thank you, everyone.

Article of January 31, 2021, "'It's a mess': Biden's first 10 days dominated by vaccine mysteries," by Tyler Pager, Adam Cancryn and Joanne Keenen, Politico, Submitted by Ms. Eshoo

Biden's team is still trying to locate upwards of 20 million vaccine doses that have been sent to states — a mystery that has hampered plans to speed up the national vaccination effort.

[14] The information appears at the conclusion of the hearing, except for five documents that have been retained in committee files and are available with the other material at https://docs.house.gov/Committee/Calendar/ByEvent.aspx?EventID=111136.

Joe Biden promised he'd bring in a competent, tested team to run the pandemic response, set ambitious vaccination targets and impose strict public health guidelines.

His team arrived at the White House with a 200-page response plan ready to roll out. But instead, they have spent much of the last week trying to wrap their hands around the mushrooming crisis — a process officials acknowledge has been humbling, and triggered a concerted effort to temper expectations about how quickly they might get the nation back to normal.

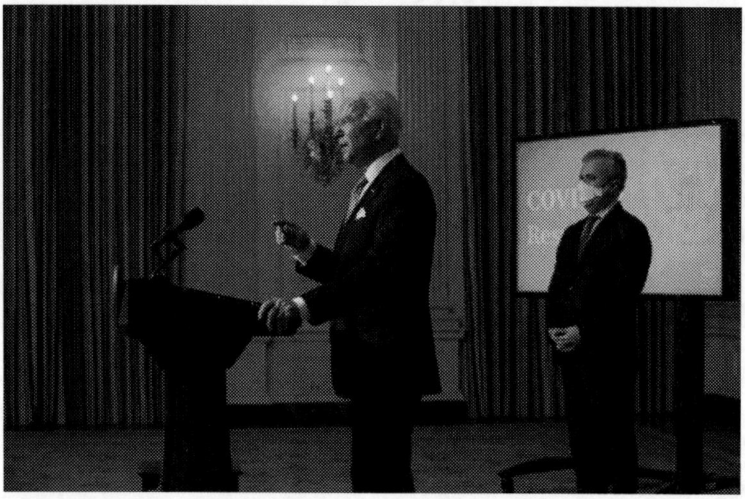

U.S. President Joe Biden speaks about the coronavirus pandemic in the State Dining Room of the White House on January 26, 2021 in Washington, DC. | Doug Mills, Pool/Getty Images.

After a week on the job, Biden's team is still trying to locate upwards of 20 million vaccine doses that have been sent to states — a mystery that has hampered plans to speed up the national vaccination effort. They're searching for new ways to boost production of a vaccine stockpile that they've discovered is mostly empty. And they're nervously eyeing a series of new Covid-19 strains that threaten to derail the response.

"It's the Mike Tyson quote: 'Everybody's got a plan until they get punched in the mouth,'" said one person with knowledge of the vaccine effort who's not authorized to discuss the work. "They are planning. They are competent. It's just the weight of everything when you sit down in that chair. It's heavy."

Biden officials leading the coronavirus response launched a series of regular briefings this week to keep the public informed on the state of the pandemic and government efforts to contain it and rush vaccines out to as many Americans as possible.

But the briefings were short on details. And behind the scenes, officials say, the team was still struggling to get a handle on basic information, liaise with the career government workers who have been running the response and build out a long-term strategy for bringing — and then keeping — the virus under control.

Biden Administration Readies Battle Plan as Covid Variants Reach the U.S.

By Sarah Owermohle

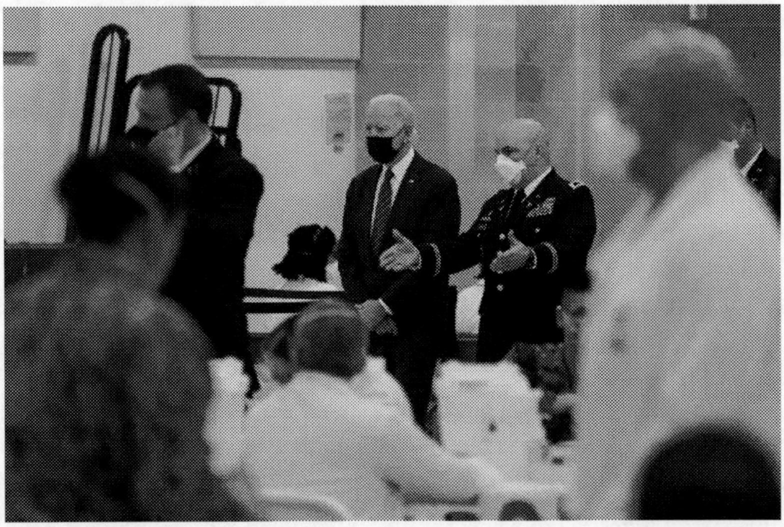

"One of the virtues of a well-run transition is that by the time you take the reins, you have developed some rapport and trust with the career people you're working with," the person familiar with the administration's work said. The "courtship has been unnaturally short," the person added.

"Nobody had a complete picture," said Julie Morita, a member of the Biden transition team and executive vice president at the Robert Wood Johnson Foundation. "The plans that were being made were being made with the assumption that more information would be available and be revealed once they got into the White House."

It's a steep challenge that Biden officials said they'd been anticipating for weeks, amid a rocky transition period that left them scrambling to piece together vaccine distribution plans and coordinate with state health officials.

Yet in the days since taking over, the Covid response team has confronted a situation that officials described as far worse than expected — and that has prompted public assessments so dour they surprised some who had worked on the administration's former transition team.

On Tuesday, Biden warned that the "vaccine program is in worse shape than we anticipated or expected," echoing complaints from his chief of staff, Ron Klain, that a "plan didn't really exist."

Biden's Covid response team has since made a concerted effort not to heap blame on the Trump administration, one official said — even as their vague allusions to a worse-than-expected situation have prompted speculation about what specific problems they've encountered.

But people with knowledge of the response detailed fresh concerns that are centered largely on the federal government's vaccine supply. Biden's team is still trying to get a firm grasp on the whereabouts of more than 20 million doses of Covid-19 vaccine that the federal government bought and distributed to states but has yet to record as being administered to patients.

Only a small percentage of those unaccounted for doses — roughly 2 million, two officials said — is due to lags in data reporting, the Biden team believes. That would mean the rest of the crucial supply is boxed away in warehouses, sitting idle in freezers or floating elsewhere in the complex distribution pipeline that runs from the administration to individual states.

That's a dilemma that predated the Biden team's arrival, with Biden himself hammering the vaccine rollout's first weeks under the Trump administration as a "dismal failure."

Yet the response team underestimated at the outset how difficult it would be to fix.

The Biden transition had only received high-level briefings on the distribution effort in the runup to the inauguration on Jan. 20, a transition official said, and was largely kept out of detailed discussions about the on-the-ground operation. The team didn't get granular access to Tiberius — the central government system used for tracking vaccine distribution — until the transition's final days.

It was not until after Biden was sworn in that the Covid response team discovered the system was blinded to much of the route that vaccines traveled from the government's distribution hubs to people's arms.

Instead, once the vaccine shipments are delivered to the states, responsibility for tracking them has been left up to states' individual public health systems. The administration then only gets an update once the doses are actually administered and an official record is submitted.

"I think they were really caught off guard by that," said one adviser. "It's a mess."

Top Biden officials have stressed that the missing doses are spread out across the states, which remain largely responsible for getting them to the health providers charged with vaccinating the tens of millions of people waiting in line for shots.

But the Covid team has since had to spend hours on the phone with various state officials trying to manually track down the unused doses, a time-consuming task that's sapped resources and has yet to give officials a full picture of where exactly supplies are going.

They've also sought to persuade health providers to stop holding doses in reserve, a practice borne out of concerns people wouldn't be able to get the second shot of their two-dose regimen — but one that's no longer necessary and has only contributed to the confusion, according to two people with knowledge of the discussions.

On a call with White House officials Tuesday, Arkansas Republican Gov. Asa Hutchinson vented that some states are bearing the brunt of the blame for the uneven rollout because of those reserves — a nuance not reflected in the federal numbers, according to notes of the call obtained by POLITICO.

The complaint prompted a pledge from Centers for Disease Control and Prevention Director Rochelle Walensky to issue clearer guidance for how states should manage their allocated vaccines.

Illinois Democratic Gov. J.B. Pritzker later blamed a Trump administration program that designated pharmacies to distribute vaccines to long-term care facilities for "bringing our numbers way down" because of how slow it has been to get shots in arms.

The White House has since given states permission to seize unused doses from the pharmacy program and reallocate them elsewhere.

"There is no doubt they are doing a better job," George Helmy, the chief of staff for New Jersey Democratic Gov. Phil Murphy, said about the Biden administration. "We have a true partner who is being transparent and collaborative."

As they grapple with the immediate distribution issues, federal officials have also raced to build out detailed plans for eventually distributing the shots to broader populations beyond health care workers and older Americans — a project that people familiar with the effort say the Trump administration never even started on.

And though the Biden team had planned to boost the pace of vaccine manufacturing over time, some Biden officials said they were shocked to learn soon after Inauguration Day that there was little in the federal vaccine reserve — and that the companies producing the shots were nowhere near capable of churning out as many doses as the Trump administration had projected in the preceding months.

The Biden administration has since warned that supplies will remain limited until the summer, raising the possibility of ongoing shortages even as the nation's daily vaccination rate picks up.

The White House cheered promising data on a new single-dose vaccine from Johnson & Johnson on Friday. But production obstacles have dampened expectations for its immediate impact, with one federal official likening the anticipated early flow of shots to "a trickle."

That has turned the Covid team's first days into something closer to a triage operation than the more orderly rollout that the administration had hoped for, especially as much of the federal health department operates on a skeleton staff made up of career officials and a handful of early political appointees.

And though the Biden administration is still pressing ahead with building mass vaccination sites and long-planned preparations for the long-term response effort, officials said the time lost navigating this early set of difficulties has set back a response already likely to consume much of Biden's first year in office.

"This isn't over any time soon," said Craig Fugate, a former Obama administration FEMA administrator who worked on the transition. "There may not be a bright red line where when we cross that line we're done, we're finished and everything's going to be great."

Statement by the Association of American Medical Colleges on "Road to Recovery: Ramping up COVID-19 Vaccines, Testing, and Medical Supply Chain" Submitted for the Record to the Energy and Commerce, Subcommittee on Health, United States House of Representatives, February 2, 2021

The Association of American Medical Colleges (AAMC) thanks the Subcommittee for convening the February 3 hearing, "Road to Recovery: Ramping Up COVID-19 Vaccines, Testing, and Medical Supply Chain" and for the opportunity to provide written comment for inclusion in the record.

The AAMC is a not-for-profit association dedicated to transforming health through medical education, health care, medical research, and community collaborations. Its members are all 155 accredited U.S. medical schools; more than 400 teaching hospitals and health systems, including Department of Veterans Affairs medical centers; and more than 70 academic societies. Through these institutions and organizations, the AAMC leads and serves America's medical schools and teaching hospitals and their more than 179,000 full-time faculty members, 92,000 medical students, 140,000 resident physicians, and 60,000 graduate students and postdoctoral researchers in the biomedical sciences.

Major teaching hospitals, medical schools, teaching physicians, and scientists at academic medical centers have mobilized on all fronts to contain and mitigate COVID-19. In partnership with their physician faculty from affiliated medical schools, AAMC-member teaching hospitals provide 25% of the nation's medical and surgical intensive care beds, 36% of cardiac intensive care beds, 61% of pediatric intensive care beds, and 69% of all Level I Trauma Centers. As well-established and respected regional referral centers and centers for tertiary care, they have worked in collaboration with their state and local departments of health, regional emergency management systems, and all other major players in emergency response to develop and activate surge and crisis response plans at their own institutions and throughout their broader communities.

In addition to their role in clinical care, AAMC-member institutions are major centers of cuttingedge medical research, with scientists and clinicians at medical schools and teaching hospitals conducting over 50% of extramural research funded by the National Institutes of Health (NIH). Many of our member institutions have developed much-needed tests for COVID-19, a fluid and rapidly changing area as they bring new equipment online, try to source materials, and stand up reporting procedures in extremely challenging conditions. They are also at the forefront of research efforts to identify and advance clinical care protocols, viable therapeutics, and new vaccines to blunt the pandemic's impact.

Drawing on the expertise of the AAMC's staff and the frontline experience of our member institutions, in July, the AAMC released "The Way Forward on COVID-19: A Road Map to Reset the Nation's Approach to the Pandemic," a blueprint containing 11 evidence-based actions to establish a comprehensive, coordinated plan to respond to the pandemic. The report included a major emphasis on remedying critical supply and drug shortages; increasing availability and accessibility of testing; coordinating distribution of COVID-19 vaccines; and promoting health equity throughout the nation's response, among other recommendations.

While many of the road map's recommendations unfortunately still are needed urgently today, we are encouraged that President Biden's "American Rescue Plan" and "National Strategy for the COVID-19 Response and Pandemic Preparedness" align with many elements of the strategy that the AAMC and other experts have outlined. As the Subcommittee considers opportunities to accelerate and scale up vaccinations and testing, as well as related supply chain issues, the AAMC offers the following observations and recommendations from the experience of academic medical centers across the country:

Ramping up COVID-19 Vaccines

- There is urgent need to ensure both that vaccine supply continues to increase and that teaching hospitals have direct access to transparent and advance communications about timing and quantity of vaccine allocations to allow for efficient planning.
- There should be appropriate flexibility in applying vaccination prioritization guidance.
- Ongoing and additional support is need for:
    - Community-based partnerships to address hesitancy.
    - Ensuring all individuals receive the vaccine without incurring any cost.
    - Offsetting expenses that teaching hospitals, health departments, and others are incurring in their vaccination efforts.

  - Strengthening and rebuilding core public health infrastructure.
- Policymakers should engage vendors of electronic health records (EHR) systems to ensure that any potential record-keeping solutions are compatible with institutions' existing EHRs and other existing systems.

Ramping up COVID-19 Testing

- The national pandemic response should seek sustained and regular testing targets for effective diagnosis and screening and should ensure dedicated funding; continued investment in technology and test development; and more strategic use of resources.
- While commercial labs and an increase in rapid tests for screening play an important role in increasing the nation's testing capacity, hospitals and health systems also must be able to perform on-site diagnostic testing for patients.
- Maximizing testing capacity requires fully transparent federal coordination of all aspects of the testing supply chain.
- The government should maintain a centralized system to ensure a stockpile of testing supplies and to quickly assess U.S. testing capacity based on all available testing components across sectors and geographic regions.
- We encourage the new federal interagency COVID-19 Pandemic Testing Board to engage the academic medicine community and other stakeholders to inform its efforts.
- The AAMC strongly recommends a robust investment in the nation's sequencing and surveillance capacity to ensure that our testing, vaccines, therapeutics, and other countermeasures remain reliable tools against the virus as new strains emerge.

The Medical Supply Chain

- In the short term, we strongly support efforts to accelerate domestic production of critical supplies to address all these needs.
- There should be clear guidance from the federal government regarding the quantity and types of supplies states and hospitals should have on hand.
- Federal funding for hospitals to establish and maintain inventories of recommended supplies will be important.
- A real-time dashboard that is kept up-to-date and takes into consideration other state, local, private-sector, and hospital supplies should be shared with key stakeholders.

The following addresses these observations and recommendations in greater detail.

Ramping up COVID-19 Vaccines

Even before the Food and Drug Administration (FDA) issued emergency use authorizations (EUA) for the first vaccines, academic medical centers were working with state and local officials to prepare for the large-scale vaccination campaigns. They purchased ultra-cold freezers to store the vaccines, developed agreements to serve as hubs for distribution to other vaccine providers, and worked with community leaders and liaisons to conduct outreach, among other preparations, even as they were forced to respond to surging cases. As vaccine doses have become available, the experience has varied widely as a result of the variation in distribution plans from state to state and even within states.

Universally, however, the limited supply of vaccines has posed major challenges for facilities. Because of the low supply, reliable and early communication about the timing and volume of vaccines to be delivered to facilities is essential but has been elusive. Abrupt cancellations and reductions of shipments have been extraordinarily disruptive both to the individuals who had been scheduled to be vaccinated and to the clinicians, staff, volunteers, and administrators coordinating the large-scale vaccination clinics. In addition to inconvenience, when planned vaccination clinics need to be cancelled or rescheduled, the resulting confusion may lead the public to cast doubt on the vaccination program – and even the vaccine itself – if they perceive this critical undertaking is not well organized.

The AAMC welcomes the recent White House announcement that jurisdictions will be receiving an increase in their weekly supply of vaccines and that the Department of Health and Human Services (HHS) will be providing a three-week look ahead of supply allocation estimates for states, Tribes, and territories. We encourage Congress and the Administration to act with urgency to ensure both that supply continues to increase and that teaching hospitals and others coordinating vaccination clinics have direct access to transparent and advance communications about timing and quantity of vaccine allocations to allow for efficient planning. Without access to accurate information about expected supply, logistical planning is substantially more difficult, a challenge that only will increase as additional vaccine candidates – including one whose dosage and storage requirements differ from the two current products – become available.

Changing, inconsistent, and unclear guidance at the federal, state, and local levels also affects planning and leads to gaps in vaccination strategies. At the same time, overly rigid prioritization directives in some states could force facilities to discard doses unnecessarily and may also inadvertently be exacerbating inequities. For example, in many parts of the country, life expectancy for some populations is well below 75 years, so strict adherence to age-based priority eligibility for individuals 75 years and older likely excludes high-risk individuals from initial vaccination rounds. In other cases, states have adopted a model that progresses through prioritization categories by closing eligibility for earlier categories – for example, prohibiting health care workers who delayed seeking vaccination in phase 1a from receiving the vaccine once the jurisdiction has advanced to phase 1b. As another example, hospitals in some states are not able to include cancer patients in the early priority groups, despite their susceptibility.

To ensure efficient distribution of the vaccine, it is important to allow teaching hospitals to apply the issued prioritization guidance in a manner that allows them the appropriate flexibility to vaccinate high-risk patients and preserves their ability to continue providing care to their greater communities – including priority eligibility for physicians and other clinicians but also non-clinical staff. Food service staff, registration staff, environmental services staff, IT staff, and others at academic medical centers are essential to supporting continuity of clinical operations at teaching hospitals. Additionally, because medical students interact with patients and may be involved in clinical care, the AAMC supports vaccinating medical students with other frontline workers; however, not all states allow facilities to include students in their initial eligibility categories.

While uptake among faculty and staff at academic medical centers is generally high, some – including non-clinical staff – have delayed vaccination. Some of this hesitancy is rooted in historic mistrust as a result of racial bias in health care and unethical research practices in the past. In other cases, women of childbearing age have expressed concerns. Frequent and extensive outreach and education efforts are underway at medical schools and teaching hospitals nationwide and in partnership with community leaders. The Centers for Disease Control and Prevention (CDC) recently awarded the AAMC the Building Confidence in COVID-19 Vaccines Cooperative Agreement. We will be working with the CDC to build trust and confidence in the COVID-19 vaccine among health care personnel and individuals from communities disproportionately impacted by COVID-19 around the country. The AAMC strongly supports ongoing and additional efforts to support community-based partnerships to address hesitancy and promote vaccinations among those populations disproportionately impacted by the pandemic. In addition to the immediate benefit of encouraging higher vaccination rates among these populations, such efforts may also lay the groundwork for connecting individuals who have not previously sought preventive care to a medical home over the long term.

As AAMC-member institutions extend vaccination efforts beyond their campuses to the general population, additional challenges are emerging and are expected to increase. For example, vaccination clinics are pulling the health care workforce away from other clinical duties, which is especially challenging during the current COVID-19 surge in many regions. Many institutions are training and leveraging medical students, other health professions students, and other health professionals to assist with administering vaccines. Because individuals must be monitored for 15 minutes after vaccination, in addition to having a sufficient number of clinicians to administer the vaccine, facilities must ensure that attending physicians and/or other qualified staff are on site to monitor and respond to any potential adverse events, rare as they may be. Additional personnel are needed for other responsibilities such as scheduling, collecting needed consents, taking medical histories, and providing other logistical support. As the scale of the vaccination clinics increases, the workforce needs will expand as well.

Securing a space that can accommodate such a massive operation while allowing for the necessary social distancing is also a challenge. Existing venues on teaching hospital campuses are unlikely to meet the need. Ensuring accessibility and geographic proximity will be another key consideration to make the vaccine available to the general population, and in some cases mobile units may be necessary.

The expenses associated with these efforts far exceeds the reimbursement providers may receive for administering the vaccine, and the reimbursement process only adds to the administrative burden providers are facing. The AAMC strongly supports ensuring all individuals receive the vaccine without incurring any cost. Additionally, we encourage development of a mechanism to offset the expenses that teaching hospitals are incurring in administering large-scale vaccination clinics and/or in storing vaccine supplies for their communities. Such support should, to the extent possible, minimize administrative burdens to the providers, and should supplement, not replace, aid to state and local health departments for their vaccine distribution expenses. Ensuring ongoing support for health departments is also key.

Developing an easy, efficient process for supporting these clinics is especially critical as teaching hospitals begin vaccinating individuals beyond their own patients. Establishing accessible and efficient scheduling and tracking systems to accommodate appointments for large-scale vaccination clinics has been challenging even within the institution's own patient population. Extending these efforts to individuals who are not affiliated with their health systems will pose extensive logistical and administrative challenges, including corresponding paperwork, data entry, and tracking challenges. As policymakers consider potential federal strategies to support such work, the AAMC encourages engaging vendors of electronic health records (EHR) systems to identify solutions that are compatible with institutions' existing EHRs.

Additionally, we support additional investment in and attention to existing public health data systems and other core public health infrastructure, which has languished after years of underinvestment. Understaffed and under-resourced public health functions at all levels of government and nationwide have complicated the already complex response to the novel coronavirus and vaccination efforts specifically. Robust, sustained support for foundational capabilities at health departments will be necessary to rebuild this critical infrastructure and help stabilize the nation's response.

Ramping up COVID-19 Testing

Laboratories in the United States obtained the genetic sequence for the virus soon after it was identified in China, allowing for the rapid development of the probes and reagents required to develop highly sensitive diagnostic tests for the virus. However, the infrastructure and coordination to ramp up testing capacity and have a clear picture of where to direct supplies did not exist and has not yet been entirely implemented. In conducting polymerase chain reaction (PCR) tests to diagnose COVID-19 in all stages of infection, hospitals and academic labs continue to be hampered by inconsistent and sporadic changes in access to reagents, nasopharyngeal swabs, transport media, testing machines, and other equipment. These shortfalls have impeded the ability to expand diagnostic testing capacity to fulfill community and national needs and improve testing access for all individuals, particularly those from underserved communities. While commercial labs and an increase in rapid tests for screening play an important role in greatly increasing the nation's testing capacity, hospitals and health systems also must be able to perform on-site diagnostic testing for patients to ensure patient and health care worker safety and efficiency of care.

While many institutions have developed workarounds to the extent possible and have sought to diversify their testing capacity to minimize the impact of test-specific shortages, demand is likely to increase as spikes in new cases continue to occur across the country. Additionally, the ability for hospitals, physician practices, and other health care providers to resume delivering non-emergent care and for schools and businesses to reopen safely will depend on a robust, reliable testing capacity.

To help meet this goal, the AAMC recommends that the national pandemic response should seek sustained and regular testing targets for effective diagnosis and screening. Improvements in testing technology and availability have increased daily test rates to nearly 1 million per day, but we are far short of the number of tests that should be administered daily under current conditions. A commitment to increasing the number of tests and suppressing the virus requires dedicated funding; continued investment in technology and test development; and smarter, more strategic use of our resources.

To better prepare for diagnostic test development for the next pandemic, we must pre-determine how to secure a reliable, functional supply chain for all testing components. Maximizing testing capacity requires a better and fully transparent federal coordination of all aspects of the testing supply chain, including ensuring that all suppliers do not rely on a single manufacturer. In addition, the government should maintain a centralized system that is ready to be deployed at any time to ensure a stockpile of testing supplies specifically and to quickly assess U.S. testing capacity based on all available testing components across sectors and geographic regions. This will give organizations, academic institutions, and private companies a roadmap of how to pivot quickly to access and/or generate the needed equipment and reagents and implement a plan with specific directions for test development and deployment.

We welcome the establishment of the federal interagency COVID-19 Pandemic Testing Board via the president's recent Executive Order, and we applaud its commitment to harmonizing the nation's approach to testing. As the group begins its work, we encourage the Board to engage the academic medicine community, who can help inform the Administration's efforts to reverse testing supply shortfalls and to expand short- and long-term lab capacity, as described in the president's National Strategy.

In addition to addressing specific testing and supply chain issues, to contain the pandemic, we must be more agile in responding to the virus as it changes. Paramount in this effort is the need to better understand which existing or emerging variants of the virus are infecting people in the U.S. Currently, we are sequencing only a small fragment of the nation's confirmed cases, leaving us vulnerable to wide infection by undetected variants. We cannot know if tests are detecting new variants or if vaccines are protective against those variants without greatly increased sequencing. The AAMC strongly recommends a robust investment in the nation's sequencing and surveillance capacity to ensure that our testing, vaccines, therapeutics, and other countermeasures remain reliable tools against the virus as new strains emerge. We are pleased that the president's Rescue Plan proposes "to dramatically increase" funding for these efforts, and we encourage Congress to provide the necessary resources without delay.

The Medical Supply Chain

Early in the pandemic, hospitals began feeling additional strain on their existing and stockpiled supplies as visits to the emergency room increased. While shortages of personal protective equipment (PPE) – including N95 and other respirators, gloves, gowns, and other equipment – have been pervasive, our members also encountered difficulty acquiring a number of critical products, including hand sanitizer, disinfectants, and other supplies. In many cases, turning to their states and the federal Strategic National Stockpile (SNS) offered little relief, as the effects of an under-resourced SNS and a patchy supply chain became apparent. For example, the nation's just-in-time systems of inventory management did not adequately take into account the possibility of international disruptions, leaving the country ill-prepared to backstop suppliers dependent on overseas manufacturing. In addition to hospitals, which regularly use PPE, other entities, such as long-term care facilities, private physician practices, and urgent care settings suddenly needed access to PPE, quickly depleting what little supply existed.

Aside from the SNS, facilities also faced difficulty in procuring supplies through their usual channels. The distribution methodologies for allocating PPE to both states and individual facilities have been unclear and unreliable. As administrators have scoured potential leads on their own, they have encountered substantially higher prices for routine supplies, often from weak negotiating positions. Institutions have reported delays and uncertainty in whether orders that they place will be fulfilled fully, partially, or at all, and/or have needed to be resourceful in identifying ways to transport purchases successfully to the U.S.

In the short term, we strongly support efforts to accelerate domestic production of critical supplies to address all these needs. Additionally, there should be clear guidance from the federal government regarding the quantity and types of supplies states and hospitals should have on hand based on their local population and to be able to respond to different types of public health emergencies. Hospitals and states should have the appropriate level of flexibility on how they meet the recommended federal guidelines, which should also take into account PPE demand from non-hospital facilities, including long-term care facilities, testing personnel, research labs, and other entities. Federal funding for hospitals to establish and maintain inventories of recommended supplies will be important, particularly given that stockpiles would not be used for regular patient care and given space constraints facilities often face.

A real-time dashboard that is kept up-to-date and takes into consideration other state, local, private-sector, and hospital supplies should be shared with key stakeholders. States and local public health teams must work with hospitals and others to coordinate reserves of supplies. Reliable investment in the SNS to ensure its inventories are current and clear communications about the role of the SNS as a resource of last resort will help clarify confusion about its role. And the federal government should promote and enforce protections against unreasonable product pricing in times of crisis, including prices of existing and new drugs used to treat COVID-19 and other conditions.

Conclusion

The physicians, other health professionals, and scientists at the nation's medical schools and teaching hospitals are committed to defeating this virus. We are grateful for the steps Congress has taken to date to support their work, and we look forward to continuing to work with both Congress and the Administration to end this public health crisis. Thank you again for examining these issues in the Subcommittee's hearing, and please consider the AAMC a resource if additional information about vaccines, testing, medical supply chain issues, or other aspects of academic medicine's pandemic response and preparedness would be helpful. Please do not hesitate to contact AAMC Chief Public Policy Officer Karen Fisher, J.D or AAMC Senior Director Tannaz Rasouli with any questions.

February 3, 2021

The Honorable Frank Pallone
Chair
House Committee on Energy and Commerce

The Honorable Anna Eshoo
Chair
House Committee on Energy and Commerce
Subcommittee on Health

The Honorable Cathy McMorris Rodgers
Ranking Member
House Committee on Energy and Commerce

The Honorable Brett Guthrie
Ranking Member
House Committee on Energy and Commerce
Subcommittee on Health

Dear Chairs Pallone, Eshoo, and Ranking Members McMorris Rodgers and Guthrie:

Thank you for holding this important hearing to examine the COVID-19 vaccine supply chain and distribution process. Like all Americans, AARP's 38 million members urgently want to see an end to the coronavirus pandemic. We are heartened by the fact that we have two authorized vaccines to fight this deadly virus, and possibly more on the way. It is critical that these vaccines are administered as efficiently and quickly as possible, and we look forward to working with you to achieve that goal.

Since the start of the pandemic, nearly 95 percent of the deaths from COVID-19 have been among people age 50 and older. That is why it is so important that older adults be prioritized to receive these vaccines. The situation in America's nursing homes is particularly dire: although residents of long-term care facilities represent fewer than one percent of the population, residents and staff represent nearly 40 percent of the deaths.

Thankfully, millions of vaccine doses have been administered to date, with approximately one million doses delivered daily. However, we continue to hear from older adults having difficulty accessing COVID-19 vaccines. In many instances, demand has far outstripped supply. For example, during the week of January 18th, Minnesota's vaccine appointment website received over one million hits for 6,000 available appointments. Now the state is ramping up vaccine distribution, but there are over a million people in the "high-priority" category. In other states, individuals must complete multiple steps before signing up for a vaccine appointment, often with little outside guidance. An AARP member in Tennessee was unable to get through to her county's vaccine appointment line, and needed help from our AARP call center to set up an online account to get on a waiting list. We also heard from an AARP member in New Jersey who became desperate after running into multiple obstacles while trying to schedule his second appointment. We hear about these challenges every day from our members, making it clear that Americans would greatly benefit from immediate steps to increase local supplies of COVID-19 vaccines and improve distribution processes.

We strongly urge you to take immediate action to address access problems and mitigate whatever barriers may be causing these delays. Full-scale mobilization is necessary, and any slowdowns or early bottlenecks in the production and distribution systems need to be urgently addressed. We believe federal and state governments should improve the current vaccine infrastructure, while expanding the ways that individuals can receive a vaccine. We support utilizing existing vaccinators (e.g., pharmacies) to supplement vaccine administration and build upon existing vaccination systems. At the same time, we support building mass vaccination centers and utilizing mobile clinics – especially in areas with few health providers – as well as developing new, critical modes of providing in-home vaccination to home-bound individuals.

As noted above, we continue to hear from members who are struggling to make appointments, including those who do not have access to the internet. Currently, the process to make an appointment varies state to state, or even county by county. Americans over the age of 50 are unsure how to make or confirm their appointment and are deeply frustrated and increasingly desperate. Many do not have access to the internet or do not have experience using online appointment systems. In addition, some states require individuals to visit multiple websites just to monitor vaccine appointment availability. We urge the federal government to work with states to develop 1-800 numbers for scheduling vaccine appointments that are centralized, well-staffed, and offer culturally competent customer service in several languages.

We also strongly encourage the federal government to ensure that all consumers have access to a centralized, regularly-updated online tool that will allow them to use their ZIP code to search for where they can get a vaccine and what they should expect. This tool should also be available in a variety of languages and easy to use for consumers, including those Americans over the age of 50 that do not regularly use the internet. We also strongly encourage Congress and the Administration to find ways to streamline any associated processes, such as allowing individuals to review and sign necessary forms in advance, to help reduce potential barriers to vaccinations. For example, steps should be taken to standardize the information a patient needs to present when they arrive at their appointments, including issuing guidance for states to use. Finally, we urge you to pay special attention to communities that may need specific education and outreach, such as rural communities and diverse communities. AARP will continue to help share this information with people as quickly as possible.

Moreover, in order to increase public awareness of vaccine allocation decisions and improve confidence in a fair distribution process, it is important that we all have access to accurate, timely, and transparent information, including how many residents and staff of long-term care facilities have been vaccinated. We appreciate that the Biden Administration has committed to expanding the collection and reporting of vaccination data, and we urge this data be available on a state-by-state basis. In addition, we believe vaccination data needs to be broken down by age, race, and ethnicity for states, the federal government, and consumers to fully understand where the gaps are in vaccination administration. It is also of utmost importance that this information be updated as quickly as possible, even daily.

While we are pleased that Congress and the Administration have taken steps to eliminate any out-of-pocket costs for patients receiving the vaccine, we have seen unfortunate incidents where individuals receive a bill from their provider after receiving the vaccine. For example, AARP helped to resolve instances where providers in Alaska and Wisconsin billed their patients, likely for the administration fee associated with the vaccine. This is deeply confusing for Americans over the age of 50 who have been told that vaccines would be available to them at no cost. It is critical that COVID-19 vaccines be administered by health care providers who agree not to charge patients regardless of their insurance status or-—at minimum—are fully transparent about potential charges during the registration process.

Additionally, considering the horrific death toll in America's nursing homes and other long-term care facilities, we are deeply concerned about reports that many facility staff are choosing to forgo COVID-19 vaccines. We appreciate the ongoing efforts from the CDC, but more must be done to save lives and ensure that staff, residents, and their families feel confident in COVID-19 vaccines.

Finally, while some older adults remain hesitant about COVID-19 vaccines, we cannot stress enough how eager many are to receive a vaccine, which offers so much promise for a return to normalcy. We have heard so many questions from AARP members about when and how they can expect to be vaccinated, who will notify them, what information they will need to provide, and where they can sign up. Clear information on what they can anticipate and when they may have the opportunity to receive the vaccine would be of tremendous value and will help to reduce the growing frustration around the COVID-19 vaccination process.

We appreciate your efforts and stand ready to work with our federal and state governments to address these challenges. Together, we can defeat this virus and help ensure a brighter future for Americans of all ages.

Sincerely,

Nancy A. LeaMond
Executive Vice President and
Chief Advocacy and Engagement Officer

Statement of the National Immigration Law Center, House Committee on Energy and Commerce Subcommittee on Health, Road to Recovery: Ramping up COVID-19 Vaccines, Testing, and Medical Supply Chain, Tuesday February 3, 2021

Dear Members of the House Committee on Energy and Commerce Subcommittee on Health,

The National Immigration Law Center (NILC) appreciates the opportunity to submit this written statement for the record for the hearing titled, "Road to Recovery: Ramping Up COVID-19 Vaccines, Testing, and Medical Supply Chain." NILC is the leading advocacy organization in the U.S. dedicated to defending and advancing the rights and opportunities of low-income immigrants and their families. We focus on issues that promote the well-being and economic security of immigrants and their families: health care and safety net programs; education and training; workers' rights; and federal and state policies affecting immigrants. We have decades of experience advocating for policies that improve the health of immigrants and their families, as well as established relationships with immigrant and community organizations across the country for whom we provide technical, policy and advocacy assistance.

NILC urges Congress and the Biden-Harris administration to ensure that immigrants and their families have equitable access to the COVID-19 vaccine. This testimony details the many barriers, both longstanding and new to the context of this pandemic, that immigrants must overcome to obtain access health care, and specifically to testing and vaccines for Coronavirus 2019 (COVID-19). In December, NILC led a letter to the Centers for Disease Control and the Biden-Harris COVID-19 task force, outlining a number of concerns about immigrants' access to vaccines.[15] Nearly 250 organizations co-signed the letter. Given that immigrants comprise almost 14% of the US population and nearly one in five essential workers, our country cannot hope to overcome the pandemic without ensuring their access to COVID-19 testing, treatment and vaccines.[16,17]

---

[15] See letter at https://drive.google.com/file/d/1OsJtmqP232UHhLnt5YmFGWTr2hOj5t9M/view.

[16] Budiman, Abby, "Key findings about U.S. immigrants," Pew Research Center, August 20, 2020, http://www.pewresearch.org/fact-tank/2020/08/20/key-findings-about-u-s-immigrants/#:~:text=The%20U.S.%20foreign-born.

[17] "Immigrant Essential Workers are Crucial to America's COVID-19 Recovery," Fwd.us, December 16, 2020, https://www.fwd.us/news/immigrant-essential-workers/.

NILC agrees with the Members of Congress who have recognized that the equitable inclusion of noncitizens in the distribution of vaccinations is necessary to protect the lives and livelihoods of all.[18] As we detail in this testimony, the barriers to vaccine equity for immigrants are complex and interwoven.

Immigrants confront lack of reliable information in languages they speak or write, misinformation spread in communities and on social networks, fears of being detained by immigration enforcement or having their personal information shared with immigration authorities, concerns that accessing public services will undermine their ability to obtain permanent resident status, barriers because of the industry they work in and limited familiarity with our uniquely complex healthcare system – before they take the initial step to obtain a vaccination or other healthcare service.

NILC appreciates the steps the Biden-Harris administration has taken toward ensuring equity in vaccine distribution. President Biden's National Strategy for the COVID-19 Response and Pandemic Preparedness includes multiple references to immigrants.[19] His "Executive Order on Ensuring an Equitable Pandemic Response and Recovery" created a task force for "mitigating the health inequities caused or exacerbated by the COVID-19 pandemic and for preventing such inequities in the future."[20] The President's "Executive Order on Improving and Expanding Access to Care and Treatments for COVID-19" directed the Department of Health and Humans Services to "facilitate the equitable and effective distribution of therapeutics."[21] The American Rescue Plan proposal includes access to vaccines without immigration status restrictions.[22] However, more work lies ahead to make these promises real.

We highlight key areas in need of improvement below.

Insufficient Funding for Community Focused Outreach and Assistance

NILC's partners, which include organizations that work with immigrants directly, report that the scarcity of resources available to conduct culturally and linguistically competent outreach and education is a major barrier to a successful vaccination campaign. Misinformation about the vaccine is spreading online through social media, including through networks and applications used primarily by non-English language speakers. Particularly among immigrants from nations with repressive governments, these rumors amplify fear and exacerbate their distrust of government authorities.

---

[18] Grijalva, Raul, U.S. Representative, et al. "An equitable distribution of COVID-19 vaccine must include noncitizens," The Hill, January 26, 2020, https://thehill.com/blogs/congress-blog/healthcare/535901-an-equitable-distribution-of-covid-19-vaccine-must-include.

[19] "National Strategy for the COVID-19 Response and Pandemic Preparedness," The White House, January 21, 2021, https://www.whitehouse.gov/wp-content/uploads/2021/01/National-Strategy-for-the-COVID-19-Response-and-Pandemic-Preparedness.pdf.

[20] "Executive Order on Ensuring an Equitable Pandemic Response and Recovery," The White House, January 21, 2021, https://www.whitehouse.gov/briefing-room/presidential-actions/2021/01/21/executive-order-ensuring-an-equitable-pandemic-response-and-recovery/.

[21] "Executive Order on Improving and Expanding Access to Care and Treatments for COVID-19," The White House, January 21, 2021, https://www.whitehouse.gov/briefing-room/presidential-actions/2021/01/21/executive-order-improving-and-expanding-access-to-care-and-treatments-for-covid-19/.

[22] "President Biden Announces American Rescue Plan," The White House, January 20, 2021, https://www.whitehouse.gov/briefing-room/legislation/2021/01/20/president-biden-announces-american-rescue-plan/.

The Kaiser Family Foundation has estimated that the Department of Health and Human Services (HHS) may have over $1 billion available that could be used for consumer assistance programs.[23] HHS should use some of this funding to make an immediate and significant investment in the Navigator program, prioritizing funding for community-based organizations with established connections to immigrant and limited English proficient (LEP) populations. Navigators play an essential role in enrollment and beyond, particularly in helping consumers learn how to use health insurance.

While the announcement of the 3 month Open Enrollment period is an important and positive step, the $50 million allocated for outreach and education is insufficient to overcome immigrants' concern and convince them to enroll in health coverage and use it to obtain COVID vaccinations.[24] Navigators generally require an average of 90 minutes to enroll a consumer in health care.[25] S More time is typically needed to enroll immigrant families because of complex situations like multi-generational households and seasonal work, as well as the need to verify immigration status. Congress should ensure a sustainable funding source for this work by passing the ENROLL Act, which would reverse the Trump administration's sabotage of the Navigator program and ensure it has adequate funding in the future and the MORE Health Education Act, which would fund culturally appropriate advertising. Both these bills were included in the House-passed Patient Protection and Affordable Care Enhancement Act (H.R. 1425 in the 116th Congress).

Congress should also work with the Center for Disease Control and Prevention (CDC) and other agencies to ensure that COVID-19 outreach funding includes dedicated resources for community-based organizations that serve immigrant populations. The inclusion of trusted community messengers is essential for the success of any vaccination campaign that targets immigrants. Congress should empower the CDC to take creative steps such as proactively reaching out to community-based organizations or using larger immigrant-serving organizations as pass-throughs, because the organizations with the closest ties to immigrant communities often lack the administrative infrastructure to apply for federal funding.

States Are Not Allowed to Discriminate against Immigrants in Distribution

The governor of at least one state has stated that it will deprioritize immigrants in vaccine distribution.[26] The CDC should publicly confirm unequivocally that states and other jurisdictions may not use immigration status as a basis to deny the vaccine or to establish priorities for its distribution and administration. Such discrimination should be prohibited in

---

23 Pollitz, Karne and Jennifer Tolbert, "Opportunities and Resources to Expand Enrollment during the Pandemic and Beyond," January 25, 2021, https://www.kff.org/health-reform/issue-brief/opportunities-and-resources-to-expand-enrollment-during-the-pandemic-and-beyond/.

24 "2021 Special Enrollment Period in response to the COVID-19 Emergency," Center for Medicare and Medicaid Services, January 28, 2021, https://www.cms.gov/newsroom/fact-sheets/2021-special-enrollment-period-response-covid-19-emergency.

25 Pollitz, Karen Jennifer Tolbert and Ashley Semanskee, "2016 Survey of Health Insurance Marketplace Assister Programs and Brokers," June 8, 2016, https://www.kff.org/health-reform/report/2016-survey-of-health-insurance-marketplace-assister-programs-and-brokers/.

26 Armus, Teo, "Nebraska governor says citizens, legal residents will get vaccine priority over undocumented immigrants," Washington Post, January 6, 2021, https://www.washingtonpost.com/nation/2021/01/06/nebraska-covid-vaccine-immigrants-meatpacking/.

explicit policies that include the prohibition of practices with a disparate impact, such as limiting vaccination sites in predominantly immigrant neighborhoods.

The CDC should uplift state practices that proactively enhance immigrant inclusion and encourage other states to follow suit, providing technical assistance and connections. For example, Illinois and Utah have stated proactively that immigration status does not affect one's ability to get a vaccine.[27,28] Arizona health officials are planning immigrant specific outreach campaigns.[29]

Everyone, Regardless of Their Immigration Status, Should Have Access to Free COVID-19 Testing, Vaccinations and Treatment

Immigrants are uninsured at substantially higher rates than the US-born. Among lawfully present immigrants, 23% are uninsured, compared to nine percent of U.S. citizens. For undocumented immigrants, the uninsured rate rises to 45%.[30] The sources of these disparities include policy decisions to exclude many immigrants from Medicaid and federally supported health insurance programs. While we call on Congress and the Biden Administration to begin the long process of unwinding those exclusions, in this moment there is an urgent need to ensure that neither immigration status nor a lack of health insurance is a barrier to COVID-19 testing, treatment and vaccination.

In addition to other funding for healthcare providers, Congress should ensure that Federally Qualified Health Centers and other non-profit providers have robust funding. Needed actions include modifying the Health Resources and Services Administration reimbursement process to reimburse all claims in a timely manner and specifically the eliminate delays in reimbursement processing for providers treating patients without identity verification documents. Congress should also pass the Stronger Medicaid Response Act to ensure that states have the flexibility to use Medicaid funding to cover the costs of all uninsured individuals, regardless of status.

Protecting Sensitive Data and Addressing Privacy Concerns

Fears that their personal information will be shared with immigration enforcement frequently deter immigrants from seeking public services and undermine efforts to administer the vaccine. The CEO of a company that makes an application aimed at connecting immigrants to social services has stated that, "a key vaccine concern among some users was that their personal information could be used against them."[31] In New Mexico, concerns that information could be

---

27 "COVID-19 Vaccine," Illinois Department of Public Health, https://www.dph.illinois.gov/covid19/vaccine-faq.

28 "Frequently Asked Questions," State of Utah, January 19, 2021, https://coronavirus-download.utah.gov/Health/Coronavirus_Vaccine_FAQ.pdf.

29 Casey, Matthew, "As Vaccinations Expand, More Undocumented Arizonans to Become Eligible," Fronteras, January 7, 2021, https://fronterasdesk.org/content/1648613/vaccinations-expand-more-undocumented-arizonans-become-eligible.

30 "Health Coverage of Immigrants," Kaiser Family Foundation, March 18, 2020, https://www.kff.org/racial-equity-and-health-policy/fact-sheet/health-coverage-of-immigrants/.

31 https://www.marketwatch.com/story/just-because-were-undocumented-does-not-mean-were-worth-less-than-other-people-will-undocumented-immigrants-get-covid-19-vaccines-11611064883.

shared with law enforcement are a major reason that immigrants are hesitant to get the vaccine.[32]

We appreciate that the President's National Strategy specifically declares its intent to "safeguard privacy and ensure that these data will be used exclusively for public health services, and that it will not be shared with or used by any federal or state law enforcement activities, including actions by the U.S. Immigration and Customs Enforcement."[33] However, Congress needs to act to limit the information collected by healthcare providers to that which is necessary for public health purposes and to ensure that personally identifiable information is protected from use or disclosure. These limitations need to be unambiguous and readily understood by consumers.

In some states, either the jurisdictional government or providers require vaccine patients to provide documentation of identity or residency before they receive the vaccine; in other cases, patients must use an email address to register in the system.[34] For example, Florida's major hospital system requires either a driver's license or two alternative documents to prove residency.[35] In at least one instance, providers are using credit agencies to verify the identity of patients for the vaccine.[36] In order to ensure there are no immigration barriers to the vaccine, Congress should restrict the information state and local jurisdictions and healthcare providers can require for vaccination.

Congress and the Administration Should Ensure That Language Access Is Prioritized and Protected

Title VI of the Civil Rights Act of 1964 makes it unlawful to discriminate against individuals based on their national origin. Courts have affirmed that this protection includes equity in language access.

Executive Order 13166 applied this principle across the federal government and Section 1557 of the Affordable Care Act applies it to all federally funded and operated health programs. Yet many health care providers fail to inform immigrants with limited English proficiency (LEP) of their right to be assisted, at no cost, by a qualified interpreter. In addition, many lack access to translated materials on the pandemic. States, including Massachusetts, Oregon, and

---

[32] https://www.krqe.com/health/coronavirus-vaccine/advocacy-groups-say-immigrants-in-new-mexico-hesitant-to-register-for-covid-19-vaccine/.

[33] "National Strategy for the COVID-19 Response and Pandemic Preparedness," The White House, January 21, 2021, https://www.whitehouse.gov/wp-content/uploads/2021/01/National-Strategy-for-the-COVID-19-Response-and-Pandemic-Preparedness.pdf.

[34] Visram, Talib, "How will undocumented immigrants get the COVID-19 vaccine?," Fast Company, January 22, 2021, https://www.fastcompany.com/90595912/how-will-undocumented-immigrants-get-the-covid-vaccine.

[35] Claudia Chacin, Ana, Bianca Pardo Ocasio and Taylor Dolven, "Florida now requiring proof of state residency for COVID vaccines," January 21, 2021, https://www.miamiherald.com/news/coronavirus/article248671090.html.

[36] Cole, Samantha, "Vaccine Site Uses Credit History to Verify Patients' Identities," Motherboard, January 15, 2021, https://www.vice.com/amp/en/article/y3gq9j/nyc-vaccine-site-credit-history-experian-identity-rejected?twitter_impression=true.

the District of Columbia have pledged that all public resources will be translated into multiple languages and the federal government should follow their lead.[37,38,39]

Some states and localities have used unsophisticated tools, such as Google Translate, in an attempt to translate COVID-19 materials, resulting in to critical translation errors.[40] In Virginia, it produced a Spanish translation that stated the vaccine was "not necessary," and a correction was not issued more than three weeks after community members had identified the error.[41] Immigrant community advocates tell NILC that appeals to their state and local governments for improved in-language materials have been rebuffed due to a lack of resources or an inaccurate assumption that what has already been produced is sufficient.

Public and private insurers generally require providers to subsume language access services as part of their administrative costs but historically do not enforce these requirements. As a result, providers often fail to hire in-person interpreters, despite their link with better health outcomes, or even establish contracts with telephonic interpretation services.[42]

Congress should work to address language access systematic issues in the long term, and during this pandemic, work with the administration ensure that important information being provided to patients on the COVID vaccine is translated into the languages (other than English) most commonly spoken in the United States. It could accomplish this by passing the Coronavirus Language Access Act (S. 4526 in the 116th Congress).

Front-Line Immigrant Workers Must Have Equitable Access to Vaccines

We appreciate the President's recognition that, "Healthcare workers and other essential workers, many of whom are people of color and immigrants, have put their lives on the line during the coronavirus disease 2019 (COVID-19) pandemic."[43] Immigrants are disproportionately represented among food and agricultural workers in the United States.[44] Food production industries, such as meatpacking, have experienced many outbreaks, which

---

[37] "COVID-19 Vaccination Plan," Massachusetts Department of Public Health, October 16, 2020, https://www.mass.gov/doc/massachusetts-interim-draft-plan/download.

[38] "COVID-19 Vaccination Plan," Oregon Health Authority, November 6, 2020, https://www.oregon.gov/oha/covid19/Documents/COVID-19-Vaccination-Plan-Oregon.pdf.

[39] "COVID-19 Vaccination Plan," DC Health, November 27, 2020, https://coronavirus.dc.gov/sites/default/files/dc/sites/coronavirus/page_content/attachments/DC_COVID-19%20Vaccination%20Plan%2011.27.pdf.

[40] Stanmyre, Matthew, "N.J. immigrant communities were hard hit by COVID. Now, they may not have ready access to vaccines, experts fear," January 24, 2021, https://www.nj.com/coronavirus/2021/01/nj-immigrant-communities-were-hard-hit-by-covid-now-they-may-not-have-access-to-vaccines-experts-fear.html.

[41] Moreno, Sabrina, "Virginia uses Google Translate for COVID vaccine information. Here's how that magnifies language barriers, misinformation," Richmond Times-Dispatch, January 14, 2021, https://richmond.com/news/local/virginia-uses-google-translate-for-covid-vaccine-information-heres-how-that-magnifies-language-barriers-misinformation/article_715cb81a-d880-5c98-aac5-6b30b378bbd3.html.

[42] Chandrika, Divi et al, "Language proficiency and adverse events in US hospitals: a pilot study," Int J Qual Health Care, April 2007, 19(2):60-7 https://pubmed.ncbi.nlm.nih.gov/17277013/.

[43] "Executive Order on Protecting Worker Health and Safety," The White House, January 21, 2021, https://www.whitehouse.gov/briefing-room/presidential-actions/2021/01/21/executive-order-protecting-worker-health-and-safety/.

[44] "The Essential Role of Immigrants in the U.S. Food Supply Chain," Migration Policy Institute, April 2020, https://www.migrationpolicy.org/content/essential-role-immigrants-us-food-supply-chain.

have disproportionately impacted communities of color.[45] New research shows that they are among the deadliest industries to work in during the pandemic, second only to health care.[46] Organizations representing agricultural and food production industries have requested they be prioritized for a vaccine.[47]

Advocates have told NILC that the lack of access to paid leave is a major barrier to eligible immigrants' access to vaccinations. The Families First Coronavirus Response Act ("FFCRA") required certain employers to provide their employees with emergency paid sick leave ("EPSL") or expanded family and medical leave ("EFMLA") for specified reasons related to COVID-19. While this employer mandate expired on December 31, 2020, the Coronavirus Response and Relief Supplemental Appropriations Act enacted on December 27, 2020, gave employers covered by FFCRA the option to obtain a tax credit if they extended EPSL and EFMLA leave benefits through March 31, 2021. Congress must extend an expansive paid leave policy that does not exclude industries and is broad enough to cover both taking the vaccine and recuperating from any side effects.

Immigrants Must Not Fear Immigration Consequences from Vaccination

NILC's networks, as well as the media, report that fears related to the Trump Administration's public charge regulations are deterring immigrants from seeking vaccinations.[48] While the Department of Homeland Security (DHS) has stated that COVID-19, "treatment or preventive services will not negatively affect any alien as part of a future Public Charge analysis," the information was not disseminated in a consumer-friendly format, so that predictably this understanding has eluded many immigrant communities[49]. Ultimately, DHS and related agencies must fully repeal the Trump Administration's public charge regulations, and we appreciate yesterday's Executive Order from President Biden requesting DHS review of the public charge rule. In the meantime, all effort must be made to communicate to immigrants in an accessible, linguistically and culturally competent manner.

---

[45] Waltenburg, Michelle, et all, "COVID-19 Among Workers in Meat and Poultry Processing Facilities — United States, April–May 2020," Centers for Disease Control and Prevention Morbidity and Mortality Weekly Report, July 10, 2020, https://www.cdc.gov/mmwr/volumes/69/wr/mm6927e2.htm.

[46] Chen, Yea-Hung, "Excess mortality associated with the COVID-19 pandemic among Californians 18–65 years of age, by occupational sector and occupation: March through October 2020," medRxiv, January 21, 2021, https://www.medrxiv.org/content/10.1101/2021.01.21.21250266v1.full.

[47] See letter from United Food and Commercial Workers and North American Meat Institute https://www.ufcw.org/wp-content/blogs.dir/61/files/2020/12/UFCW-and-NAMI-Governor-Letter.pdf.

[48] Bedford, Tori, "Fear Of Deportation Prompts Undocumented Immigrants To Resist COVID-19 Vaccine," GBH, January 5, 2021, https://www.wgbh.org/news/local-news/2021/01/05/fear-of-deportation-prompts-undocumented-immigrants-to-resist-covid-19-vaccine.

[49] "Public Charge, U.S. Citizenship and Immigration Services, https://www.uscis.gov/green-card/green-card-processes-and-procedures/public-charge.

Immigrants in Detention Must Have Equitable Access to Vaccines

The rate of COVID-19 spread in immigrant detention facilities is significantly higher than in the general population.[50] Conditions in U.S. Immigration Customs Enforcement (ICE) detention facilities pose unacceptable health risks and Congressional investigations have revealed that ICE's widespread failure to provide adequate health care and has contributed to the death of immigrants in ICE custody.[51] Yet reporting indicates that ICE lacks a plan to vaccinate people in its custody.[52] While NILC believes that Congress must ensure that DHS works toward ending immigration detention during the pandemic and beyond, while immigrants are detained, they must be protected. Some researchers have outlined steps that ICE must take, such as outlining clear plans for vaccination.[53] Considering that ICE has not provided people in detention with adequate health care and supplies up to this point, this plan must be publicly posted with regular data on progress.[54]

We appreciate Congress is looking to improve the COVID-19 public health response. We look forward to working with you to ensure that immigrants are included at all aspects of it.

Sincerely, Ben D'Avanzo

Senior Health Policy Analyst National Immigration Law Center

Written Statement for the Record, for the Hearing Entitled "Road to Recovery: Ramping up Covid-19 Vaccines, Testing, and Medical Supply Chain," United States House of Representatives, Committee on Energy and Commerce, Subcommittee on Health, February 3, 2021

The Asian & Pacific Islander American Health Forum (APIAHF) submits this written testimony for the record for the February 3, 2021 hearing before the House Energy & Commerce, Health Subcommittee entitled "Road to Recovery: Ramping up COVID-19 Vaccines, Testing and Medical Supply Chain."

APIAHF is the nation's leading health policy organization working to advance the health and well-being of over 20 million Asian Americans, Native Hawaiians and Pacific Islanders (AA and NHPI) across the U.S. and territories. APIAHF works to improve access to and the quality of care for communities who are predominantly immigrant, many of whom are limited English proficient, and may be new to the U.S. healthcare system or unfamiliar with private or public coverage. We have longstanding relationships with over 150 community-based

---

[50] Erfani, Parsa et al, "COVID-19 Testing and Cases in Immigration Detention Centers, April-August 2020" JAMA, October 29, 2020, https://jamanetwork.com/journals/jama/fullarticle/2772627.

[51] Staff report, "The Trump Administration's Mistreatment of Detained Immigrants, " U.S. House of Representatives Committee on Oversight and Reform and Subcommittee on Civil Rights and Civil Liberties, September 2020, https://oversight.house.gov/sites/democrats.oversight.house.gov/files/2020-09-24.%20Staff %20Report%20on%20ICE%20Contractors.pdf.

[52] Montoya-Galvez, Camilo, "Questions surround COVID-19 vaccine timeline for immigrants in ICE custody," CBS News, January 18, 2021, https://www.cbsnews.com/news/covid-19-vaccine-timeline-immigrants-ice-custody/.

[53] Uppal, Nishant, Parsa Erfani, and Raquel Sofia Sandoval, "ICE must provide Covid-19 vaccines to all detained migrants," STAT, January 12, 2021, https://www.statnews.com/2021/01/12/ice-must-provide-covid-19-vaccines-to-all-detained-migrants/.

[54] "Praying for Hand Soap and Masks," Physicians for Human Rights, January 12, 2021, https://phr.org/our-work/resources/praying-for-hand-soap-and-masks/?utm_content=homepage_hero.

organizations across 34 states and the Pacific, to whom we provide capacity building, advocacy and technical assistance.

For over 32 years, we have focused our policy efforts on 1) improving access to health insurance and care for AA and NHPI and immigrant communities, 2) ensuring the collection, analysis and reporting of detailed demographic health data and 3) protecting and advancing the language rights of the 1 in 3 AAs and NHPIs who are limited English proficient.

As such, we have a strong understanding of the needs and barriers to good health that were already experienced by AA and NHPI communities across the country and ways in which COVID-19 is magnifying and exacerbating inequities among communities of color. It is imperative that Congress continue to take action to address these disparities as they threaten to undermine our collective national response and recovery.

COVID-19 National Crisis Is Disproportionately Impacting Communities of Color

The novel COVID-19 virus is a national crisis that demonstrates that public health has no boundaries. Yet the impact is being unevenly felt among communities of color who, due to a combination of structural, economic, social and environmental disparities and discrimination, are experiencing higher burdens associated with the pandemic. As a result, COVID-19 is disproportionately leading to severe illness and mortality within these communities.

We wish to emphasize that, in the face of narratives to the contrary, these communities facing disparities are in no way to blame. COVID-19 has exposed what advocates for health equity have known for decades, if not centuries: our history of racism and prejudice has led to serious health consequences that continue today. Or as put recently by journalist Zeeshan Aleem, "it's not people of color driving up America's casualties, but America that is driving up people of color's casualties."[55]

Nearly one year into the COVID-19 pandemic, the national emergency has magnified long-standing inequities that continue to undermine the health and well-being of AAs and NHPIs specially, and communities of color overall. To date, the federal response has been inadequate and has failed to identify and respond to the disproportionate impact COVID-19 is having on AAs and NHPIs nationally, and particularly within certain communities. The longstanding failure of state, federal and local governments to collect, analyze and report on detailed data have hampered our federal response at a time when the limited data that is available is clear that AAs and NHPIs are being impacted.

According to the UCLA COVID-19 Racial Data Tracker, NHPIs are the most likely to have contracted COVID-19 in 2020.[56] In at least 10 states, AAs have a case fatality rate that is disproportionately higher than the general population, while the same is true for NHPIs in 8 states.[57] Recent estimates indicate a high burden of COVID-19 deaths among AAs, with almost

---

[55] Aleem, Zeeshan, "HHS Secretary Alex Azar suggests health problems in communities of color explain coronavirus death numbers," *Vox* (May 17, 2020). Available at: https://www.vox.com/covid-19-coronavirus-us-response-trump/2020/5/17/21261708/alex-azar-coronavirus-trump-economy-african-american.

[56] https://covidtracking.com/race.

[57] Testimony from the National Council of Asian Pacific Islander Physicians to the Committee on Ways and Means (June 9, 2020). Available at: https://mcusercontent.com/d7f02dd24377959c916d14de6/files/5ebe9b24-21f8-4d67-93d2-4f218db2e323/NCAPIP_Statement_to_House_Ways_and_Means_Committee_on_COVID_19_Disparities.pdf.

14,000 excess deaths, and AAs have the second-highest increase in deaths following Hispanic Americans.[58]

APIAHF has led national efforts to ensure the federal COVID-19 response addresses the needs of AA and NHPI communities including identifying critical gaps in data and infrastructure, language access and barriers for immigrant communities. In addition, as a long-term provider to the CDC, APIAHF is supporting CDC COVID-19 Response projects including building National AA NHPI COVID19 Response Network, which builds upon networks created by APIAHF and other national partners. The network includes a National AA NHPI Healthcare Workforce Education and Training Initiative and National Partnership for Rapid Response to COVID-19.

These inequities are compounded by the dual challenges that AA and NHPI communities face of a public health emergency and a spate of violence and xenophobic hate. AA and NHPI organizations have documented at least 1,900 hate incidents in 46 states.[59]

At the same time AA and NHPI communities are experiencing the dual blow of COVID-19 and COVID-19 hate, an estimated 2,000,000 AA and Pacific Islander essential workers are staffing vital public safety sectors. These include the 21% of physicians[60] who are AA and the nearly 10% of registered nurses[61] who are Filipino, as well as 21% of critical care fellows[62] and 22% of pharmacists.[63] Dr. Chen Fu, a Chinese American doctor working in a New York City hospital recently told NBC's *The Today Show* how he faced, despite his front line work, animosity and harassment in public.[64]

While Congress has responded to the crisis, such efforts have been insufficient to address the distinct needs of communities of color, in particular immigrant and limited English proficient communities and as we enter the next phase of our response involving vaccine distribution and administration. Failing to address this oversight threatens to perpetuate existing barriers, as recent data suggests is already happening, and undermines our collective national response.

Vaccine Distribution Must be Equitable

As outlined in APIAHF and the Center for the Study of Asian American Health at NYU School of Medicine and community organizations around the nation letter to the National Academies

58 Flagg A, Sharma D, Fenn L, Stobbe M. COVID-19's Toll on People of Color Is Worse Than We Knew. *The Marshall Project.*

59 "Hate Incidents," *AAPI Emergency Response Network* (last accessed May 25, 2020). Available at: https://www.aapiern.org/hate-incidents.

60 "COVID-19 in Numbers, Physicians & Surgeons," *Data USA* (last accessed May 25, 2020). Available at: https://datausa.io/profile/soc/physicians-surgeons.

61 "COVID-19 in Numbers, Registered Nurses," *Data USA* (last accessed May 25, 2020). Available at: https://datausa.io/profile/soc/registered-nurses.

62 Lane-Fall MB, Miano TA, Aysola J, Augoustides JGT. "Diversity in the Emerging Critical Care Workforce: Analysis of Demographic Trends in Critical Care Fellows From 2004 to 2014," *Crit Care Med.* 2017;45(5):822-827. doi:10.1097/CCM.0000000000002322.

63 "COVID-19 in Numbers, Pharmacists," *Data USA* (last accessed May 25, 2020). Available at:https://datausa.io/profile/soc/pharmacists.

64 Nguyen, Vicky, "Threats against Asian Americans are on the Rise Amid Coronavirus Crisis," *The Today Show* (April 24, 2020). Available at https://www.today.com/video/threats-against-asian-americans-are-on-the-rise-amid-coronavirus-crisis-82510405969.

for Science, Engineering and Medicine,[65] equity must be a central component of our national vaccine distribution and administration efforts. This point has been echoed by leading civil rights organizations under the Leadership Conference for Civil and Human Rights Principles for COVID-19 Vaccine Development and Distribution, which call for communities to be included in vaccine distribution efforts and for affirmative steps to address vaccine hesitancy.[66] And as noted below, having detailed data is central to achieving those efforts, as well as diverse clinical trials.[67]

It is also important to understand that AANHPI communities face specific risks associated with COVID-19 that must be accounted for in distribution efforts:

Essential Workers

Essential workers face higher risks of COVID-19 infection because of increased exposure to the virus. About 10 percent of the US workforce are employed in jobs where they are exposed to infection or disease at least once per week.[68] About 30 percent of AAs and NHPIs are represented in the essential workforce, including healthcare, food preparation services, personal care, protective services, sales and production. Pacific Islanders also have a high concentration in the meat- and poultry-processing industry, another essential industry. The burden of exposure to infection or disease at least once a week was more than 75 percent among healthcare support and healthcare practitioner workers, and about 30 percent among protective services workers.[17] In some states, AAs and NHPIs make up the highest share of healthcare workers, with a large proportion who are immigrants.[69]

Among AAs and NHPIs, there are several populations that have been reported to have a greater burden of COVID-19 deaths, in addition to the higher risk of COVID-19 disease and severe higher rates of comorbid conditions.

- Filipino nurses make up a large proportion of health workers, are employed in hospital sessions (58.5 percent), and are represented in acute cute and critical care (42.5 percent) and geriatrics or gerontology (7 percent).[70] In California, almost one-fifth of

[65] Statement on Preliminary Framework of Equitable Allocation of COVID-19 Vaccine (last accessed January 28, 2021). Available at https://www.apiahf.org/resource/statement-on-preliminary-framework-for-equitable-allocation-of-covid-19-vaccine/.

[66] Leadership Conference on Civil and Human Rights, "Civil Rights Principles for COVID-19 Vaccine Development and Distribution." Available at: https://civilrights.org/resource/civil-rights-principles-for-covid-19-vaccine-development-and-distribution/.

[67] Asian & Pacific Islander American Health Forum, NYU Center for the Study of Asian American Health, Clinical Trial Diversity Factsheet. Published December 2020. Available at: https://www.apiahf.org/resource/clinical-trial-diversity-factsheet/.

[68] Krisberg K. Essential workers facing higher risks during COVID-19 outbreak: Meat packers, retail workers sickened. *The Nation's Health*. 2020;50(6):1-16. See also Baker MG, Peckham TK, Seixas NS. Estimating the burden of United States workers exposed to infection or disease: A key factor in containing risk of COVID-19 infection. *PLOS ONE*. 2020;15(4):e0232452. doi:10.1371/journal.pone.0232452.

[69] Dang E, Huang S, Kwok A, Lung H, Park M, Yueh E. COVID-19 and Advancing Asian American Recovery. *McKinsey & Company* https://www.mckinsey.com/~/media/McKinsey/Industries/Public%20and%20Social%20Sector/Our%20Insights/COVID%2019% 20and%20advancing%20Asian%20American%20recovery/COVID-19-and-advancing-Asian-American-recovery-final.pdf. *See also New American Economy Research Fund*. Asian Americans and Pacific Islander Americans on the Frontlines. Published May 21, 2020. Accessed August 31, 2020. https://research.newamericaneconomy.org/report/aapi-americans-on-the-frontlines/.

[70] Jurado L-FM, Saria MG. Filipino nurses in the United States. *Nursing Management*. 2018;49(3):36–41. doi:10.1097/01.NUMA.0000530423.71453.58.

registered nurses are Filipino and are overrepresented compared to the patient population.[71] In addition to their occupational exposures, a high proportion of Filipino nurses in the US were born in the Philippines (94.2 percent).[72]

- AAs and NHPIs make up over 71 percent of the share of all healthcare workers in Hawaii and over 26 percent of healthcare workers in California.[73]
- In the healthcare workforce in the US, Filipinos represent 18.4 percent in the share of healthcare workers compared to 9.1 percent of all AAs and NHPIs.[74]
- In the food preparation workforce in the US, Chinese, Filipino, and NHPIs represent 6.1, 4.9, and 6.8 percent, respectively, in the share of food preparation workers compared to 4.9 percent of all AAs and NHPIs.[75]

Social Determinants of Health

If a vaccine is to be equitably accessible, the social conditions and determinants of health for AA and NHPI communities must be considered.[76] This includes the rates of un- or under-insurance, immigration status, language access, cultural awareness, chronic health conditions, and more. The high prevalence of underlying health conditions like diabetes and pre-diabetes[77] are a large contributing factor to COVID-19 disparities among AAs and NHPIs. According to the CDC, among COVID-19 confirmed hospitalized adults, over 90 percent of adults had an underlying health condition that included hypertension (56.9 percent), obesity (47.6 percent), metabolic disease (41.4 percent), and cardiovascular disease (32.5 percent).[78] Additionally, COVID-19 morbidity and mortality have been associated with diabetes in several recent studies.[79] Diabetes is of particular concern for Filipino, South Asian and NHPI communities

[71] Wong T. Little noticed, Filipino Americans are dying of COVID-19 at an alarming rate. *Los Angeles Times*. https://www.latimes.com/california/story/2020-07-21/filipino-americans-dying-covid. Published July 21, 2020. Accessed September 3, 2020. See also Waneka R, Spetz J. *The Diversity of California's Registered Nursing Workforce – 2013 Update* California Board of Registered Nursing; 2013. Accessed October 2, 2011. http://0-proquest.umi.com.library.touro.edu/pqdweb?index=0&did=2166665531&SrchMode=1&sid=1&Fmt=3&VInst=PROD&VType=PQD&RQT=309&VName=PQD&TS=1317549965&clientId=31638.

[72] Jurado L-FM, Saria MG. Filipino nurses in the United States. *Nursing Management*. 2018;49(3):36–41. doi:10.1097/01.NUMA.0000530423.71453.58.

[73] Asian Americans and Pacific Islander Americans on the Frontlines. *New American Economy Research Fund*. Published May 21, 2020. Accessed August 31, 2020. https://research.newamericaneconomy.org/report/aapi-americans-on-the-frontlines/.

[74] US Census Bureau. 2018 American Community Survey 1-Year Estimates. Accessed April 21, 2020.

[75] *Id.*

[76] Written Statement for the Record for the Hearing Entitled 'The Disproportionate Impact of COVID-19 on Communities of Color' Committee on Ways and Means, *Asian & Pacific Islander American Health Forum*. Published May 27, 2020. Available at: https://www.apiahf.org/wpcontent/uploads/2020/05/5.26.2020-Asian-Pacific-Islander-American-Health-Forum-WrittenTestimony-to-Ways-and-Means-Committee-1.pdf.

[77] Ko JY, Danielson ML, Town M, et al. Risk Factors for COVID-19-associated hospitalization: COVID-19-Associated Hospitalization Surveillance Network and Behavioral Risk Factor Surveillance System. *medRxiv*. Published online July 27, 2020:2020.07.27.20161810. doi:10.1101/2020.07.27.20161810.

[78] Centers for Disease Control and Prevention. COVID-NET: COVID-19-Associated Hospitalization Surveillance Network. Accessed August 31, 2020. https://gis.cdc.gov/grasp/COVIDNet/COVID19_5.html.

[79] Apicella M, Campopiano MC, Mantuano M, Mazoni L, Coppelli A, Prato SD. COVID-19 in people with diabetes: understanding the reasons for worse outcomes. *The Lancet Diabetes & Endocrinology*. 2020;8(9):782-792. doi:10.1016/S2213-8587(20)30238-2. See also Holman N, Knighton P, Kar P, et al. Risk factors for COVID-19-related mortality in people with type 1 and type 2 diabetes in England: a population-based cohort study. *The Lancet Diabetes & Endocrinology*. Published online August 13, 2020. doi:10.1016/S2213-8587(20)30271-0.

affecting 12 percent, 11 percent and 9 percent, respectively as compared to 8.5 percent in US total.[80]

- NHPIs have disproportionately high prevalence of cardiometabolic diseases including diabetes and obesity, and are among the highest-risk populations in the US.[81]
- Studies have found that Asians as an aggregate have greater diabetes prevalence than their white counterparts[82] and have the highest proportion of undiagnosed diabetes among all racial and ethnic groups.[83]
- Furthermore, there is variation in the prevalence of diabetes when data are disaggregated by Asian subgroups. For example, a study by Uchima et al. (2019) using data from the Hawai'i Behavioral Risk Factor Surveillance System found that NHPI (9.9 percent), Filipino (11.2 percent), and Chinese (9.1 percent) adults had significantly higher prevalence of diabetes than white adults (5.4 percent).[84] Another study found that all AA women and men (Asian Indian, Chinese, Filipino, Japanese, Korean, and Vietnamese) had greater prevalence of type 2 diabetes compared to non-Hispanic whites, with Asian Indian and Filipinos reporting the highest rates among AA subgroups.[85]

Multi-Generational Homes

Living in more crowded homes, and/or multi-generational homes, may increase the risk of COVID infection, particularly among households with vulnerable populations (e.g., older adults) or essential workers and limited space to isolate.[86]

- AAs and NHPIs are more likely to live in multigenerational homes than other racial/ethnic groups.[87] More than 70 percent of AAs and NHPIs lived in multigenerational homes, with about 13 percent of AAs and NHPIs living in three-

---

[80] Wyatt LC, Russo R, Kranick J, et al. *Health Atlas 2012-2017 for AANHPI: A Comprehensive Look at Health for AANHPI in the U.S. 2020.*

[81] Mau MK, Sinclair K, Saito EP, Baumhofer KN, Kaholokula JK. Cardiometabolic Health Disparities in Native Hawaiians and Other Pacific Islanders. *Epidemiol Rev*. 2009;31:113-129. doi:10.1093/ajerev/mxp004.

[82] Menke A, Casagrande S, Geiss L, Cowie CC. Prevalence of and Trends in Diabetes Among Adults in the United States, 1988-2012. *JAMA*. 2015;314(10):1021-1029. doi:10.1001/jama.2015.10029. See also Wang EJ, Wong EC, Dixit AA, Fortmann SP, Linde RB, Palaniappan LP. Type 2 Diabetes: Identifying High Risk Asian American Subgroups in a Clinical Population. *Diabetes Res Clin Pract*. 2011;93(2):248-254. doi:10.1016/j.diabres.2011.05.025.

[83] Menke A, Casagrande S, Geiss L, Cowie CC. Prevalence of and Trends in Diabetes Among Adults in the United States, 1988-2012. *JAMA*. 2015;314(10):1021-1029. doi:10.1001/jama.2015.10029.

[84] Uchima O, Wu YY, Browne C, Braun KL. Disparities in Diabetes Prevalence Among Native Hawaiians/Other Pacific Islanders and Asians in Hawai'i. *Prev Chronic Dis*. 2019;16. doi:10.5888/pcd16.180187.

[85] Wang EJ, Wong EC, Dixit AA, Fortmann SP, Linde RB, Palaniappan LP. Type 2 Diabetes: Identifying High Risk Asian American Subgroups in a Clinical Population. *Diabetes Res Clin Pract*. 2011;93(2):248-254. doi:10.1016/j.diabres.2011.05.025.

[86] Dougherty C. 12 People in a 3-Bedroom House, Then the Virus Entered the Equation. *The New York Times*. https://www.nytimes.com/2020/08/01/business/economy/housing-overcrowding-coronavirus.html. Published August 1, 2020. Accessed August 31, 2020. *See also* Mejia MC, Cha P. Overcrowded Housing and COVID-19 Risk among Essential Workers. Public Policy Institute of California. Accessed August 31, 2020. https://www.ppic.org/blog/overcrowded-housing-and-covid-19-risk-among-essential-workers/.

[87] Cohn D, Passel JS. Record 64 million Americans live in multigenerational households. *Pew Research Center*. Published April 5, 2018. Accessed August 31, 2020. https://www.pewresearch.org/fact-tank/2018/04/05/a-record-64-million-americans-live-in-multigenerational-households/.

generational households.[88] The percent of adults 65 years and older living in multigenerational homes ranged from 4.6 percent among NHPIs to 12.1 percent among Filipinos.[89]

- Among AA and NHPI groups, Filipinos (18.7 percent) and NHPIs (16.4 percent) reported the percentages of living in three-generational households.[90]
- NHPIs have higher COVID-19 death rates than any other racial or ethnic group, especially in regions with dense populations of NHPIs like Louisiana, Arkansas and Iowa.[91]
- About 24.1 percent of NHPIs live in 19 hotspot counties where NHPI populations are disproportionately affected by COVID-19 and 5.1 percent of AAs live in 4 hotspot counties where AA residents are disproportionately affected by COVID-19.[92]

As such, given the large number of AANHPIs living in multigenerational households[93], vaccine prioritization should include family/caregivers as part of the essential and/or healthcare workers categories.

Language Access

One third of AAs and Pacific Islanders are limited English proficient (LEP), meaning they speak little to no English, creating a substantial barrier to accessing routine care, let alone critical information and access to vaccines and clinical trials. Despite existing federal law and regulation requiring protections for LEP communities, who account for 25 million Americans, including over 6 million AAs and over 100,000 NHPIs, and established language access plans of federal agencies, language remains a significant barrier for the health of AAs and NHPIs.[94]

Our concerns are furthered confirmed by a survey commissioned by APIAHF with 45 community-based partners working with AA and NHPI communities which found that 9 in 10 respondents reported that existing language resources related to COVID-19 are inadequate.[95] As such, it is critical that any vaccine framework address language access barriers and advocate for allocation of resources, at the trial, distribution and public education of any COVID-19 vaccine.

---

[88] US Census Bureau. 2018 American Community Survey 1-Year Estimates.

[89] *Id.*

[90] *Id.*

[91] Chang RC, Penaia C, Thomas K. Count Native Hawaiian And Pacific Islanders In COVID-19 Data—It's An OMB Mandate. *Health Affairs Blog*. doi:10.1377/hblog20200825.671245.

[92] Centers for Disease Control and Prevention. Demographic Trends of COVID-19 cases and deaths in the US reported to CDC. CDC COVID Data Tracker.

[93] Living in more crowded homes, and/or multi-generational homes, may increase the risk of COVID infection, particularly among households with vulnerable populations (e.g., older adults) or essential workers and limited space to isolate. AAs and NHPIs are more likely to live in multigenerational homes than other racial/ethnic groups (Cohn D, Passel JS. Record 64 million Americans live in multigenerational households. *Pew Research Center*. Published April 5, 2018. Accessed August 31, 2020. https://www.pewresearch.org/fact-tank/2018/04/05/a-record-64-million-americans-live-in-multigenerational-households/). More than 70 percent of AAs and NHPIs lived in multigenerational homes, with about 13 percent of AAs and NHPIs living in three-generational households. (US Census Bureau. 2018 American Community Survey 1-Year Estimates). The percent of adults 65 years and older living in multigenerational homes ranged from 4.6% among NHPIs to 12.1% among Filipinos.

[94] COVID-19 Language Access Letter to Congressional Leadership, *Asian & Pacific Islander American Health Forum*. Published July 23, 2020. Available at: https://www.apiahf.org/resource/covid19-lep-letter/.

[95] What Asian American, Native Hawaiian and Pacific Islander Organizations Need in the Face of the COVID-19 Pandemic, *Asian & Pacific Islander American Health Forum*. Published July 20, 2020. Available at: https://www.apiahf.org/resource/covid-19-need-to-know/.

Immigration Status

While the Affordable Care Act (ACA) has resulted in more than 20 million Americans gaining coverage through Medicaid and the Health Insurance Marketplace, coverage remains unequal with millions of immigrants ineligible for Medicaid and other public health insurance programs.[96] Federal restrictions, dating back to the 1996 Personal Responsibility and Work Opportunity Reconciliation Act of 1996, bar many categories of immigrants from coverage while undocumented immigrants are not even able to buy unsubsidized insurance on the ACA marketplaces. As a result, 31% of noncitizens are uninsured, compared to 8% of naturalized citizens and 7% of native-born citizens.[97]

Finally, it is extremely important to look at the underlying conditions (racism, poverty, co-morbidities, lack of access to health info/care/insurance), homelessness, institutionalization, and systemic inequality. Racism is a consequence of systemic inequalities and our national vaccine distribution and administration strategy must acknowledge the potential impact on vaccine allocation and public health.

Detailed Demographic Data about Vaccine Administration Is Needed

As the United States has confirmed more than 25 million COVID-19 cases[98] and more than 23 million doses[99] of vaccines have been administered as of January 2021, we remain concern that detailed demographic data continues to not be available about vaccine distribution and administration.

Disparities in COVID-19 impact are also present in vaccine distribution and administration efforts. According to new analysis by Kaiser Health News, Black Americans, for example, are being vaccinated at disproportionately lower rates than whites.[100] This analysis was based on 16 states that have reported race and ethnicity for vaccine distribution and raises serious concerns given that Asian American and non-Hispanic Black health care workers are more likely to contract COVID-19 and die compared to their white counterparts.[101] While many factors may be contributing to lower vaccination rates in communities of color, it is impossible to equitably address them without the collection, analysis and regular public reporting of detailed demographic data.

APIAHF and Trust for America's Health recently outlined these concerns to the Centers for Disease Control and Prevention, appreciating that CDC is working to support our whole-of-government response to COVID-19 and that there was a lack of data collected under the last

---

[96] Chartbook: Accomplishments of Affordable Care Act, *Center on Budget and Policy Priorities*. Published March 19, 2020. Available at: https://www.cbpp.org/research/health/chart-book-accomplishments-of-affordable-care-act.

[97] APIAHF analysis of 2018 American Community Survey data.

[98] Johns Hopkins University COVID-19 Data Tracker, available here: https://gisanddata.maps.arcgis.com/apps/opsdashboard/index.html?utm_source=newsletter&utm_medium=email&utm_campaign=newsletter_axiosvitals&stream=top#/bda7594740fd40299423467b48e9ecf6.

[99] Centers for Disease Control & Prevention, COVID-19 Data Tracker, available here: https://covid.cdc.gov/covid-data-tracker/#vaccinations.

[100] Kaiser Health News, Black Americans are Getting Vaccinated at Lower Rates Compared to White Americans, available here: https://khn.org/news/article/black-americans-are-getting-vaccinated-at-lower-rates-than-white-americans/?utm_source=newsletter&utm_medium=email&utm_campaign=newsletter_axiosvitals&stream=top.

[101] The Guardian, Key Findings About US HealthCare Workers To Date, available here: https://www.theguardian.com/us-news/ng-interactive/2020/dec/22/lost-on-the-frontline-our-findings-to-date.

administration which compounds those efforts, as well as the challenge of aggregating data from multiple states and immunization information systems.

Tracking demographic data for those who have received the vaccine is critical to equitable vaccination efforts, including being able to tailor culturally and linguistically accessible outreach.

It is imperative that Congress respond to the complex crisis that communities of color are experiencing due to COVID-19 and include the supports that are needed to ensure equitable distribution of COVID-19 vaccines. Thank you for receiving this testimony.

Juliet K. Choi
Chief Executive Officer
Asian & Pacific Islander American Health Forum

January 29, 2021

The Honorable Diana DeGette
Chairwoman
Subcommittee on Oversight & Investigations,
Committee on Energy & Commerce
U.S. House of Representatives
Washington, D.C.

The Honorable Morgan Griffith
Ranking Member
Subcommittee on Oversight & Investigations,
Committee on Energy & Commerce
Washington, D.C.

The Honorable Anna Eshoo
Chairwoman
Subcommittee on Health,
Committee on Energy & Commerce
U.S. House of Representatives
Washington, D.C.

The Honorable Brett Guthrie
Ranking Member
Subcommittee on Health,
Committee on Energy & Commerce
Washington, D.C.

Dear Chairwomen DeGette and Eshoo and Ranking Members Griffith and Guthrie:

On behalf of the American Academy of Family Physicians (AAFP) and the 136,700 family physicians and medical students we represent, I write in response to the two hearings: "No Time to Lose: Solutions to Increase COVID-19 Vaccinations in the States" and "Road to

Recovery: Ramping Up COVID-19 Vaccines, Testing, and Medical Supply Chain." We thank you for your attention to these timely and important issues and would like to offer our recommendations for combating COVID-19 vaccine hesitancy and ensuring efficient, equitable vaccine administration.

As vaccine distribution is accelerated, the AAFP strongly urges improved collaboration with primary care physicians and practices, including by explicitly incorporating them in distribution plans and empowering them to administer vaccines across the country.

Family physicians provide preventive services and comprehensive primary care to patients across the lifespan. Family physicians are also integral members of their communities and see firsthand how pervasive health inequities contribute to poor health outcomes, with COVID-19 being just the latest example. As such, they play a critical role in the fight against COVID-19 by diagnosing and treating their patients, as well as counseling patients and administe ring vaccines.

According to data from the Medical Expenditure Panel Survey, primary care physicians provided 54 percent of all clinical visits for vaccinations, which made them more likely to administer vaccines than other stakeholders, such as pharmacies or grocery stores.[102] In other words, patients already rely on their primary care physicians to educate them about vaccines and administer vaccines. Evidence confirms that health care professionals are the most trusted advisor for vaccination decisions.[103] Indeed, family physicians report that their patients are contacting them for information on the COVID-19 vaccines and, in many cases, asking when they can receive the vaccine from their current primary care physician.

Unfortunately, 85 percent of independent practices are unable to obtain COVID-19 vaccines for their patients. Most practices are also not receiving information from their state or local governments about where their patients can access the vaccine. Many small and independent physician practices are in rural and other under resourced areas that lack large retail pharmacies or other mass immunizers. Primary care physicians are well-equipped to administer the vaccine and are eager to help improve access to COVID-19 vaccines in their communities.

We call on the federal, state, and local governments to take immediate steps to supply community-based primary care physicians with COVID-19 vaccines. Leveraging health care distributors who already supply physicians with flu and other vaccines could help more health care providers access vaccines and ultimately accelerate the pace of immunizations.

COVID-19 vaccination strategies should leverage trusted primary care physicians to combat vaccine hesitancy. Early data suggests that Black and Hispanic populations are being vaccinated at a slower rate than White populations, despite being disproportionately impacted by COVID-19 cases and deaths. Further, a significant proportion of rural residents report vaccine hesitancy and rural residents remain much more likely than those in urban areas to indicate that they will not get the vaccine. As trusted members of their communities, and the primary source of comprehensive health services in rural and under resourced areas, community primary care physicians play an integral role to ensuring equitable vaccination rates across the nation.

---

[102] Analysis conducted by the Robert Graham Center. Publication forthcoming.

[103] Paterson P, Meurice F, Stanberry LR, Glismann S, Rosenthal SL, Larson HJ. Vaccine hesitancy and healthcare providers. Vaccine. 2016 Dec 20;34(52):6700-6706. doi: 10.1016/j.vaccine.2016.10.042. Epub 2016 Oct 31. PMID: 27810314.

1133 CONNECTICUT AVE., N.W., STE. 1100 | WASHINGTON, DC 20036-4305 | (800) 794-7481 | (202) 232-9033

The AAFP commends the committee's attention to ensure equity in the distribution of the COVID-19 vaccines. We strongly believe that incorporating primary care physicians and practices into vaccination plans, as well as enhancing coordination and communication with physicians, will advance our shared goal of ensuring equitable access to vaccines for all. We look forward to engaging with you further as you examine the COVID-19 response and develop legislative solutions. Should you have any questions, please contact John Aguilar, Legislative Affairs Manager at jaguilar@aafp.org.

Sincerely,

Gary L. LeRoy, MD, FAAFP Board Chair
American Academy of Family Physicians

Written Testimony of the American Psychological Association, by Arthur C. Evans, Jr, PhD, Chief Executive Officer and Executive Vice President American Psychological Association, Submitted to the Subcommittee on Health, of the Committee on Energy and Commerce, Hearing: on Road to Recovery: Ramping up Covid-19 Vaccines, Testing, and Medical Supply Chain, Wednesday, February 3, 2021-11:00am

The American Psychological Association (APA) is the leading scientific and professional organization representing psychology in the United States, with over 121,000 researchers, educators, clinicians, consultants, and students. APA's mission is to make a positive impact on critical societal issues through the application of psychological science and practice. APA applauds the Sub-committee for examining the nation's evolving response to COVID-19. As of February 2nd, there are over 26 million COVID-19 cases and over 440,000 deaths attributable to COVID-19.

Legislative Priorities in the 117th Congress

APA recommends that the Subcommittee do all that is within its jurisdiction to support the following congressional actions:

- Enact the $1.9 trillion COVID Relief Plan proposed by the Biden administration, which includes $4.5 billion for mental and behavioral health care.
- Support robust investments in national recovery efforts and sound public health measures through FY 2022 appropriations.
- Enact legislation to address the racial and ethnic disparities in access to mental health care exacerbated by the COVID-19 public health emergency.
- Enact legislation allowing Medicare to continue to pay for a broad range of mental and behavioral health services furnished through audio-only telephone after the public health emergency ends.

- Enact legislation requiring Employee Retirement Income Security Act (ERISA) health plans to cover tele-mental health, at parity, and through multiple access modalities to ensure equitable access to essential mental and behavioral health care.
- Ensure that the functions of the National Vaccine Program Office at the Centers for Disease Control and Prevention (CDC) are restored and elevated to include acceleration and coordination of genetic sequencing of SARS-CoV-2 variants across the United States.
- Promote wide availability, usability, and use of FDA approved at-home SARS-CoV-2 test kits to ensure that that those without access to technology are not disenfranchised from participation in data-reporting systems.
- Ensure that FDA device approval requires inclusion of representative Black, Indigenous, and People of Color (BIPOC) populations and eliminates bias in device evaluation so that potentially life-saving devices, such as pulse oximeters, can accurately detect oxygen saturation levels through skin at all levels of pigmentation.
- Enact legislation protecting pregnant women, especially Black women and other women of color, during the pandemic by promoting vaccinations in a culturally competent way and providing funding to support maternal health.
- Consider federal programs to incentivize vaccination following the leadership of programs initiated by private industry.
- Call for the inclusion of behavioral scientists, including those with knowledge and expertise in psychological science, on federal agency panels and task forces advising on COVID-19 response.
- Incentivize robust investment in rapid research examining disparities among BIPOC populations, including disparities in infections and deaths, adoption of attitudes regarding safety precautions, vaccine acceptance, and clinical trials participation.

The Pathway to Recovery

We ask the Subcommittee to consider the following key points in fulfilling its oversight role, and to direct the Department of Health and Human Services (HHS) and its counterparts among the states to implement policies accordingly.

Equity

Data show diverse racial and ethnic groups are being disproportionately affected by COVID-19. Inequities in the social determinants of health affecting these groups are interrelated and influence a wide range of health and quality-of-life outcomes and risks. The pandemic highlighted long-standing systemic health and social inequities that put many racial and ethnic minorities at increased risk of contracting the coronavirus and of becoming ill and dying from COVID-19.[1] While it is true that underlying comorbidities contribute to disparities in COVID-19 diagnoses and worse outcomes among racial and ethnic minorities, this analysis overlooks

[1] Centers for Disease Control and Prevention. (04, July 2020). Health Equity Considerations and Racial and Ethnic Minority Groups. https://www.cdc.gov/coronavirus/2019-ncov/community/health-equity/race-ethnicity.html#fn1.

the root causes of the heath gap: historic and contemporary racism and discrimination.[2] Social and economic inequality, discrimination, stigma, and marginalization are at the root of the differences we see among racial and ethnic minorities. Research documents that even when these groups can access care, a variety of factors – including providers' implicit biases and the inequitable distribution of health care resources – contribute to a lower overall quality of care and worse outcomes for these groups relative to white patients.[3,4] These factors, combined with higher risks for chronic health conditions, put racial and ethnic minorities at greater risk. The Subcommittee and HHS should work together to mitigate these observed inequities, engaging hard-hit groups while doing so. Psychological research demonstrates that communities that work together to address the needs of all members can flatten the curve faster than those fraught with division and distrust.[5]

Vaccines

APA believes that building a community of trust is necessary for successful vaccine engagement. The COVID-19 pandemic has magnified long embedded racial, ethnic, and socioeconomic inequities across the public health sector. Community leaders, grassroots activists, and health care providers need to be able to recognize barriers to vaccination acceptance, while at the same time maintaining respect for the factors underlying these barriers. Out of such understanding, it is hoped that culturally competent interventions and deployment strategies will promote positive individual health choices and civic responsibility.

Psychological science indicates that vaccine acceptance is an outcome behavior that can be influenced by a wide array of factors.[6] Mistrust concerning vaccines has become directed at public health systems, the media, and pharmaceutical companies. This mistrust derives in large part from prior histories of unethical practices by public health systems directed at BIPOC; religious traditions that prohibit routine vaccinations across the life cycle, vocal interest groups and movements known as anti-vaxxers, and the politicization of vaccine development in the past election cycle by both parties. These barriers contribute to vaccination hesitancy characterized by a delay in acceptance or refusal of vaccines despite availability.

Yet, we are guided by previous research on vaccine acceptance in society. The CDC concluded that only 47% of adults in the U.S. between July 2018 and May 2019 participated in flu immunization[7]. Social norms can also influence vaccine acceptance behaviors. In a study focused on flu vaccination among adults, decisions to vaccinate were influenced by their social circles' actions and the consequences of the flu without immunization.[8] Unfortunately, persistent gaps and racial disparities still exist in vaccine uptake. Preliminary CDC data shows

---

[2] Smedley BD. (2019). Multilevel interventions to undo the health consequences of racism: The need for comprehensive approaches. *Cultural Diversity and Ethnic Minority Psychology, 25*(1), 123-125.

[3] Williams, D. R., & Mohammed, S. A. (2013). Racism and health I: Pathways and scientific evidence. American Behavioral Scientist, 57, 1152-1173.

[4] Institute of Medicine. (2003). Unequal Treatment: Confronting Racial and Ethnic Healthcare Disparities. Smedley B.D., Stith, A.S., & Nelson, A.R. (Eds.). Washington, DC: National Academies Press.

[5] Miller PK, and Weller BE. (2019). Uncovering profiles of economic, social, and cultural capital to explore depression across racial groups. *Journal of Racial and Ethnic Health Disparities*, 6(6), 1167–1181. https://doi.org/10.1007/s40615-019-00618-4.

[6] Hornsey, M. J., & Fielding, K. S. (2017). Attitude roots and Jiu Jitsu persuasion: Understanding and overcoming the motivated rejection of science. American Psychologist, 72(5), 459–473. https://doi-org.libdata.lib.ua.edu/10.1037/a0040437.

[7] cdc.gov/flu/fluvaxview/coverage-1819estimates.htm.

[8] Ibid.

Black and Latinx people are getting vaccinated at much lower rates than white people, despite being disproportionately impacted.[9] Research has demonstrated that trust building borne of effective and respectful communication can influence communities and individuals to participate in immunization. APA, through the attached "Building Vaccine Confidence through Community Engagement" document, has developed information that can be used to facilitate transparent and thoughtful conversations between community leaders and individuals to foster informed decisions about vaccine behaviors.

APA would also like to highlight the recently released report by the National Institutes of Health (NIH) Behavioral and Social Sciences Research Coordinating Committee. The report "COVID-19 Vaccination Communication: Applying Behavioral and Social Science to Address Vaccine Hesitancy and Foster Vaccine Confidence," was developed in consultation with leading experts in social and behavioral sciences and public health. This important contribution to the discussion outlines evidence-informed communication strategies designed to support COVID-19 distribution. The report's recommendations provide useful information to public health officials, policymakers, and the public in responding to the unique challenges the U.S. currently faces in responding to the COVID-19 pandemic. We are including it as an attachment to this testimony [along with APA's Council of Representatives' statement on *Psychology's Understanding of the Challenges Related to the COVID-19 Global Pandemic in the United States*]. Further, novel collaborations between science agencies and the National Academies of Science, Engineering, and Medicine should be encouraged and expanded. The Societal Experts Action Network (SEAN) has provided essential rapid consultation to provide real-time advice on pandemic-related issues informed by the social, behavioral, and economic sciences. A permanent program like SEAN could have broad impact beyond this pandemic by applying behavioral and social science to a wide range of societal problems as did the Social and Behavioral Science Team in the Obama administration.

Ultimately, there remain several obstacles to an effective and equitable vaccine engagement and deployment apparatus in the U.S. The authoritative national vaccine distribution platform is underperforming. The Vaccine Administration Management System (VAMS) is supported by the CDC but has been plagued by a multitude of problems and abandoned for alternatives by most states.[10] An effective national distribution dashboard should contain up-to-date evidence on vaccine distribution, efficacy, and safety in addition to issues involving racial, ethnic, and socioeconomic status. Psychological science can be useful in the design of a vaccine distribution platform, helping to ensure usability and characterizing performance in decision-related terms.

The vaccine distribution system is also severely flawed. Greater resources were needed at the outset of this effort, and insufficient federal funding has led to an outsourcing of distribution. Unfortunately, this may contribute to access issues with communities most in need unable to receive the vaccines meant for them. Vaccine hesitancy further compounds information deficits, vaccine scheduling issues, and transportation barriers that shrink the number of available individuals. Comprehensive reviews of the psychological literature reveal that successful vaccination campaigns involve understanding how people think and feel about vaccination, the multitude of social processes leading to vaccination, and optimizing

---

[9] https://khn.org/news/article/black-americans-are-getting-vaccinated-at-lower-rates-than-white-americans/.
[10] https://www.technologyreview.com/2021/01/30/1017086/cdc-44-million-vaccine-data-vams-problems/.

approaches to changing vaccination behavior directly.[11] Promotional materials, informed by psychological science and empirical evidence, can mitigate these obstacles and increase vaccine uptake during this crucial period. There is limited data about the extent of viral shedding following vaccination, so science-based health promotion programs should be instituted to guide post-vaccination behavior to mitigate community spread of SARS-CoV-2, and research programs should be instituted to better understand it.

Testing and Contact Tracing

While APA applauds the efforts among states to distribute vaccines in a prompt and reasoned manner, at the same time we hope that this Subcommittee will seek transparency from states on their plans to distribute vaccines in an equitable manner. With the assistance of APA's "Equity Flattens the Curve" network, APA staff analyzed the state COVID-19 testing plans required under the Paycheck Protection Program and Health Care Enhancement Act. Overall, APA's analysis found that many of these plans rely on overly broad categories of these communities, such as "racial," "ethnic," and/or "minority" rather than specifying an outreach strategy that considers the unique characteristics of the state's Black, Latino/a/x, or other underrepresented communities. Additionally, although a significant portion of the deaths attributable to COVID-19 derive from congregate settings, many of these plans failed to identify a testing strategy for them. For example, while prison populations—including individuals who have been convicted of a crime, defendants awaiting trial, and prison staff—are infected at a five times higher rate and die at a significantly higher rate than the overall national rate, a plan for testing in "jails," "prisons," or "correctional" facilities only appears in 14% of state plans. These deficiencies call into serious question whether states have a strategy to address the vaccination needs of these communities and calls into question the role of Congress to ensure state plans uniformly address these inequities.

APA's findings, summarized in the letter circulated to the bipartisan leadership of the House Oversight and Appropriations Committees, also found certain inconsistencies in the systematic collection and reporting of data concerning the spread of COVID-19. Further, the CDC reports that only 20 states include race and ethnicity data on their vaccine dashboards, even though people of color make up a large segment of the health care workforce and the long-term care workforce whom many states identify as priority populations for vaccination.[12] We also understand that contact tracing data is not systematically collected or reported publicly, which misses an opportunity to obtain and disseminate data identifying the sources of infections. Using last summer's Sturgis motorcycle rally in South Dakota as an example, as of October 17th, 2020, 330 cases were linked to the rally. However, many experts believe this drastically understates the actual number of infections, which they estimate to be in the tens of thousands, and that the lack of interstate cooperation on contact tracing undermined any individual state's efforts to collect this information.

---

[11] Brewer, N. T., Chapman, G. B., Rothman, A. J., Leask, J., & Kempe, A. (2017). Increasing vaccination: putting psychological science into action. Psychological Science in the Public Interest, 18(3), 149-207.

[12] Painter EM, Ussery EN, Patel A, et al. Demographic Characteristics of Persons Vaccinated During the First Month of the COVID-19 Vaccination Program — United States, December 14, 2020–January 14, 2021. MMWR Morb Mortal Wkly Rep. ePub: 1 February 2021. DOI: http://dx.doi.org/10.15585/mmwr.mm7005e1external icon.

APA thanks the Subcommittee for taking its recommendations into consideration.

Statement from the American Society for Microbiology, in Response to the House Energy & Commerce, Subcommittee on Health, Hearing: "Road to Recovery: Ramping up COVID-19 Vaccines, Testing, and Medical Supply Chain," February 3, 2021

New, comprehensive and transparent testing approaches are needed to get the COVID-19 pandemic under control in the weeks and months ahead. The persistent testing challenges the American Society for Microbiology (ASM) and its members have been communicating to policymakers still remain. Left unaddressed, they will continue to hinder our efforts to maximize vaccine distribution, restart the economy, and begin getting back to everyday life.

ASM has been tracking shortages in our member laboratories and can contribute data to inform a more comprehensive strategy. The Clinical Microbiology Supply Shortage Collection (CMSSC) tool provides real time, geographically diverse information demonstrating that many labs lack the supplies necessary to maximize their testing capacity. In addition, the supply chain issues that have plagued COVID-19 testing are affecting other routine microbial l tests for a wide range of infectious diseases. For example, recent CMSSC data indicates 47.5% of labs surveyed have a shortage of supplies for detection of routine bacteria (including the bacteria causing strep throat, pneumonia, bronchitis and urinary tract infections).

ASM thanks Chairwoman Anna Eshoo, Ranking Member Brett Guthrie, and members of the House Energy & Commerce Subcommittee on Health for holding this hearing to discuss our nation's continued response to and efforts toward recovery from the COVID-19 pandemic. We appreciate the focus on key areas where we have faced ongoing challenges for months such as testing and supply chain failures. We encourage Congress to provide additional emergency funding in the coming weeks to ensure we can continue to respond and tackle new challenges such as emerging SARS-CoV-2 variants.

In addition to addressing supply shortages, ASM and its members have identified two other urgent priorities:

Increase Testing Capacity and Access

While the overall numbers of COVID-19 tests have increased since the beginning of the pandemic, so too has the need, and that will continue to grow. Disparities in testing access must be addressed given the disproportionate burden of COVID-19 borne by segments of our society.

A coordinated plan to test asymptomatic individuals will be a key part of reopening schools and offices, allowing travel, and rescheduling long-delayed medical procedures. As the massive effort to roll out vaccines takes hold, on-going testing for public health surveillance will also be a key element of that effort. For surveillance to be effective in light of new variants that have emerged, the testing capacity must be followed by boosting capacity to obtain samples for sequencing.

The Biden Administration's efforts to develop a national strategy for testing and or vaccines to respond to COVID-19 addresses a need that is long overdue, and which was highlighted in a the latest GAO bimonthly report. ASM concurs with the recommendations made in the GAO report, which include a call for a national, comprehensive and publicly-available testing strategy, and a warning about continued critical gaps in the medical supply chain.

Increase Transparency

In addition to ramping up production of these critical supplies, the federal government needs to be transparent about the state of testing supply distribution, something that has been lacking since the beginning of the pandemic. With line of sight to the entire testing ecosystem, we will not be able to effectively manage supplies and ensure that laboratories have certainty for planning purposes.

ASM reiterates our commitment to assisting the Committee, its members, the Congress, and the Biden Administration as the U.S. continues to respond to the COVID-19 pandemic.

The American Society for Microbiology is one of the largest professional societies dedicated to the life sciences and is composed of 30,000 scientists and health practitioners. ASM's mission is to promote and advance the microbial sciences.

ASM advances the microbial sciences through conferences, publications, certifications and educational opportunities. It enhances laboratory capacity around the globe through training and resources. It provides a network for scientists in academia, industry and clinical settings. Additionally, ASM promotes a deeper understanding of the microbial sciences to diverse audiences.

Statement of Steven C. Anderson, President and Chief Executive Officer, The National Association of Chain Drug Stores (NACDS), for United States House of Representatives, Committee on Energy and Commerce, Subcommittee on Health, on “Road to Recovery: Ramping up COVID-19 Vaccines, Testing and Medical Supply Chain,” February 3, 2021

The National Association of Chain Drug Stores (NACDS) appreciates the opportunity to offer a statement for the record for the Committee on Energy and Commerce’s hearing titled, *Road to Recovery: Ramping up COVID-19 Vaccines, Testing and Medical Supply Chain*. NACDS represents nearly 40,000 pharmacies (traditional drug stores, supermarkets and mass merchants with four or more pharmacies) who employ nearly 3 million individuals, including pharmacists, technicians, and nurse practitioners, among others.

Executive Summary

Retail pharmacies are playing a critical role in the nation’s COVID-19 response and recovery efforts, supporting public health at the federal, state and local levels, and serving the needs of their communities during this unprecedented time. Indeed, retail pharmacies offer trusted, accessible, and convenient healthcare access. Ninety percent of Americans live within 5 miles of a pharmacy. Importantly, retail pharmacies have ramped up healthcare operations to build, execute, and surge COVID-19 testing sites, flu vaccine clinics, and an array of COVID-19 vaccination models (in-store, mass stations, mobile clinics et al.). These efforts are supported by robust infrastructures from inventory management, storage and handling, online eligibility and appointment scheduling tools to detailed data reporting to states and the federal government. Of great interest to Congress is the tremendous value of ongoing public-private partnerships between public health and retail pharmacies.[13] The value of these partnerships in COVID-19 recovery efforts is extraordinary as public health leaders continue to leverage community pharmacies to execute national and local COVID-19 testing and pandemic immunization plans among other efforts. Retail pharmacies are deeply committed to engage in recovery efforts to re-open America by accelerating COVID vaccinations, expanding COVID testing, administering preventative vaccines, and promoting better community health. To this end:

- Retail pharmacies can safely, swiftly, and equitably *administer 100 million vaccine doses in 30 days* assuming available vaccine supply and patient demand;[14]
- Retail pharmacies employ highly trusted pharmacists to serve their communities, e.g., *72% of Hispanics and 66% of Black Americans trust pharmacists to provide COVID-19 vaccines; and*
- Retail pharmacies can expand COVID-19 testing capabilities to re-open local businesses and schools along with providing preventative vaccines to promote better community health.

To support the nation's recovery trajectory, NACDS strongly urges Congress to ensure that retail pharmacies continue their critical role in the pandemic recovery by taking the following actions:

Recommendation 1: Maintain important authorities established under the Public Readiness and Preparedness (PREP) Act declaration, which have expanded America's access to vaccination and testing services at local retail pharmacies.

Recommendation 2: Sustain the ability for retail pharmacies to continue to provide vaccination, testing, and other preventative services by helping to establish clear and permanent coverage and frictionless reimbursement pathways.

Recommendation 3: Ensure critical patient access to pharmacy services by expanding the Federal Pharmacy Partnership Program to serve Medicare and Medicaid populations.

---

[13] Serving the Greater Good. Public Health & Community Pharmacy Partnerships. Johns Hopkins Bloomberg School of Public Health Center for Health Security, October 2017, *available at* https://www.centerforhealthsecurity.org/our-work/pubs_archive/pubs-pdfs/2017/public-health-and-community-pharmacy-partnerships-report.pdf.

[14] This conservative modeling is extrapolated from CDC pandemic modeling from H1N1 under the Obama/Biden Administration. Adding one more vaccinator per store cuts the time to 15 days; and placing three vaccinators in each store, cuts the time by one-third.

Discussion

Accessible and Trusted Retail Pharmacies Are Boosting Critical Access to COVID-19 Vaccines and Testing in Communities across the Nation

With 60,000 locations across the nation, community pharmacies (chain and independents) are the most accessible healthcare destination, offering the public access to professional care, close to home, and during expanded hours. Pharmacies provide trustworthy access to care for so many Americans, sometimes as the only healthcare destination within walking or driving distance. In this way, pharmacies are seamlessly integrated into the neighborhoods they serve. In fact, 90% of Americans live within 5 miles of a community pharmacy. Longstanding evidence demonstrates that access to pharmacy care is a fundamental component to vital and sustainable communities.[15] For instance, high-risk Medicaid patients tend to be sicker and require more healthcare services but are less mobile than the general population as they rely more heavily on public transportation and have fewer options for traveling to providers that are not conveniently located. Studies have shown that Medicaid patients visit their pharmacies about 35 times a year,[16] and an analysis of 680,000 Medicare beneficiaries (including more than 65,000 Black and more than 16,500 Hispanic beneficiaries), showed pharmacy visits significantly outnumber primary care encounters (13 pharmacy visits to 7 primary care encounters per year), with the difference in rural areas being even more profound (14 compared to 5).[17]

Pharmacists are particularly valued by those in the greatest need, and their impact to those individuals is further amplified by a supporting pharmacy infrastructure, including pharmacy staff. As a result, pharmacies, pharmacists, and pharmacy staff have played a large role in the success of public health campaigns. This history of trust cannot be overstated and should be leveraged significantly to support efforts to streghten public confidence in the safety and efficacy of the COVID-19 vaccines. In fact, in a 2020 poll conducted by Morning Consult (commissioned by NACDS), three-in-four adults said they trust pharmacists to administer a COVID-19 vaccination, and nearly one-third of adults say they are more likely to get a COVID-19 vaccination if it is available at a pharmacy.[18]

---

[15] Dalton K, Byrne S., Role of the pharmacist in reducing healthcare costs: current insight, Integr Pharm Res Pract. 2017;6:37–46, Published 2017 Jan 25 doi:10.2147/IPRP.S108047, *available at* https://www.ncbi.nlm.nih.gov/pmc/articles/PMC5774321/; Newman TV, Hernandez I, et al., Optimizing the Role of Community Pharmacists in Managing the Health of Populations: Barriers, Facilitators, and Policy Recommendations, J Manag Care Spec Pharm. 2019 Sep;25(9):995-1000, doi: 10.18553/jmcp.2019.25.9.995, available at https://www.ncbi.nlm.nih.gov/pubmed/31456493. Armistead LT, Ferreri SP., Improving Value through Community Pharmacy Partnerships. Population Health Management, 2018, available at https://www.liebertpub.com/doi/abs/10.1089/pop.2018.0040?journalCode=pop; Milosavlijevic A, et al., Community pharmacist-led interventions and their impact on patients' medication adherence and other health outcomes: a systematic review, International Journal of Pharmacy Practice, June 2018, *available at* https://onlinelibrary.wiley.com/doi/full/10.1111/ijpp.12462.

[16] Gaskins RE. Innovating Medicaid: the North Carolina Experience, NC Med J. 2017, available at https://www.ncbi.nlm.nih.gov/pubmed/28115558.

[17] Berenbrok LA, Gabriel N, Coley KC, Hernandez I., Evaluation of Frequency of Encounters with Primary Care Physicians vs Visits to Community Pharmacies Among Medicare Beneficiaries, JAMA Netw Open. 2020;3(7):e209132, available at doi:10.1001/jamanetworkopen.2020.9132.

[18] This poll was conducted by Morning Consult and commissioned by the National Association of Chain Drug Stores. It was conducted between August 13-August 16, 2020 among a national sample of 2,200 Adults. The interviews were conducted online and the data were weighted to approximate a target sample of Adults based on gender, educational attainment, age, race, and region. Results from the full survey have a margin of error of plus or minus 2 percentage points.

What's more, the pharmacy infrastructure is contributing to vaccine confidence for populations at increased risk of COVID-19 and its complications. Indeed, 66% of Black Americans and 72% of Hispanics trust pharmacists to provide COVID-19 vaccines. Further, opinion research suggests that for many in these communities the pharmacy itself is preferred over mass vaccination sites, and that mass vaccination sites would do well to include local healthcare professionals such as trusted pharmacists.

Retail Pharmacies Play a Key Role In Expanding Access to COVID-19 Vaccines

After the 2009 H1N1 pandemic, the Obama/Biden Administration called on public health experts to model pandemic vaccination planning, and research the impact that community pharmacies may have on efficient and safe pandemic vaccinations.[19,20] This research found that when retail pharmacist vaccination capacity was included in pandemic modeling, the time to achieve 80% vaccination coverage nationally was reduced exponentially.[21] In extrapolating this modeling to today, America's retail pharmacies can readily administer *100 million vaccine doses in 30 days* with the requisite vaccine supply. This is a conservative estimate that leverages the nation's existing infrastructure of 40,000 retail pharmacies with one (1) vaccinating pharmacist per store to reach this goal. Of course, the solution could readily be ramped up even further as stores deploy more pharmacy vaccinators – pharmacists, pharmacy technicians, nurses, and others. Thus, one of the critical rate-limiting steps to the nation's recovery is the availability of supply of COVID-19 vaccines – not vaccinators. Retail pharmacies stand ready to meet the challenge and are prepared to do more to ensure that Americans are vaccinated proficiently, safely, and equitably.

Recent federal actions taken under the PREP Act[22,23,24] have leveraged pharmacies to provide enhanced public access to COVID-19 vaccines and other preventative vaccines by unleashing pharmacists, pharmacy technicians, and pharmacy interns from onerous state and federal barriers that had historically prohibited them from providing such services. These actions have helped foster the development of two federal COVID-19 vaccine programs aimed at meaningfully enhancing nationwide public access. The programs are: the Federal Pharmacy Partnership Program consisting of 21 chains and networks of independents, and the Federal – State Jurisdiction Transfer Program for Phase 1.[25] Further, pharmacies are also supporting their

---

[19] For example, influenza modeling found adding pharmacies saving $1.0–2.8 billion in direct costs and $4.1–99.8 billion in overall costs by averting 11.9–16.0 million influenza cases and 23,577–210,228 deaths.

[20] Pharmacist involvement in administering immunizations is correlated with higher rates of immunizations, compared to administration of vaccines by traditional providers, and the authority for pharmacists to immunize flourished following the important role of pharmacies in providing vaccines during the 2009 H1N1 pandemic. In 2018, community pharmacies delivered the influenza vaccination to an estimated 32% of adults. In the current flu season (2020-21), flu vaccinations administered at pharmacies are significantly higher.

[21] Schwerzmann J, Graitcer SB, Jester B, Krahl D, Jernigan D, Bridges CB, Miller J., Evaluating the Impact of Pharmacies on Pandemic Influenza Vaccine Administration. Disaster Med Public Health Prep, 2017 Oct, 11(5):587-593, *available at* https://www.ncbi.nlm.nih.gov/pubmed/28219461.

[22] U.S. Department of Health and Human Services, August 2020, *available at* HHS Expands Access to Childhood Vaccines during COVID-19 Pandemic.

[23] U.S. Department of Health and Human Services, October 2020, *available at* Advisory Opinion 20-03 on the Public Readiness and Emergency Preparedness Act and the Secretary's Declaration under the Act.

[24] U.S. Department of Health and Human Services. (December 2020). Fourth Amendment to the Declaration Under the Public Readiness and Emergency Preparedness Act for Medical Countermeasures Against COVID–19 and Republication of the Declaration, *available at* https://www.phe.gov/Preparedness/legal/prepact/Pages/4-PREP-Act.aspx.

[25] HHS Press Releases, *available at* https://www.hhs.gov/about/news/2020/10/16/trump-aministration-partners-cvs-walgreens-provide-covid-19-vaccine-protect-vulnerable-americans-long-term-care-facilities-nationwide.html and

state health department COVID-19 vaccine responses directly to help meet local needs. Pharmacies are committed to helping the nation at this critical point, gearing up to expeditiously expand equitable access to COVID-19 vaccinations as they become available and support the nation to eventually recover from the pandemic and emerge stronger than ever. We therefore urge Congress to continue to ensure retail pharmacies' considerable access, reach, expertise and capabilities are utilized to help in the critical national recovery effort.

Outside of Vaccinations, Retail Pharmacies Are Reshaping the Public Health Infrastructure to Provide Additional Services, Like COVID-19 Testing, to Patients on a Larger Scale

Federal actions taken under the PREP Act[26,27,28] have also accelerated the availability of new COVID-19 testing access at pharmacies and helped spearhead efforts to break down undue, longstanding barriers to pharmacy-based testing across many states. As a result, community pharmacies have been able to leverage their unique accessibility and clinical expertise to enhance COVID-19 testing capacity by offering thousands of additional access points to testing, as a key partner in the national public/private testing partnership.[29] In fact, between May and December 2020, more than 3,100 local pharmacy locations received new approval to provide point-of-care tests, which includes COVID-19 testing.[30]

The role of pharmacies in COVID-19 testing is critical considering the immense challenges in reaching the capacity needed to meet testing goals. One analysis indicates that "54% of US counties, including 68% of rural counties, do not have a single COVID-19 testing site. What's more, even among those counties with testing sites, 58% do not have sufficient capacity to meet recommended testing levels. Access to testing is even more limited by racial disparities: ZIP codes where the population is at least 75% white have an average of one testing site for every 14,5000 people, as compared to ZIP codes that are at least 75% people of color have an average of one testing site per 23,300 people."[31]

Pharmacies have been fortifying the national testing infrastructure by helping to fill gaps in testing access. Indeed, a myriad of evidence demonstrates the strong ability of pharmacy-

---

https://www.hhs.gov/about/news/2020/11/12/trump-administration-partners-chain-independent-community-pharmacies-increase-access-future-covid-19-vaccines.html.

26 Guidance for Licensed Pharmacists, COVID-19 Testing, and Immunity under the PREP Act, April 2020, *available at*https://www.phe.gov/Preparedness/legal/prepact/Documents/pharmacist-guidance-COVID19-PREP-Act.pdf.

27 HHS General Counsel's Office, Advisory Opinion, *available at* https://www.hhs.gov/guidance/sites/default/files/hhs-guidance-documents/advisory-opinion-20-02-hhs-ogc-prep-act.pdf.

28 U.S. Department of Health & Human Services Office of the Assistant Secretary for Health October 20, 2020 Guidance for PREP Act Coverage for Qualified Pharmacy Technicians and State-Authorized Pharmacy Interns for Childhood Vaccines, COVID-19 Vaccines, and COVID-19 Testing, *available at* https://www.hhs.gov/sites/default/files/prep-act-guidance.pdf.

29 Community Based Testing Sites for COVID-19, *available at* https://www.hhs.gov/coronavirus/community-based-testing-sites/index.html.

30 NASPA, *available at* https://naspa.us/resource/covid-19-testing/.

31 Health Affairs, Expand COVID-19 Testing with Real-Time Processing through Community Pharmacies, July 1, 2020, *available at* https://www.healthaffairs.org/do/10.1377/hblog20200629.567658/.

based testing models to improve patient access to care[32,33,34,35] and the nation observed this ability first-hand as pharmacies stepped up as quickly as they could to buttress testing capacity in neighborhood locations nationwide. Through these innovative models, pharmacies across the country have supported patients through the end-to-end testing process, thereby increasing access to care, even for rural and medically underserved populations.[36] Looking forward, retail pharmacies' key locations and capacity to serve communities will continue to prove beneficial for the public health infrastructure with the prevalence of asymptomatic transmission[37] and emergence of new variants of the virus.

Recommendations to Ensure Retail Pharmacies Have the Authorities to Continue to Help Fight This Pandemic and Strengthen the Public Health Infrastructure Moving Forward

Through their role in this pandemic, retail pharmacies will continue to strive to strengthen the public health infrastructure and bolster the response for future public health emergencies and national disasters. To help empower and sustain retail pharmacies in doing this work, NACDS urges Congress to immediately take the following actions.

Recommendation 1: Maintain Important Authorities Established under the PREP Act Declaration, Which Have Expanded Patient Access to Vaccination and Testing Services at Local Retail Pharmacies

As described above, authorities granted under the current PREP Act declaration have established a clear path for pharmacists, pharmacy technicians, and pharmacy interns to provide vaccination and testing services to patients, all within the backdrop of the current pandemic. Yet, the PREP Act authorities remain tenuous as they are set to expire at the conclusion of the public health emergency. The ability for qualified pharmacy professionals to provide much-needed patient care services, including screening and testing, and recommended vaccines, at trusted, local pharmacy locations should not be contingent on a public health crisis. Indeed, policymakers should maintain the ability for these services to continue to be provided at pharmacies at any time because the services hold high value to improve the health of the nation, no matter the presence of an emergency. As a matter of good public policy, NACDS urges policymakers to consider statutory and regulatory mechanisms to preserve access to testing and vaccination services at pharmacies permanently, to strengthen the nation's healthcare

---

[32] San-Juan-Rodriguez A, Newman TV, Hernandez I, et al., Impact of community pharmacist-provided preventive services on clinical, utilization, and economic outcomes: An umbrella review, Preventive Medicine, 2018, *available at* https://www.ncbi.nlm.nih.gov/pubmed/30145351.

[33] Isho N, et al., Pharmacist-initiated hepatitis C virus screening in a community pharmacy to increase awareness and link to care at the medical center,Journal of the American Pharmacists Association, March 2017, *available at https:*//www.japha.org/article/S1544-3191(17)30136-X/pdf.

[34] Darin KM, et al., Pharmacist-provided rapid HIV testing in two community pharmacies, Journal of the American Pharmacists Association, Feb. 2015, *available at* https://www.japha.org/article/S1544-3191(15)30015-7/pdf.

[35] Buss V.H., Naunton M. Analytical quality and effectiveness of point of care testing in community pharmacies: A systematic literature review, Res. Soc. Adm. Pharm, 2019.

[36] Broughel J, Yatsyshina Y., Relax Pharmacy Regulations to help with COVID-19 Testing and Treatment, March 2020, *available at* https://www.mercatus.org/publications/covid-19-policy-brief-series/relax-pharmacy-regulations-help-covid-19-testing-and.

[37] https://www.nejm.org/doi/full/10.1056/NEJMoa2029717.

infrastructure and capacity, and in preparation for any future public health emergencies or disasters.

Recommendation 2: Sustain the Ability for Retail Pharmacies to Continue to Provide Vaccination, Testing, and Relevant Preventative Services by Establishing Clear Coverage and Reimbursement Pathways

Although pharmacies are providing accessibility to vaccination and testing services, restrictive coverage and billing requirements at the state and federal levels have acted as a barrier for pharmacies to be compensated for such services in a streamlined way, which hinders scalability, sustainability, and further healthcare access expansion for the public. For example, pharmacies are unable to bill Medicare Part B for testing-related services (e.g., specimen collection) conducted by a pharmacist unless the collection is done “incident to” a physician. Such a barrier is nonsensical as pharmacists are already autonomously performing specimen collection under current PREP Act declaration authorities. Yet, these billing barriers go beyond just COVID-19 testing. Pharmacies should be reimbursed for the care provided and services performed by a pharmacist at their stores, whether it is related to vaccinations, testing, or other preventative services. Pharmacies need reliable, sustainable infrastructure to more comprehensively provide consistent public access to much needed preventive care. NACDS urges policymakers to remove barriers that undermine the ability for pharmacies to expand access to clinical care and to be reimbursed for such services.

Recommendation 3: Ensure Critical Patient Access to Pharmacy Services by Expanding the Federal Pharmacy Partnership Program to Serve Medicare and Medicaid Populations

Grant funding from early in the pandemic has provided the Biden Administration with the ability to continue the Federal Pharmacy Partnership Program. And the Administration has indicated that it will “turn on” this Program shortly to accelerate the stagnant vaccination campaign. NACDS thanks and applauds the Biden Administration for supporting this program as a key part of the broader COVID vaccination strategy. Pharmacies are honored to be part of this unified and coordinated response program, with the goal of extending access to COVID-19 vaccines from coast to coast. NACDS urges the Congress to explore how the program can be expanded to reach the vulnerable Medicaid and Medicare populations by aligning federal funding for such programs with the ability for pharmacists to provide services at pharmacies in order to end this pandemic in the short-term and provide better access to much needed preventive care in the long-term to strengthen and improve the health and wellness of the nation.

Conclusion

NACDS thanks the committee for this opportunity to offer our comments and recommendations on how retail pharmacy is providing and can continue to provide contributions to the nation’s COVID-19 response and recovery strategy and beyond.

Statement for the Record, American Nurses Association, Road to Recovery: Ramping up COVID-19 Vaccines, Testing, and Medical Supply Chain, House of Representatives, Committee on Energy and Commerce, Subcommittee on Health, February 3, 2021

The American Nurses Association (ANA) commends the House Energy and Commerce Subcommittee on Health for convening this hearing on the Road to Recovery: Ramping up COVID-19 Vaccines, Testing, and Medical Supply Chain, and thanks you for the opportunity to submit this statement for the record.

ANA is the premier organization representing the interests of the nation's 4.2 million registered nurses (RNs), through its state and constituent member associations, organizational affiliates, and individual members. ANA members also include the four advanced practice registered nurse roles (APRNs); nurse practitioners (NPs), clinical nurse specialists (CNSs), certified nurse-midwives (CNMs) and certified registered nurse anesthetists (CRNAs). ANA is dedicated to partnering with health care consumers to improve practices, policies, delivery models, outcomes, and access across the health care continuum.

Medical Supply Chain

Last year, ANA President Dr. Ernest Grant, PhD, RN, FAAN, testified before the Senate Finance Committee on a hearing entitled "Part 2: Protecting the Reliability of the U.S. Medical Supply Chain During the COVID-19 Pandemic." Dr. Grant provided the Committee with detailed recommendations ANA had submitted to former Health, Education, Labor, and Pensions (HELP) Committee Chairman Lamar Alexander and the HELP Committee in response to a white paper request. Below are some of the highlights of ANA's recommendations.

- To ensure health care providers are never again faced with a personal protective equipment (PPE) shortage, Congress should request an annual report on the state of the Strategic National Stockpile (SNS) with respect to PPE, vaccines, medicines, and other supplies. The report must include when items are expiring and what items need to be replaced. When items are approaching expiration, they should be offered to underserved medical facilities such as federally qualified health centers, rural hospitals, and clinics based on need.
- Health care facilities should be required to report monthly on their levels of these supplies so the agency in charge has up-to-date information on where shortages may be most acute in the early stages of an emergency. A formulary should be developed by the National Academy of Sciences, Engineering, and Medicine on what levels of PPE, vaccines, and other supplies health care facilities should have in their own stockpiles. In addition, manufacturers of these items should also be reporting on production and capabilities.
- The federal government must take appropriate steps to plan coordination efforts. Many states do not have the resources or expertise to carry out preparations or coordination without federal assistance. Hospitals and facilities with more capital will likely benefit

while rural and underserved areas will suffer. We need to ensure states are not pitted against each other when it comes to resources.

- The federal government needs to do more to incentivize and prioritize the manufacturing of PPE, medications, and other supplies in the United States, even if that means carrying out production itself. We cannot allow our citizens to be put at a health risk because businesses view manufacturing elsewhere better for their bottom line.

Vaccines

Vaccines are critical to the control and prevention of infectious disease transmission. This has been underscored as development and administration of COVID-19 vaccines is recognized as a critical component of addressing the ongoing pandemic. ANA has established key principles to guide nurses and other health care professionals' consideration for COVID-19 vaccines[38]. The nursing workforce not only plays a vital role in educating the public but is integral to safe and effective administration of COVID-19 vaccines to other health care professionals and patients. In a letter sent on January 27, 2021 to Congressional Leadership, ANA requests continued federal investment in vaccine development, distribution, and administration.

Vaccine Equity

Ensuring the equitable distribution of COVID-19 vaccines will be vital to ending the pandemic and building public confidence in vaccines for the future. According to a recent Kaiser Family Foundation study of early data from states collecting racial and ethnic demographic data, there is a disconnect between those who have received vaccinations and the makeup of those states' populations. The Kaiser report found that to date, vaccination patterns by race and ethnicity appear to be at odds with who the virus has affected the most.[39] Unfortunately, this data is not yet being collected by a majority of states. It will be necessary for states and localities to provide a clearer picture to inform efforts to mitigate the disproportionate impact of COVID-19 on people of color. Further, data is critical to understanding racial equity concerns in vaccination distribution plans and identifying any disparities that can be addressed through policies, changes in strategy, and education.

Conclusion

Thank you for giving nurses the opportunity to provide input on the need to ramp up COVID-19 vaccines, testing, and the medical supply chain. ANA stands ready to work with the Energy and Commerce Committee to find sustainable solutions regarding these vital mechanisms for getting the pandemic under control and getting our nation on the road to recovery. If you have questions, please contact Ingrida Lusis, Vice President of Policy and Government Affairs, at (301) 628-5081 or Ingrid.Lusis@ana.org.

[38] https://www.nursingworld.org/practice-policy/work-environment/health-safety/disaster-preparedness/coronavirus/what-you-need-to-know/covid-19-vaccines/.

[39] https://www.kff.org/policy-watch/early-state-vaccination-data-raise-warning-flags-racial-equity/.

January 27, 2021
Docket No. CDC-2021-0002
c/o Attn: January 25, 2021 ACIP Meeting
Centers for Disease Control and Prevention
Re: COVID-19 Vaccine Prioritization, Distribution and Administration; CDC-2021-0002
To Whom It May Concern:

On behalf of the food industry and the 12,000 supermarket pharmacies operated by our member companies, we at FMI – the Food Industry Association thank the Advisory Committee on Immunization Practices (ACIP) for its ongoing work to provide guidance to the Centers for Disease Control and Prevention (CDC) and the Department of Health and Human Services regarding the development, distribution and use of COVID-19 vaccines. The importance of the COVID-19 vaccine and a convenient, efficient, and safe delivery of the vaccine cannot be overstated.

As the food industry association, FMI works with and on behalf of the entire industry – from retailers who sell to consumers, to producers who supply the food and other products sold in grocery venues, as well as a variety of related critical services, including supermarket pharmacies – to advance safer and more efficient consumer supply chains for both food and pharmaceuticals. In total, FMI member companies operate roughly 33,000 grocery stores and 12,000 pharmacies, ultimately touching the lives of more than 100 million U.S. households on a weekly basis and representing an industry with nearly 6 million employees. Importantly, as part of an industry deemed essential to the nation's COVID-19 response, FMI's members have been and continue to be a critical component of ensuring the availability of food, pharmacy and health care services in communities across this nation, beginning in the initial days of the pandemic. www.fmi.org

FMI appreciates the opportunity to offer the following suggestions and feedback:

1. FMI strongly supports the ACIP's recommendations to prioritize health care personnel, including pharmacists, in the initial phase of COVID-19 vaccine allocation as well as food and agriculture industry essential workers in Phase 1b.
   However, to achieve consistent and equitable COVID-19 vaccination, the ACIP and CDC should strongly encourage states and immunization jurisdictions to adhere to the federal COVID-19 vaccine allocation recommendations. We appreciate the rigorous and scientific approach applied to the development of the federal guidelines, and state variation or divergence from those guidelines dilutes that work. While local application of national guidance may be appropriate, the CDC-ACIP should strongly encourage jurisdictions receiving allocations of COVID-19 vaccine to use and follow national prioritization guidance.
   As a result of the uneven experience across state lines, with many states reworking their vaccine prioritization frameworks in the face of federal guidance, food industry essential workers – from manufacturing/production employees working in close proximity and grocery workers who have a higher contact rate with the public, to certain transportation workers and food safety auditors who ensure food, beverages, and packaged goods are safe for consumer consumption – are struggling to access vaccinations. Our industry's essential workforce has gone above and beyond in demonstrating their continued resilience, but to keep supply chains operating and

Americans nourished until all can receive the vaccine, it is imperative these workers receive vaccinations. Furthermore, as supermarket pharmacies across the country are stepping up their support of national and state plans to provide vaccinations, modifications to federal prioritization guidelines across states are impeding efficiency in vaccine delivery, causing confusion and undermining the national COVID-19 vaccination effort.

With that in mind, FMI urges the Biden Administration to designate a Federal Coronavirus Vaccine Coordinator in each state and jurisdiction to coordinate at all levels of government and to help ensure the rapid, efficient deployment of vaccines among priority populations. Separately, to the extent that jurisdictions have already made revisions to federal COVID-19 vaccine allocation guidance, FMI respectfully requests that the CDC compile and store all such state guidance so the information is easily accessible by all stakeholders.

2. FMI member companies operate roughly 12,000 supermarket pharmacies nationwide, with pharmacists providing in-depth patient counseling and comprehensive immunization services. Supermarket pharmacies administered roughly 25% of the nation's influenza vaccinations last year, and now they stand ready to play an expanded role in increasing access to COVID-19 vaccinations. A number of FMI pharmacy members have been providing COVID-19 vaccinations via the federal pharmacy partnerships and a majority of our pharmacy members are enrolled as providers in the states where they operate. All these companies have pharmacists prepared to administer COVID-19 vaccinations in their stores and many have pharmacists available and ready to provide vaccinations off-site as well. Additionally, many of our members are utilizing their parking lots and outdoor tent-covered areas as COVID-19 vaccination clinics capable of administering nearly 1,000 shots per day. However, our members are not yet receiving vaccine supplies equal to their capacity.

   Serving as knowledgeable and trusted wellness partners within their communities, supermarket pharmacies are essential to any successful COVID-19 vaccination plan. Consumers' ability to receive a COVID-19 vaccination at the same location where they already purchase food and other essential items is not only a convenience, it also is safer and reduces the risk of exposure in the midst of a pandemic. In addition to having large footprints and parking lots that allow social distancing, many FMI pharmacy members have additional/extended store hours to provide times for seniors and immunocompromised patients to receive vaccinations. Also, being such trusted health care providers, supermarket pharmacists could play a key role in addressing patient concerns and highlighting the importance of being vaccinated. FMI members are utilizing the CDC toolkits for these communications.

3. In order for vaccine providers and healthcare professionals to fully utilize the limited supply of vaccines they receive, they must have visibility into the expected availability of future doses. To expedite vaccinations, FMI respectfully requests the federal government share with states and providers, the anticipated lot release dates for vaccine doses.

   Mass administration of vaccines requires significant staff resources and logistics coordination. Currently, FMI pharmacy members lack transparency into the number of doses that will be available and the timing on their availability. This makes planning and communicating with patients about vaccination scheduling very difficult.

Additionally, both the Pfizer and Moderna vaccines require the administration of two doses for the vaccines to be fully effective in protecting individuals from COVID-19. In order for providers to administer an initial dose of these vaccines, they must have confidence that sufficient supply will be available to administer the second dose, based on the timing indicated in the Food and Drug Administration's emergency use authorizations. Sharing anticipated lot release dates from manufacturers would give providers more clarity as they plan mass administration efforts and greater confidence that second doses will be available when their patients need them.

Again, FMI thanks the ACIP for the opportunity to provide input on this critically important initiative.

Sincerely, Leslie G. Sarasin
President and CEO

Demographic Characteristics of Persons Vaccinated During the First Month of the COVID-19 Vaccination Program — United States, December 14, 2020–January 14, 2021

Elizabeth M. Painter, Emily N. Ussery, Anita Patel, Michelle M. Hughes, Elizabeth R. Zell, Danielle L. Moulia, Lynn Gibbs Scharf, Michael Lynch, Matthew D. Ritchey, Robin L. Toblin, Bhavini Patel Murthy, LaTreace Q. Harris, Annemarie Wasley, Dale A. Rose, Amanda Cohn and Nancy E. Messonnier

In December 2020, two COVID-19 vaccines (Pfizer-BioNTech and Moderna) were authorized for emergency use in the United States for the prevention of coronavirus disease 2019 (COVID-19).[40] Because of limited initial vaccine supply, the Advisory Committee on Immunization Practices (ACIP) prioritized vaccination of health care personnel[41] and residents and staff members of long-term care facilities (LTCF) during the first phase of the U.S. COVID-19 vaccination program [1]. Both vaccines require 2 doses to complete the series. Data on vaccines administered during December 14, 2020–January 14, 2021, and reported to CDC by January 26, 2021, were analyzed to describe demographic characteristics, including sex, age, and race/ethnicity, of persons who received ≥1 dose of COVID-19 vaccine (i.e., initiated vaccination). During this period, 12,928,749 persons in the United States in 64 jurisdictions and five federal entities[42] initiated COVID-19 vaccination. Data on sex were reported for 97.0%, age for 99.9%, and race/ethnicity for 51.9% of vaccine recipients. Among persons who received the first vaccine dose and had reported demographic data, 63.0% were women, 55.0% were aged ≥50 years, and 60.4% were non-Hispanic White (White). More complete reporting

[40] https://www.cdc.gov/vaccines/covid-19/eua/index.html.

[41] Health care personnel include persons working in settings such as hospitals, long-term care facilities, outpatient clinics, public health clinics, emergency medical services, and pharmacies.

[42] Sixty-four jurisdictions include 50 states, the District of Columbia, five cities (Chicago, Philadelphia, San Antonio, Houston, and New York City), and eight territories or freely associated states; five federal entities also received a direct allocation of vaccine (Federal Bureau of Prisons, U.S. Department of Defense, U.S. Department of State, Indian Health Services, and Veterans Health Administration) and report administration data to CDC.

of race and ethnicity data at the provider and jurisdictional levels is critical to ensure rapid detection of and response to potential disparities in COVID-19 vaccination. As the U.S. COVID-19 vaccination program expands, public health officials should ensure that vaccine is administered efficiently and equitably within each successive vaccination priority category, especially among those at highest risk for infection and severe adverse health outcomes, many of whom are non-Hispanic Black (Black), non-Hispanic American Indian/Alaska Native (AI/AN), and Hispanic persons [2, 3].

Data on COVID-19 vaccine doses administered in the United States are collected by vaccination providers and reported to CDC through multiple sources, including jurisdictions, pharmacies, and federal entities, who use various reporting methods including immunization information systems,[43] Vaccine Administration Management System,[44] and direct data submission. Data on first vaccine doses administered during December 14, 2020–January 14, 2021, and reported to CDC by January 26, 2021, were analyzed to describe demographic characteristics, including sex, age, and race/ethnicity among persons who received ≥1 dose of COVID-19 vaccine. Age was calculated based on date or year of birth and date of vaccine administration and was categorized as <18, 18–29, 30–39, 40–49, 50–64, 65–74, or ≥75 years. Race and ethnicity were combined and categorized as Hispanic/Latino, White, Black, non-Hispanic Asian (Asian), AI/AN, non-Hispanic Native Hawaiian or other Pacific Islander (NH/PI), non-Hispanic multiple/other,[45] or unknown (if either race or ethnicity was reported as unknown[46] or not reported because of jurisdictional policy or law).[47] Analyses were conducted using SAS (version 9.4; SAS Institute).

During the first month of the U.S. COVID-19 vaccination program, 12,928,749 persons received at least 1 dose of COVID-19 vaccine (Figure). Vaccination was initiated by persons in all 64 jurisdictions and five federal entities reporting data to CDC. Among 12,537,841 (97.0%) vaccine recipients with reported sex, 63.0% were women and 37.0% were men (Table). Among 12,924,116 (99.9%) persons whose age was known, 55.0% were aged ≥50 years, 16.8% were aged 40–49 years, and 28.2.% were aged 18–39 years. Among 6,706,697 (51.9%) persons whose race/ ethnicity was known, 60.4% were White and 39.6% represented racial and ethnic minorities, including 14.4% categorized as multiple or other race/ethnicity, 11.5% Hispanic/Latino, 6.0% Asian, 5.4% Black, 2.0% AI/AN, and 0.3% NH/PI. Race/ethnicity was unknown or not reported for 6,222,052 (48.1%) persons initiating vaccination. Across jurisdictions and federal entities, the percentage of persons initiating vaccination with race/ethnicity that was unknown or not reported ranged from 0.2% to 100% (median = 39.6%; interquartile range = 25.3%–66.1%).

---

[43] https://www.cdc.gov/vaccines/programs/iis/index.html.

[44] https://www.cdc.gov/vaccines/covid-19/reporting/vams/program-information.html.

[45] Represents persons identified as being non-Hispanic and having multiple race categories selected or non-Hispanic and "other race" selected.

[46] If ethnicity was identified as Hispanic and race was unknown, the person was classified as Hispanic.

[47] Race/ethnicity was not reported because of jurisdictional policy or law or was unknown for all persons initiating vaccination in six jurisdictions.

Discussion

During the first month of the U.S. COVID-19 vaccination program, 12,928,749 persons received ≥1 dose of COVID-19 vaccine, representing approximately 4% of the total U.S. population and 5% of the U.S. population aged ≥16 years.[48] If vaccination was only provided to persons in the Phase 1a priority groups (health care personnel and LTCF residents), coverage among the 24 million persons included in these groups might have been as high as 50% (*1*). However, this is likely an overestimate because persons outside of the 1a priority group were vaccinated because of variation in implementation of national guidance at the jurisdictional and local levels (e.g., Florida and Texas expanded vaccination to all persons aged ≥65 years).[49]

Among persons who received the first vaccine dose and had available data for the respective demographic characteristic variable, 63.0% were women, 55.0% were aged ≥50 years, and 60.4% were White, which likely reflects the demographic characteristics of the persons (health care personnel and LTCF residents) recommended to be vaccinated in the Phase 1a priority group [4, 5]. Data from the 2019 American Community Survey show that 60% of health care workers were White, 16% were Black, 13% were Hispanic, and 7% were Asian; however, race and ethnicity varied widely by occupation and setting [6]. Women also account for approximately three fourths of persons employed in the health care industry [7]. In addition, the 2015–2016 National Study of Long-Term Care Providers found that 65% of nursing home residents were women, 75% were White, 14% were Black, and 5% were Hispanic [8].

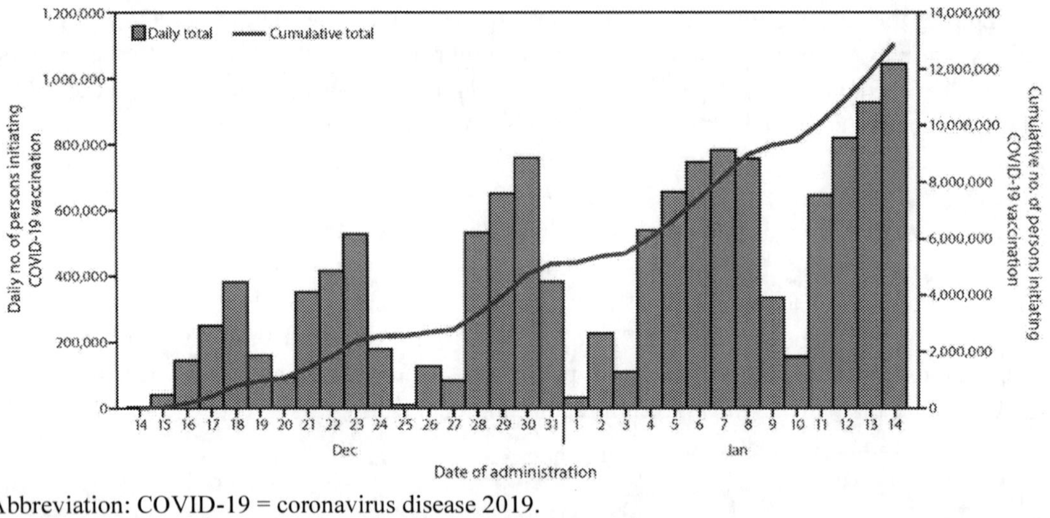

Abbreviation: COVID-19 = coronavirus disease 2019.

* Vaccines administered December 14, 2020–January 14, 2021, and reported to CDC by January 26, 2021.

Figure. Number of persons initiating COVID-19 vaccination, by date of vaccine administration (N = 12,928,749) — United States, December 14, 2020–January 14, 2021.[*]

[48] Population denominator data from U.S. Census Bureau 2019 American Community Survey 1-year population estimates. 2018 population estimates are used for American Samoa, Federated States of Micronesia, Guam, Marshall Islands, Northern Mariana Islands, Palau, and U.S. Virgin Islands.

[49] http://www.floridahealth.gov/newsroom/2020/12/122920-2046-covid-vac.pr.html; https://dshs.texas.gov/news/releases/2020/20201221.aspx.

Table. Demographic characteristics of persons initiating COVID-19 vaccination — United States, December 14, 2020–January 14, 2021*

Characteristic (no. [%] with available information)	No. (%)†
Overall	12,928,749 (100.0)
Sex (12,537,841 [97.0])	
Male	4,639,073 (37.0)
Female	7,898,768 (63.0)
Age group,§ yrs (12,924,116 [99.9])	
<18	4,837 (<0.1)
18–29	1,433,086 (11.1)
30–39	2,207,222 (17.1)
40–49	2,175,305 (16.8)
50–64	3,350,610 (25.9)
65–74	1,732,522 (13.4)
≥75	2,020,534 (15.6)
Race/Ethnicity¶ (6,706,697 [51.9])	
White, non-Hispanic	4,047,795 (60.4)
Hispanic/Latino	773,858 (11.5)
Black, non-Hispanic	359,934 (5.4)
Asian, non-Hispanic	405,227 (6.0)
AI/AN, non-Hispanic	134,127 (2.0)
NH/PI, non-Hispanic	20,585 (0.3)
Multiple/Other, non-Hispanic**	965,171 (14.4)

Abbreviations: AI/AN = American Indian/Alaska Native; COVID-19 = coronavirus disease 2019; NH/PI = Native Hawaiian or Other Pacific Islander.

* Vaccines administered December 14, 2020–January 14, 2021, and reported to CDC by January 26, 2021.

† Percentages were calculated among persons with available demographic characteristics.

§ Pfizer-BioNTech COVID-19 vaccine is authorized for persons aged ≥16 years, and Moderna COVID-19 vaccine is authorized for persons aged ≥18 years under Food and Drug Administration Emergency Use Authorizations. Ages that were outside of the expected range (<16 years or >120 years) were treated as unknown, which represented <0.1% of persons initiating vaccination.

¶ Race/ethnicity was not reported or was unknown for all persons initiating vaccination in six jurisdictions. The six jurisdictions not reporting race/ethnicity have a total population of approximately 18.9 million, which represents nearly 6% of the overall U.S. population.

** Represents persons identified as being non-Hispanic and having multiple race categories selected or being non-Hispanic and having "other race" selected.

Summary

What is already known about this topic?

In December 2020, two COVID-19 vaccines were authorized for emergency use in the United States. The first groups prioritized for vaccination included health care personnel and long-term care facility residents.

What is added by this report?

During the first month of the U.S. COVID-19 vaccination program, approximately 13,000,000 persons received ≥1 dose of vaccine. Among persons with demographic data, 63.0% were women, 55.0% were aged ≥50 years, and 60.4% were non-Hispanic White.

What are the implications for public health practice?

As the vaccination program expands, it is critical to ensure efficient and equitable administration to persons in each successive vaccine priority category, especially those at highest risk for infection and severe health outcomes.

Interpretation of data from the analysis of COVID-19 vaccination initiation is limited by the high percentage of records with unknown or missing race/ethnicity information and the unknown proportions of priority groups (health care personnel versus LTCF residents) among early vaccine recipients. Differences in how race and ethnicity data are collected and categorized, for example 14.4% of persons initiating vaccination reported as multiple or other race/ethnicity, also make comparisons difficult. The percentage of persons initiating vaccination who were Black appears lower relative to the percentage of persons who are Black among health care personnel and LTCF residents. Overall, 39.6% of persons who were vaccinated represented racial and ethnic minorities. Because persons who are Black, AI/AN, or Hispanic have been found to have more severe outcomes from COVID-19 than persons who are White, careful monitoring of vaccination by race/ ethnicity is critical [2, 9].

The findings in this report are subject to at least three limitations. First, race/ethnicity was unknown for approximately one half of the population who initiated vaccination during the first month of the COVID-19 vaccination program in the United States. In addition, the proportion of persons with unknown race/ethnicity varied across jurisdictions, including six jurisdictions that reported no race/ethnicity data.[50] In addition, a high proportion of persons receiving vaccination were categorized as non-Hispanic, multiple or other races, whereas the population estimates from the 2019 American Community Survey[51] 1-year population were 2.8% non-Hispanic, multiple or other races. Thus, the findings presented in this study might not be generalizable to all persons initiating COVID-19 vaccination in the United States. The large proportion of missing data also might result in biased estimates of race/ethnicity, particularly if some groups are more likely than others to have race/ethnicity reported as unknown. Second, vaccine administration data reported to CDC include limited data elements and did not allow for stratification by the prioritized populations (health care personnel and LTCF residents) in the initial phase of the vaccination campaign. Therefore, it was not possible to directly compare the observed demographic patterns among persons initiating vaccination to demographic characteristics of prioritized populations. Finally, implementation of the ACIP recommendations, including subprioritization, varied by jurisdiction, with some jurisdictions changing and expanding their priority populations during the first month of the vaccination program.

Although these data reflect characteristics of persons initiating vaccination during the initial phase of the U.S. COVID-19 vaccination program and have several limitations, the findings underscore the need for more complete reporting of race and ethnicity data at the provider and jurisdictional levels to ensure rapid detection of and response to potential disparities in COVID-19 vaccine administration. Jurisdictions should monitor the demographic characteristics of vaccinated persons to identify emerging disparities. In addition, as vaccination expands to include additional groups, monitoring coverage by the Social Vulnerability Index, which uses U.S. Census Bureau variables to identify communities that might need support, will be useful to ensure equity and to identify communities where focused immunization efforts might be required.[52] CDC is working with jurisdictions to use these types of analyses to help direct efforts to bring vaccines to their communities and ensure that no

[50] The six jurisdictions not reporting race/ethnicity have a total population of approximately 18.9 million, which represents nearly 6% of the overall U.S. population.

[51] https://data.census.gov/cedsci/table?q=hispanic&tid=ACSDP1Y2019. DP05&hidePreview=false.

[52] The Social Vulnerability Index uses U.S. Census variables to help local officials identify communities that might need support as the result of a disaster. https://www.atsdr.cdc.gov/placeandhealth/svi/index.html.

persons are left behind. These data from the first month of the COVID-19 vaccination program indicate substantial progress in administration of the COVID-19 vaccine. To increase coverage among persons in Phase 1a, as vaccination expands into additional populations, unvaccinated health care personnel and LTCF residents should continue to be offered COVID-19 vaccine. Equitable and sustainable COVID-19 vaccine administration in all populations requires focus on groups with lower vaccine receipt who might face challenges with access or vaccine hesitancy.

Acknowledgments

COVID-19 Vaccine Task Force; U.S. Department of Defense; immunization program managers; immunization information system managers; other staff members of the immunization programs in the 64 jurisdictions and five federal entities.

References

[1] Dooling K, McClung N, Chamberland M, et al. The Advisory Committee on Immunization Practices' interim recommendation for allocating initial supplies of COVID-19 vaccine—United States, 2020. *MMWR Morb Mortal Wkly Rep* 2020;69:1857–9. PMID:33301429 https://doi. org/10.15585/ mmwr.mm6949e1.

[2] Azar KMJ, Shen Z, Romanelli RJ, et al. Disparities in outcomes among COVID-19 patients in a large healthcare system in California. *Health Aff* (Millwood) 2020;39:1253–62. PMID:32437224 https://doi. org/10.1377/hlthaff.2020.00598.

[3] McClung N, Chamberland M, Kinlaw K, et al. The Advisory Committee on Immunization Practices' ethical principles for allocating initial supplies of COVID-19 vaccine—United States, 2020. *MMWR Morb Mortal Wkly Rep* 2020;69:1782–6. PMID:33237895 https://doi.org/10.15585/mmwr.mm6947e3.

[4] Health Resources and Services Administration, National Center for Health Workforce Analysis. Sex, race, and ethnic diversity of U.S. Health occupations (2011–2015). Rockville, MD: *US Department of Health and Human Services, Health Resources and Services Administration*; 2017. https://bhw.hrsa.gov/sites/default/files/bureau-health-workforce/data-research/diversity-us-health-occupations.pdf.

[5] Caffrey C, Sengupta M, Park-Lee E, et al. Residents living in residential care facilities: United States, 2010. *NCHS data brief*, no. 91. Hyattsville, MD: US Department of Health and Human Services, CDC, National Center for Health Statistics; 2012. https://www.cdc.gov/nchs/data/ databriefs/db91.pdf.

[6] Artiga S, Rae M, Pham O, Hamel L, Munana C. *COVID-19 risks and impact among health care workers by race/ethnicity*. Oakland, CA: Kaiser Family Foundation; 2020. https://www.kff.org/racial-equity-and-health-policy/ issue-brief/covid-19-risks-impacts-health-care-workers-race-ethnicity/.

[7] Bureau of Labor Statistics. Household data: annual averages. 18*: employed persons by detailed industry, sex, race, and Hispanic or Latino ethnicity*. Washington, DC: US Department of Labor, Bureau of Labor Statistics; 2020. https://www.bls.gov/cps/cpsaat18.htm.

[8] National Center for Health Statistics. Vital and health statistics, series 3, no. 43. Long-term care providers and services users in the United States, 2015–2016. Hyattsville, MD: *US Department of Health and Human Services, CDC, National Center for Health Statistics*; 2019. https://stacks. cdc.gov/view/cdc/76253.

[9] CDC. *COVIDView: a weekly surveillance summary of US COVID-19 activity*. Atlanta, GA: US Department of Health and Human Services, CDC; 2021. https://www.cdc.gov/coronavirus/2019-ncov/covid-data/ covidview/index.html.

Written Testimony for the House Energy and Commerce Committee: Subcommittee on Health, "Road to Recovery: Ramping up COVID-19 Vaccines, Testing, and Medical Supply Chain," February 3, 2021

Dear Chairman Pallone and Health Subcommittee Chairwoman Eshoo:

On behalf of the National Health Care for the Homeless Council, thank you for receiving this written testimony on vaccine and testing issues that have been impacting homeless population to inform the February 3rd, 2021 hearing entitled *"Road to Recovery: Ramping up COVID-19 Vaccines, Testing, and Medical Supply Chain."*

During COVID-19, people who are homeless are at very high risk of contracting the illness because of numerous vulnerabilities: many are older and/or have significant health care conditions that make them especially susceptible, they live and receive services in congregate settings, and they have very limited ability to wash their hands and maintain a sanitary environment because of limited access to bathrooms. Nearly 1.5 million people experience homelessness over the course of a year, which is more than the number of people living in nursing homes. Those without homes are rightly considered a priority group for vaccination, and issues related to their care should be getting more attention.

Below are two key issues that have created significant challenges for testing and vaccinating people experiencing homelessness. We hope that these issues can be raised during the discussion and help inform the Committee's understanding of how COVID-19 has impacted this population:

Lack of Capacity at Local and State Health Departments

As individual health care providers, we lack the authority to allocate public resources or direct public responses to COVID-19 outbreaks. Unfortunately, state and local health departments are woefully understaffed and under-resourced—the result of decades of disinvestment in public health. Hence, many are unable to fulfill their mandate to protect community public health, and are especially unable to attend to the specific needs of special populations, like those who are homeless when there is an outreach of COVID-19 in shelters or encampments. Fragmented and/or antiquated computer systems have only compounded these problems. We rely on our public health partners to help with pro-active, surveillance testing in shelters to identify and contain clusters when they occur, as well as ensuring that vaccines are able to reach this population in a systematic way.

Dual stigmas in the health care system drive vaccine hesitancy: People experiencing homelessness are often treated poorly in our health care system. They are routinely denied care, treated with disrespect, prematurely discharged (often to the street or a shelter that cannot accommodate them), and traumatized by poor experiences. This factor is compounded by long-standing racism in our public policies, which have ensured that Black, Indigenous, and other People of Color (BIPOC) are over-represented in the homeless population, comprising 41% of those in shelters and on the streets. As you know, racism in health care is well-documented. Hence, people who are both homeless and BIPOC have dual reasons for being especially hesitant to trust in the health care system and be confident in getting the COVID-19 vaccine.

We believe the changes proposed in the Administration's *National Strategy for the COVID-19 Response and Pandemic Preparedness* will increase the supply chain, improve testing activities, and better ensure successful vaccine campaigns among vulnerable populations like those experiencing homelessness. We request the Committee (and the subcommittee on Health) specifically include issues related to homelessness (and housing status in general) as it continues its work to guide the nation's response to COVID-19.

Thank you for the opportunity to outline some of our concerns

Sincerely,
G. Robert Watts, MPH, MS,
CPH Chief Executive Officer

About the National Health Care for the Homeless Council

The National Health Care for the Homeless Council is a membership organization representing Health Care for the Homeless (HCH) federally qualified health centers (FQHCs) and other organizations providing health care to people experiencing homelessness. Our members offer a wide range of services to include comprehensive primary care, mental health and addiction treatment, medical respite care, supportive services in housing, case management, outreach, and health education. Last year, 300 HCH programs served over 1 million patients in 2,000+ locations across the country. We work every day to help our patients access health care, housing, and food assistance so they can meet their basic needs and escape homelessness.

Trump's Operation Warp Speed Promised a Flood of Covid Vaccines. Instead, States Are Expecting a Trickle

The administration pledged several hundred million doses in 2020. Companies will actually ship about 10 percent of that.

By Christopher Rowland, Lena H. Sun, Isaac Stanley-Becker and Carolyn Y. Johnson
Dec. 5, 2020 at 6:08 p.m. EST

Federal officials have slashed the amount of coronavirus vaccine they plan to ship to states in December because of constraints on supply, sending local officials into a scramble to adjust vaccination plans and highlighting how early promises of a vast stockpile before the end of 2020 have fallen short.

Instead of the delivery of 300 million or so doses of vaccine immediately after emergency-use approval and before the end of 2020 as the Trump administration had originally promised, current plans call for availability of around a tenth of that, or 35 to 40 million doses.

Two vaccines, from manufacturers Pfizer and Moderna, which both use a n ovel form of mRNA to help trigger immune response, are on the verge of winning Food and Drug Administration clearance this month. Approval would cap an unprecedented sprint by government and drug companies to develop, test and manufacture a defense against the worst pandemic in a century — part of the Operation Warp Speed initiative that promised six companies advance purchase orders totaling $9.3 billion.

As planning accelerated for distributing supplies, the government began to further lower expectations. To make sure supplies don't run out and leave some people only partially immunized, the government said it would stagger deliveries to ensure that states have enough supply for the second shot, required 21 days later for the Pfizer vaccine, which is expected to be first to gain approval.

Lower-than-anticipated allocations have caused widespread confusion and concern in states, which are beginning to grasp the level of vaccine scarcity they will confront in the early going of the massive vaccination campaign.

"I come from a family of seven siblings, and best practice was always to have seven of everything being given out," said Joe Sullivan, a senior health adviser in Oregon, which is expecting about 35,000 doses in the initial wave from Pfizer. "But we know that's not possible in this case."

Maine, meanwhile, saw its allotment fall from a previous estimate of 36,000 to just 12,675 doses, officials in the state said. "This is far less than what is needed for Maine and proportionally for other states as well," Gov. Janet Mills (D) said at a news conference this past week.

The gap reflects the disconnect between Trump's campaign promises, as well as the optimistic estimates from some drug companies, and scientific and manufacturing realities.

The drop-off is a product of manufacturing problems, bottlenecks in the supply of raw materials and other hurdles in ramping up clinical-trial production of 5 liters of protein-based vaccine at a time to commercial-scale fermentation of 2,000-liter batches, the companies and the Trump administration said.

"There were a couple of our vaccine candidates that took significantly longer, in terms of failed batches, in terms of not having the purity we sought," Paul Mango, deputy chief of staff for policy at the Department of Health and Human Services, said in an interview. He declined to say which company experienced batch failures.

"We have cracked the code on these things but we're two months behind on some of them," Mango said. Several states said they were expecting an allocation from Moderna about twice the size of the initial wave from Pfizer, roughly a week later.

The flow is expected to accelerate in January and February but still will not meet the bold predictions of Trump and the leader of Operation Warp Speed, pharmaceutical executive Moncef Slaoui, who said in the White House Rose Garden in May that he was confident "several hundred million" doses of vaccine would be ready by the end of December.

Instead, Slaoui said this past week that officials are now planning to ship 35 to 40 million doses by the end of the year, enough for up to 20 million people under a two-shot regimen.

Pfizer is expected to win emergency authorization for its vaccine soon after an FDA advisory committee meets on Dec. 10. In November, the company cut its manufacturing projection for 2020 from 100 million doses to 50 million doses. It said it remains on track to produce 1.3 billion doses in 2021.

The company's lower estimate got little notice at the time, tucked at the bottom of a Nov. 9 news release announcing the stunning news that its vaccine was more than 90 percent effective. The news buoyed stock markets and triggered optimism that a solution to the pandemic was in sight.

As Pfizer began large-scale production, the company said, it encountered difficulties procuring sufficient amounts of raw ingredients. A number of specialized materials are required to create the vaccine, including nucleotides, the building block of the mRNA.

"Bringing it all together in a first-time, very large-scale operation, is no simple feat," said company spokeswoman Amy Rose. "It's as complicated as the research-and-development piece."

Moderna, a Massachusetts biotech company that has never before had a product on the market, did not make early public predictions of how much of its mRNA vaccine it would produce by the end of 2020. The company said it is now on track to have 20 million doses available in December and between 500 million to 1 billion available by the end of 2021. As with Pfizer, Moderna's vaccine is a two-shot regimen.

"The swing factor between 500 million and 1 billion [doses] is raw materials," Moderna chief executive Stephane Bancel said in an interview, adding that as the company massively ramped up its production by a factor of 1,000 this year, the demand strained its supply chain. "Some of our suppliers were not ready for that, of course," Bancel said.

Moderna's vaccine supply chain depends critically on the availability and high quality of each component, including the lipids used to encapsulate the mRNA, bags and laboratory equipment used in production, the chemical components of mRNA itself and enzymes.

"If one ingredient is missing we have to wait," Bancel said.

AstraZeneca s aid earlier in the year it would begin delivering the first of 300 million doses of viral-vector vaccine to the United States in September, an ambitious prediction that passed unfulfilled. AstraZeneca declined to comment. Other companies have either declined to say how much vaccine they expect to have available or won't report phase 3 clinical data until later in 2021.

Americans and state officials are already having to adjust their expectations to a slower rollout of vaccines.

Operation Warp Speed officials said that, within 24 hours of the Pfizer vaccine winning clearance, the government would begin releasing 6.4 million doses, in two stages: enough for the first shot, followed three weeks later by enough for the second shot. Once the Moderna vaccine is authorized, perhaps a week after Pfizer's, 12.5 million doses would begin to be released, under a similar schedule.

Army Gen. Gustave Perna, the logistical chief of Operation Warp Speed, has said those initial bursts of vaccine would be followed by a weekly "cadence" of shipments.

Health officials in numerous states said they expected to vaccinate fewer people than they had originally anticipated with the first wave of the Pfizer vaccine. The sharp decrease in expected doses reoriented their planning in the final stages of preparation for a logistical ordeal as complex as a military campaign.

Some of the calculations were technical — whether to send the shots to an even narrower set of hospitals or to include the same number of facilities but restrict immunization to the most at-risk health care workers. Other decisions involved more fundamental questions of access and how to balance public awareness with limited supply.

In Maine, the current proposed allotment "would barely enable us to vaccinate emergency department and ICU front line staff," said Nirav Shah, director of Maine's Center for Disease Control and Prevention and president-elect of the Association of State and Territorial Health Officials.

Maine has about 6,000 emergency department and intensive-care front line staff who would meet the criteria to be vaccinated in the initial round, state officials said.

State and local officials said they always expected vaccine supply would be limited in the early weeks after authorization. But the increased constraints are compounding the allocation and implementation challenges of getting doses to people in the first priority groups, said Jeff Duchin, a top official at the Seattle and King County Health department.

"We will need to make decisions on where to send a very limited supply initially that will leave many unsatisfied until the supply improves to meet demand. For example, is it preferable to give more sites a smaller number of doses, or a few sites more doses, when all serve people in the first tier to be offered vaccine?" Duchin said.

A CDC advisory committee recommended this past week that health-care personnel and residents of long-term care facilities be the first to get the limited doses once a vaccine is authorized. Because of the limited supply, the advisory committee's work group suggested a standardized approach for health-care systems to prioritize their personnel even further. They could stagger vaccinations by individual units, such as emergency departments, and prioritize those with direct patient contact and those who handle infectious material.

Few officials seemed to know exactly why they are receiving fewer doses.

"There has been some lack of clarity in terms of what states are going to get," said Rachel Levine, Pennsylvania's health secretary and president of the state health official association. "We're not crystal clear."

The initial supply "will not even touch all of our hospitals," said Mandy Cohen, secretary of the North Carolina Department of Health and Human Services. "We knew this was going to be a process, and we've tried to set expectations on the front end."

The government's decision to hold back the booster shot, Cohen said, adds a new layer of complexity.

"I think one of the hardest pieces of this is the matching of that first dose to the second dose and getting that timing exactly right," she said. "In the trial setting, when Pfizer and Moderna did that, it's a very controlled setting. We don't have data to say what happens if you come in on day 22. We'll be working very hard to follow the protocols."

Randall Williams, Missouri's health director, said he's confident the state will be able to complete the initial phase of immunization by early in the new year. A sharp drop-off in the initial allocation from Pfizer — from 180,000 to 51,000 in Missouri's case — just means the doses will be more spaced out through the first month, rather than arriving immediately after the FDA grants approval, Williams said.

The shots will even be sufficient to cover residents of long-term care facilities, whom he had not originally factored into planning for the first priority group. "In some ways, this puts us ahead of where we thought we were going to be," Williams said.

Federal officials, acclaiming the expected arrival of vaccines, are also begging people to be patient. "We will have more and more people getting vaccinated," said Adm. Brett Giroir, the assistant secretary of health and human services during a visit Wednesday to Louisiana, saying "most Americans" might have to wait until May or June.

Experts agreed the administration's plan to pay companies billions of dollars in advance to spur manufacturing in parallel to the initiation of clinical trials — a strategy never attempted on such a massive scale — must still be considered a success. The advance payments eliminated or reduced financial risk for the companies, which have raced to ramp up production of doses that are still in the pipeline, if coming slower than originally pledged.

"They have done better than I could have imagined they could have done," said Barry Bloom, a professor and expert in immunology and infectious diseases at the Harvard T.H. Chan School of Public Health.

Each of the coronavirus vaccine manufacturers contracted by the government, with the exception of Pfizer, will get paid for delivery stockpiles of vaccine even if they fail to win emergency authorization, according to Operation Warp Speed. Together, the six received advance purchase orders of $9.3 billion, according to a tally by analysts at the Wall Street firm Bernstein. Some received additional subsidies of hundred of millions of dollars for research and development.

"This money certainly has been important in helping these companies build out their manufacturing capacity ahead of time. It's just that it's really hard to do so," said Rachel Sachs, a law professor and specialist in pharmaceutical pricing at Washington University in St. Louis.

Coronavirus: What you need to read

The Washington Post is providing some coronavirus coverage free, including:

Coronavirus maps: Cases and deaths in the U.S. | Cases and deaths worldwide
Coronavirus variants: What you need to know
Vaccine tracker: See how many doses will be available in your state

What you need to know: Vaccines FAQ | Covid-19 symptoms guide | Coronavirus etiquette | Your life at home | Personal finance guide | Make your own fabric mask | Follow all of our coverage and sign up for our free newsletter

Got a pandemic question? We answer one every day in our coronavirus newsletter
How to help: Your community | Seniors | Restaurants | Keep at-risk people in mind

U.S. CDC Says 41.4 Million Doses of COVID-19 Vaccines Distributed, 20.5 Million Administered

By Reuters Staff

(Reuters) - The U.S. Centers for Disease Control and Prevention said it had administered 20,537,990 doses of COVID-19 vaccines in the country as of Saturday morning and distributed 41,411,550 doses.

The tally of vaccine doses are for both Moderna and Pfizer/BioNTech vaccines as of 6:00 a.m. ET on Saturday, the agency said.

The agency said 17,390,345 people had received one or more doses, while 3,027,865 people got the second dose as of Saturday.

A total of 2,437,670 vaccine doses have been administered in long-term care facilities, the agency said.

According to the tally posted on Jan. 22, the agency had administered 19,107,959 doses of the vaccines, and distributed 39,892,400 doses.

Reporting by Rama Venkat in Bengaluru; editing by Diane Craft

'Pixie Dust': Why Some Vaccine Sits on Shelves While Shortages Intensify Nationwide

Confusion over set-asides for nursing homes and reluctance to order vaccine that might go unused mean some doses remain in warehouses.

By Isaac Stanley-Becker and Lena H. Sun
Jan. 21, 2021 at 7:44 p.m. EST

Please Note:
The Washington Post is providing this important information about the coronavirus for free. For more, sign up for our daily Coronavirus Updates newsletter where all stories are free to read. To support this work, please subscribe to the Post.

In a phone call with the four-star Army general overseeing the distribution of coronavirus vaccines, Tennessee's top health official laid out what she saw as the No. 1 obstacle to getting more shots into people's arms.

"The only limitation is supply," Health Commissioner Lisa Piercey recalled telling the general, Gustave F. Perna, earlier this month.

From Miami to Manhattan, hospital leaders and public officials have been equally emphatic. But in one of the most puzzling aspects of the early vaccine rollout, the shortages are intensifying in some jurisdictions, while others have yet to use all their vaccine. The bottleneck isn't just in administering the vaccines; some states are not ordering everything they've been allotted.

The result is widespread confusion about how much vaccine is available from one week to the next, and how much supply states actually need to inoculate residents in priority groups. Both areas of confusion are barriers to the national immunization campaign that President Biden pledged to mount in his first days in office.

The president's advisers have said they were left no plan by the Trump administration. But what they inherited this week was more like a black box than a bare cupboard — the result of fractured communication among federal, state and local officials and a juggling act between manufacturers making a new product and thousands of providers, from big hospital systems to tiny clinics, struggling to plan around an unknown amount of vaccine.

"We don't have the visibility that we would hope to have into supply and allocations," Jeff Zients, the Biden administration's coronavirus coordinator, acknowledged in a Wednesday briefing.

The delays in ordering and distribution have many causes, including uncertainty about vaccine supply and the status of second doses as well as the hesitancy of some people to get the shots. Also at issue are the logistical hurdles of performing immunizations in long-term-care facilities and the ultracold storage requirements and batch size of the product developed by Pfizer and German company BioNTech. That vaccine, one of two authorized for emergency use in the United States, comes in a minimum order of 975 doses. Once vials are opened, doses must be used within six hours.

Perversely, limited supply is sometimes the obstacle to faster distribution, health officials say, because there is reluctance to set up vaccination sites and mobilize beleaguered medical workers only to perform a meager number of inoculations.

Kentucky's public health commissioner, Steven J. Stack, likened apportioning limited supply to sprinkling "pixie dust" across his state.

"The people who are willing to give it and administer it don't get enough of it to plan their staffing and their operations and to tell the public when they're likely to be able to provide it," he said.

Asked why federal and state officials often give conflicting accounts about supply, Anthony S. Fauci, a top Biden adviser and director of the National Institute of Allergy and Infectious Diseases, said Thursday at a White House briefing, "I don't know the answer."

David Kessler, a top Biden adviser who now leads the federal government's vaccine accelerator effort, has made few immediate changes to how vaccines will be allocated to 64 jurisdictions and five federal agencies. The new administration has vowed to set up federally run mass vaccination sites but does not anticipate new federal allocations, instead drawing on supply already made available to states, according to an administration official who spoke on the condition of anonymity to discuss ongoing deliberations.

Zients said there was not yet a decision on whether to move ahead with a change announced by the Trump administration to give slightly more vaccine to states with larger elderly populations, to encourage immunization of adults 65 and older, along with front-line workers.

He said his team has heard "over and over" from governors about the need for more precise projections on vaccine supply, but state health officials are quickly recognizing that this expectation is not realistic.

"Please know we've never promised a steady stream of vaccine to anybody, even to ourselves," Mississippi's top health official, Thomas Dobbs, said Thursday.

Of Biden's promise to shift Trump's strategy, Dobbs said all the state has heard are "rumors of rumors of rumors."

The pace of vaccine administration became politically charged in recent weeks as Biden's advisers blamed the sluggish national rollout on the Trump administration, which in turn pressured states to dispense their supplies more quickly and held up certain states, such as Florida, as examples. Last week, the outgoing administration proposed rewarding states giving shots at a rapid clip with additional doses, a system Biden officials say they will scrap.

The situation deepened anxiety among providers and state officials about requesting doses that might ultimately go unused, potentially endangering their future supplies.

"I don't want to be the small practice responsible for wasting a valuable resource," said Macdonald M. DuBose, a geriatric medicine specialist and the chairman of the South Carolina Medical Association.

That some jurisdictions aren't ordering all available vaccine while others beg for more goes to the heart of the disjointed immunization effort underway in the United States. It also helps explain why the federal government has liquidated its reserve of second doses at the same time that Pfizer maintains it has millions of doses in reserve — as many as 5 million by the end of last week, or about 25 percent of what had been made available to the United States at that point, according to former federal officials.

Those are not doses earmarked for booster shots, according to multiple people knowledgeable about the process, some of whom spoke on the condition of anonymity because they were not authorized to address it. Rather, those are doses that have accumulated week after week because some states are not ordering up to their limit or are putting aside a set amount of their vaccine supply for purposes including inoculations in nursing homes or mass vaccination clinics.

Ordering limits are set for states twice a week, on Thursday and Sunday. They reflect updated allocations, so the actual number of unclaimed doses is a moving target. The ordering is spaced out both to ease the burden on distributors and to help states distinguish between first and second doses, with priority given to the latter.

As of early this week, states not ordering up to their limits included Illinois, Kansas, Mississippi, Nevada, South Carolina and Texas, according to Michael Pratt, a former Health and Human Services spokesman. Data c ompiled by the Centers for Disease Control and Prevention indicates the fewest doses per capita have been distributed in Nevada, South Carolina and Texas. By the end of the week, Mississippi had ordered all the vaccine available to the state, officials said.

The discrepancy is so glaring in South Carolina that the public health director, Brannon Traxler, affirmed Wednesday that the state is receiving its "fair and appropriate allocation." She was responding to concerns that South Carolinians were being shortchanged in favor of people in other parts of the country.

The reason so much of South Carolina's allocation has gone unused, she said, is that the state had set aside the entire amount needed for long-term-care facilities rather than parceling that out in increments, as other states have done. CVS and Walgreens pharmacies are handling immunizations at long-term-care facilities as part of a federal partnership, which has been slow to get off the ground in some places. Maine recently redirected nearly 2,000 doses from Walgreens to two hospitals because the pharmacy had no immediate plans to administer the shots, according to state officials.

But doctors and public health experts said the supply problems in South Carolina and elsewhere go beyond the need to stockpile doses for nursing homes.

DuBose said too few providers have the cold-storage capacity for Pfizer's product. He also said communication from the state and the federal governments has been inadequate, both in identifying who is eligible for vaccination and persuading those people to take the vaccines.

"There's just an assumption that this is something everybody is going to wait hours in the rain to receive," he said.

Mixed messages about the status of second doses, meanwhile, created uncertainty about supply, said Harris Pastides, an epidemiologist and former president of the University of South Carolina who advised the state on earlier phases of its pandemic response.

The Trump administration was never clear about whether states were supposed to maintain reserves of second doses, he said, especially as Britain began to experiment with spacing out the doses to deliver some protection to more people more quickly.

When federal officials announced last week that they were no longer maintaining a stockpile at the national level because of increased confidence in manufacturing — not because they were changing the approach to second doses — they led states to believe they would see a windfall in supply. It turned out that much of the reserve had already been shipped out, making it all the more difficult for state and local officials to instill confidence in their populations that there would still be enough for booster shots.

Melaney Arnold, a spokeswoman for the Illinois Department of Public Health, pointed to confusion over the release of second doses and said the gap between what was available to the state and what it had ordered would be eliminated "as more residents become eligible for second doses and our providers put in those orders."

Officials in other states, including Texas, said they had already increased their orders substantially and were mystified by federal figures showing their allotments not being fully distributed.

The only time Texas ordered less than its full allotment was during the week of Christmas, when Moderna doses were first shipped to the states, said Chris Van Deusen, a spokesman for the Texas Department of State Health Services. The next week, he said, "we pulled that down and haven't done that since." The state places its orders several days each week, said Van Deusen, suggesting that the full scope of its requests may not be immediately clear to federal officials.

To add to the confusion, starting next week, each state's allocation will reflect an updated number of doses contained in each Pfizer-BioNTech vial — six instead of the current five. Given Pfizer's packaging, that means the minimum order will be 1,170 doses instead of 975.

Thousands of Vaccine Appointments Canceled as Supply Lags

Last Updated Feb. 1, 2021, 5:54 a.m. ET

Doctors in Peru are staging a hunger strike to protest a lack of pandemic equipment. As Biden and Harris were sworn at the Capitol, masks were the order of the day. Crowds weren't.

This briefing has ended. Follow our live Covid-19 coverage.

Here's what you need to know:

- 'It's such a lottery': Disappointment and frustration as vaccine offers melt away.
- On Biden's first day in charge, swift action on Covid-19 and the economy is a priority.
- A new president takes office: the view from an I.C.U.
- Without big galas, an inauguration so small, it fit on your phone.
- A company vaccinating Ohio nursing-home residents lets 890 doses go bad.
- Doctors in Peru stage a hunger strike over the government's pandemic response.
- Convinced that they are immune, many Iraqis take heedless risks.
- Biden restores ties with the World Health Organization that were cut by Trump.

'It's Such a Lottery': Disappointment and Frustration as Vaccine Offers Melt Away

That Covid-19 vaccine appointment may not just be hard to get — it may not even be all that secure.

Thousands of people across the country learned that their appointments had been abruptly canceled in the last few days, after vaccine shipments to local health departments and other distributors fell short of what was expected.

The health department in Erie County, N.Y., which includes Buffalo, canceled seven days of appointments this week, affecting 8,010 people, saying the state had sent far fewer doses than the county ordered. All future appointments should be considered "tentative, and are subject to vaccine availability," the department said in a statement on Wednesday.

"We made appointments based on our hope and expectation that we would be able to fill those," said Kara Kane, a department spokeswoman. "There's a lot of confusion, a lot of questions, a lot of concern."

Dianne Bennett, 78, lost a first-dose appointment at the Erie County Medical Center because of the cancellations, as did her husband. They were told to try again later, but Ms. Bennett said they had no idea when another appointment would be available.

"It's such a lottery," she said. "I just think it's outrageous."

Similar issues have cropped up across the country, as demand far outpaces supply and vaccine providers struggle to predict how many doses will arrive.

At Beaufort Memorial Hospital in South Carolina, hospital officials canceled 6,000 scheduled appointments through March 30 after they were notified that thousands of vaccine doses they expected were not coming.

San Francisco's public health department expects to run out of vaccine on Thursday, The Los Angeles Times reported, because the city's allocation dropped sharply from a week ago and the state did not replace doses that had to be discarded.

Local health officials throughout California say they have trouble scheduling appointments because they are unsure how much vaccine they will receive from week to week, the paper said.

In New York City, 23,000 vaccination appointments scheduled for Thursday and Friday were postponed because of a shipping delay, Mayor Bill de Blasio said on Wednesday, a day after warning that the city's supply would soon be exhausted.

"We already were feeling the stress of a shortage of vaccine," the mayor said at a news conference. "Now the situation has been made even worse."

Recent moves to open up eligibility have aggravated the situation.

Tracking the Coronavirus ›

United States ›	On Feb. 1	14-day change
New cases	139,830	–29%
New deaths	2,010	–2%

Risk in your area ›

Washington, D.C., is at a **very high risk** level. See more detail ›

Choose a different county

U.S. vaccinations ›

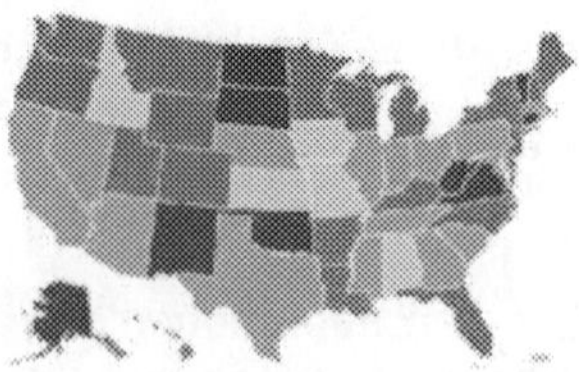

Fully vaccinated	1.8%
At least one dose	8.0%

Other trackers: Choose your own places to track

Hospitals | Global cases | Global vaccinations

State restrictions | U.K. cases | Vaccine development

After the state of Georgia announced that anyone 65 or older could get the vaccine, the 10-county Northwest Health District was swamped with more than 10,000 appointment requests in one weekend — far more than it could satisfy with the supply it had on hand. So it shut down its scheduling website, and told people to call their local health department to arrange an appointment instead, frustrating many people who thought they had already secured a slot.

> "We're having to schedule appointments at least a week out, based on anticipated delivery, but we don't know what will show up on a daily basis," said Logan Boss, the spokesman for the health district. "It's difficult to explain that to the public."

— *Lucy Tompkins*

On Biden's First Day in Charge, Swift Action on Covid-19 and the Economy Is a Priority

Within hours of his inauguration on Wednesday, President Biden signed 17 executive orders, memorandums and proclamations, five of which were aimed at helping the country bring the pandemic to heel.

In an effort to strengthen the nation's response to the coronavirus, which as of this week, has claimed more than 400,000 lives, Mr. Biden signed an executive order appointing Jeffrey D. Zients the official Covid-19 response coordinator, reporting to the president. Mr. Zients was the co-chairman of the Biden transition team, and led the National Economic Council under President Barack Obama.

That order also restores the National Security Council's Directorate for Global Health Security and Biodefense, a group disbanded under President Donald Trump in 2018.

Though Mr. Biden has not ordered a national mask mandate, which would probably face legal challenges, he is requiring social distancing and the wearing of masks by federal employees, contractors and others on federal property. He is also starting a "100 days masking challenge" urging all Americans to wear masks and state and local officials to implement public measures to prevent the spread of the coronavirus.

Mr. Biden is also reinstating ties with the World Health Organization after the Trump administration withdrew the nation's membership and funding last year.

Mr. Biden also took action to help Americans who are struggling economically as a result of the pandemic.

He is moving to extend a federal moratorium on evictions and has asked agencies, including the departments of Agriculture, Veterans Affairs and Housing and Urban Development, to prolong a moratorium on foreclosures on federally guaranteed mortgages. The extensions all run through at least the end of March.

Frustrations Boil at Pace of Vaccinations at Long-Term Care Facilities

The Trump administration raised hopes of a speedy process for nursing homes and assisted living facilities. Patience is wearing thin.

By Rebecca Robbins

Jan. 16, 2021

In mid-December, a top Trump administration official floated an enticing possibility: All nursing home residents in the United States could be vaccinated against the coronavirus by Christmas. "It's really a remarkable, remarkable prospect," Alex M. Azar II, the secretary of health and human services, declared.

It turned out to be a fantasy.

A month later, vaccinations of some of the country's most vulnerable citizens are going more slowly than many state officials, industry executives and families expected. Their hopes had been buoyed when government officials said long-term care facilities would be at the front of the line for vaccines.

CVS and Walgreens, which are largely responsible for vaccinating residents and workers in long-term care facilities, are on track to make at least initial vaccination visits to nearly all nursing homes they are working with by Jan. 25. The two pharmacy chains have already given out more than 1.7 million vaccine doses at long-term care facilities.

But the progress is uneven across the country and not nearly as comprehensive for different types of long-term care. For example, thousands of assisted living facilities — for older people who need less care than those in nursing homes — do not yet even have an appointment for their first visit from the pharmacy teams, in large part because states have given such facilities lower priority in their vaccine-distribution plans.

"I've had facilities call me, and I've had people cry, I've had people curse, because this was the first sign of hope that they've had in many, many months," said Betsy Johnson, who leads a group that represents Kentucky's nursing homes and assisted living facilities.

"It's just human nature to think, 'OK, but I was supposed to be first — and I don't even know when my clinic is going to happen,'" Ms. Johnson said.

In Pennsylvania, teams from CVS or Walgreens are not scheduled to visit some nursing homes until February, and the vast majority of the state's assisted living facilities have not yet been scheduled for a first visit, said Zach Shamberg, president of the Pennsylvania Health Care Association.

"There's a great deal of frustration, there's a great deal of apprehension, as to when or if this vaccine will come," Mr. Shamberg said.

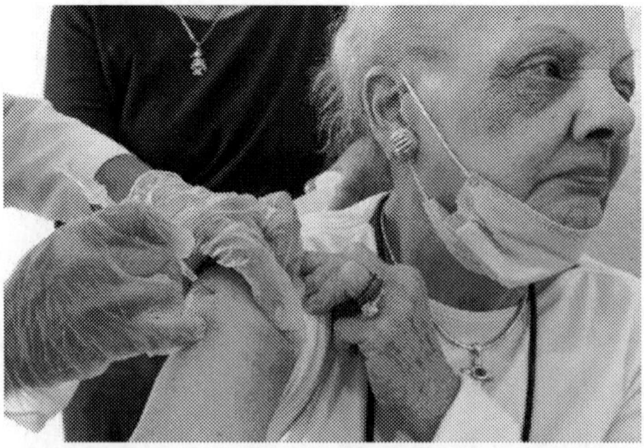

Dana Sweeny receiving a Covid-19 vaccination on Tuesday at a senior community in Coral Gables, Fla. Cristobal Herrera-Ulashkevich/EPA.

The pace of the vaccination program has taken on greater urgency as the rapidly spreading virus continues to decimate nursing homes and similar facilities. The virus's surge since November has killed about 30,000 long-term care staff and residents, raising the total of virus-related deaths in these facilities to at least 136,000, according to a New York Times tracker. Since the pandemic began, long-term care facilities have accounted for just 5 percent of coronavirus cases but 36 percent of virus-related deaths.

Even as the vaccination campaign accelerates, the suffering is unlikely to wane. The coming months could be "the deadliest of the pandemic" for people living and working in long-term care, according to an analysis released on Thursday by the Kaiser Family Foundation.

The Trump administration announced in October that it had teamed up with CVS and Walgreens to lead a federal effort to vaccinate residents and workers at long-term care facilities, among the first eligible groups.

On Friday, CVS said it had given out just over one million doses in more than 12,000 initial visits to long-term care facilities. Nearly 8,000 visits are scheduled for the coming week. Walgreens said it had given out nearly 750,000 doses in nearly 9,000 visits to facilities, mostly nursing homes. The number of visits that Walgreens has scheduled with assisted living facilities "continues to accelerate," a company spokeswoman, Rebekah Pajak, said.

The vaccinations by CVS and Walgreens were always expected to take several months because of the need to visit tens of thousands of facilities three times. The first two visits are for most residents and staff to get the two doses of the vaccine, with the third visit as a backup for people who missed the first clinic.

The idea that all nursing home residents could get their first doses by Christmas was not a realistic prospect even when Mr. Azar, the health secretary, floated it 12 days before the holiday. By that point, some states had told the Centers for Disease Control and Prevention that they would not activate the federal program to vaccinate their nursing homes until Dec. 28. The logistics would have been challenging even if states had put a priority on getting their first doses to nursing homes.

Michael Pratt, a spokesman for the Health and Human Services Department, said Mr. Azar had been speaking only aspirationally about what states were capable of doing, since they had enough vaccine doses to cover all nursing home residents by Christmas. But that would have required that states place less of a priority on vaccinating high-risk groups like heath care workers.

T.J. Crawford, a spokesman for CVS, said the chain was making first visits to all facilities within four weeks of each state's activating its vaccination program for nursing homes or assisted living facilities.

"This isn't a drive-through or stadium vaccination effort," Mr. Crawford said. "We're visiting more than 40,000 facilities with an average of less than 100 residents, in some cases going room to room." He said CVS was "on track and delivering on goals established and communicated early in the process."

But a growing number of governors and state health officials have voiced frustration with CVS's and Walgreens' speed.

In Mississippi, some long-term facilities won't get their first visit until Feb. 11, the state health officer, Dr. Thomas Dobbs, said this month. "We're clearly disappointed with the progress in the long-term care program," he said.

Some states and cities are exploring ways to hasten the inoculations.

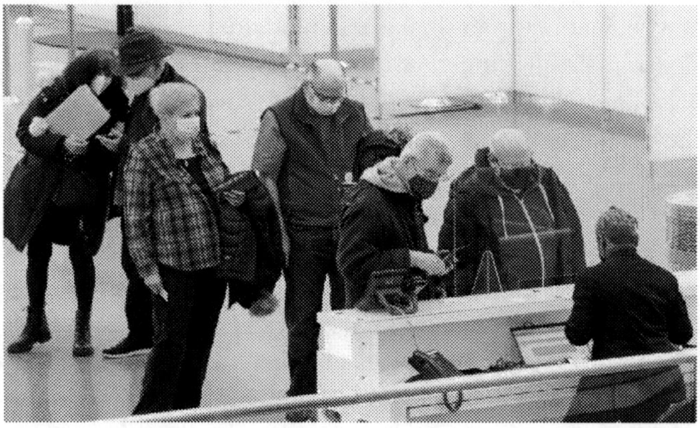

Seniors at a vaccination site in the Javits Convention Center in Manhattan. Mary Altaffer/Associated Press.

Covid-19 Vaccines ›

Answers to Your Vaccine Questions

Am I eligible for the Covid vaccine in my state?

Currently more than 150 million people — almost half the population — are eligible to be vaccinated. But each state makes the final decision about who goes first. The nation's 21 million health care workers and three million residents of long-term care facilities were the first to qualify. In mid-January, federal officials urged all states to open up eligibility to everyone 65 and older and to adults of any age with medical conditions that put them at high risk of becoming seriously ill or dying from Covid-19. Adults in the general population are at the back of the line. If federal and state health officials can clear up bottlenecks in vaccine distribution, everyone 16 and older will become eligible as early as this spring or early summer. The vaccine hasn't been approved in children, although studies are underway. It may be months before a vaccine is available for anyone under the age of 16. Go to your state health website for up-to-date information on vaccination policies in your area

Is the vaccine free?

Can I choose which vaccine I get?

How long will the vaccine last? Will I need another one next year?

Will my employer require vaccinations?

Where can I find out more?

Seattle is using its Fire Department to vaccinate nearly 1,000 residents and staff at adult family homes, a type of long-term care, by the end of January. Florida hired an emergency services company, CDR Maguire, to give out doses at 1,900 assisted living facilities that had not been scheduled for visits by CVS and Walgreens teams before Jan. 24.

In Michigan, officials have asked the federal government to let them work with other pharmacies, such as the supermarket chains Meijer and Kroger, to speed up the vaccination effort in long-term care facilities, said Bobby Leddy, a spokesman for Gov. Gretchen Whitmer.

West Virginia is the only state that has not activated the federal program involving CVS and Walgreens, though Walgreens is separately working with West Virginia to vaccinate 32 of its long-term care facilities. Relying mostly on local independent pharmacies, the state said on Dec. 30 that it had wrapped up the first round at its 214 long-term care facilities.

Some of the initially feared problems that could slow down the vaccine rollout in nursing homes have not emerged as serious obstacles, at least so far, according to facility operators and industry researchers.

Despite widespread worries that the vaccines' side effects — which can include fevers, chills and fatigue — would cause staff to miss work and residents to need more care, that has not happened to any significant degree. And while there was early confusion about how nursing homes should get consent from residents or their families, that process has largely gone smoothly.

But other things are slowing the campaign. A significant number of long-term care workers have balked at receiving the vaccine. The virus's spread is also delaying the process. People should not be vaccinated while they still have Covid-19 symptoms or are isolating, according to the C.D.C.

Outbreaks and cases of Covid-19 in some long-term care communities have led Walgreens to delay scheduling initial visits or to reschedule them, said Rick Gates, an executive leading the company's long-term care vaccinations.

CVS has encountered the same issue, though it has not been widespread. The company has left the decision about whether to proceed with visits in such cases to local clinic team leaders and officials at the facilities, Mr. Crawford said.

Another factor is that some states did not quickly activate their programs to vaccinate people at assisted living facilities and similar communities. In some cases, they waited until weeks after they began vaccinations at nursing homes.

But many long-term care facilities include both nursing homes and assisted living. In those cases, pharmacy teams have been able to vaccinate only a subset of residents.

In Prairie du Chien, Wis., for example, a team from Walgreens on Thursday made its first visit to the local nursing home, Prairie Maison, to inject nearly all of its roughly 50 residents with the Moderna vaccine.

But Prairie Maison is part of a larger senior community, which includes about 50 assisted living residents. Because Wisconsin did not activate its vaccination program for assisted living until Friday, those residents weren't offered the vaccine — even though they are in the same building as the nursing home residents.

"Vaccinating one group and not the other doesn't make a lot of sense," said Dr. Mark Grunwald, the chairman of Prairie Maison's board.

Abby Goodnough contributed reporting.

Trump Officials Actively Lobbied to Deny States Money for Vaccine Rollout Last Fall

By Nicholas Florko

January 31, 2021

WASHINGTON — Top Trump officials actively lobbied Congress to deny state governments any extra funding for the Covid-19 vaccine rollout last fall — despite frantic warnings from state officials that they didn't have the money they needed to ramp up a massive vaccination operation.

The push, described to STAT by congressional aides in both parties and openly acknowledged by one of the Trump officials, came from multiple high-ranking Trump health officials in repeated meetings with legislators.

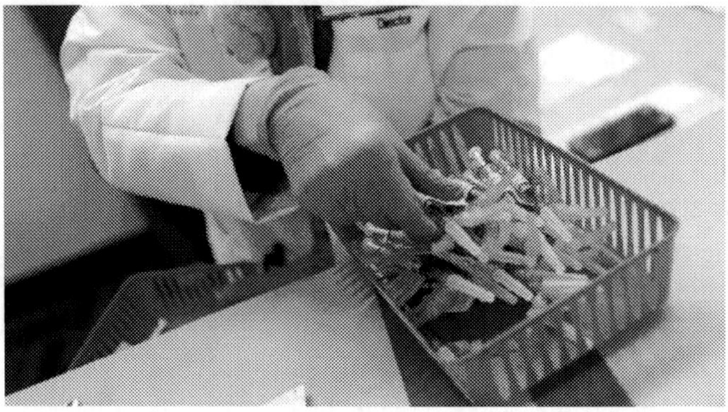

Technicians sort doses of the Pfizer Covid-19 vaccine at the Virginia Hospital Center in Arlington. *Win McNamee/Getty Images.*

Without the extra money, states spent last October and November rationing the small pot of federal dollars they had been given. And when vaccines began shipping in December, states seemed woefully underprepared.

The previously unreported lobbying efforts underscore that even after the Trump administration spent billions helping drug makers develop Covid-19 vaccines, it not only dismissed states' concerns about the help they would need to roll them out, but actively undermined their efforts to press Congress to get the funding they needed.

Much of the lobbying push came from Paul Mango, the former deputy chief of staff for policy at the Department of Health and Human Services. He argued, repeatedly, that states hadn't demonstrated they needed additional funding because, at least as of last October, they hadn't spent the $200 million that the Centers for Disease Control and Prevention sent to states in September.

Far from denying his efforts, Mango doubled down in an interview with STAT — and even accused states of pressing for the money to bolster their empty tax coffers.

"A lot of them had shut down their economies and they weren't getting tax revenue," he said.

"I'm sure they could use money — that's not in dispute — what's in dispute is whether they needed money given all they hadn't used to actually administer vaccines," Mango added, suggesting that his lobbying efforts were an attempt to protect taxpayers from wasteful government spending.

Mango and other Trump officials started lobbying Congress to deny states the money last fall. At the time, states were working with the Trump administration and the CDC to craft plans to administer the first Covid-19 vaccines, which were expected to be authorized in November. Meanwhile, Congress was busy negotiating a Covid-19 response package that was almost guaranteed to include some funding for the vaccination effort. On Oct. 15, states formally asked congressional leadership for $8.4 billion in funding.

On Oct. 27, Mango told congressional staff, including those working for the House Appropriations Committee, that states did not need more federal funding because they had not yet spent the $200 million provided by the government earlier that year, a Democratic aide told STAT.

Mango also said that HHS had asked states for detailed financial plans for how they planned to spend the extra money, but that their plans were "vague." STAT was unable to obtain those plans: The Association for State and Territorial Health Officials told STAT it did not have access to them.

"Every time we got on our biweekly update with the Hill, they said, 'Don't you guys need more money for distribution?' and we said the same thing we told you: 'We've already allocated $200 million. They haven't drawn anything down, they haven't drawn down their testing [funding], and we are looking for business plans. If we get those things, we will be the first to let you know and we will be happy to give them more money," Mango told STAT.

It's true that the states hadn't spent most of the money by October. State health departments, for their part, say there are several good reasons why. For one, they hadn't begun vaccinating anyone yet. States were also drawing down other sources of funding that were set to expire. And they were reluctant to immediately spend the new funding because they were unsure when new funding would be appropriated by Congress.

STAT was unable to independently confirm how much of the $200 million has since been spent by states. Mango insisted that as of Dec. 31, states had only "drawn down 1% of the $200 million." ASTHO has claimed that the metric Mango has referenced is not a real-time metric and may take weeks or months to be reported to the federal government.

Mango also made a similar argument, repeatedly, about the CDC, according to a second Democratic aide. At the time, Trump's CDC Director, Robert Redfield, was requesting $6 billion for states' efforts on the vaccine rollout. Mango said the money Redfield requested wasn't needed, according to the aide.

Mango told STAT this week that Redfield's 2020 request was "lobbying Congress for money behind our back," referring to the Trump administration.

"I call it the mutual-admiration society — they were trying to help their friends at the state public health offices even though they didn't have any real plan to spend the money," Mango said.

Mango wasn't the only one using the argument. Russ Vought, the head of the White House budget office, likewise argued that states did not need additional funding because they had not already spent the $200 million allocated to them, a Republican Senate aide said. The Republican aide called Vought "obsessed" with the fact that states hadn't spent the money.

The Republican aide also emphasized that even staunch fiscal conservatives knew that states needed more than $200 million to vaccinate the majority of Americans.

Trump staffers were so reluctant to acknowledge that states needed additional funding that staffers negotiating the relief packages eventually gave up on asking the Trump administration how much money states needed. Instead, they went directly to associations representing state and local health departments, a second Republican aide confirmed.

The lobbying from the Trump administration prompted a flurry of defensive action from state health officials.

In a sharply worded letter on Dec. 4, ASTHO and the Association of Immunization Managers wrote to Surgeon General Jerome Adams that, "Recent communications by senior Administration officials to Congress … indicate that this Administration and some members of Congress do not support our request for substantial additional resources for vaccine administration and infrastructure."

"This is extremely unfortunate," ASTHO wrote. "We believe that it is neither a partisan nor political statement to share the very obvious fact that the vaccination of 330,000,000 Americans safely and effectively will take far more than the $340 million currently allocated to local, state, and territorial governmental public health agencies."

In addition to the missive, ASTHO requested a meeting with its members and HHS Secretary Alex Azar to discuss the situation. The meeting request, which was made on Oct. 20, was denied, according to the group's executive director Michael Fraser.

A former senior adviser to Adams told STAT that the question of whether the Trump administration should advocate for more funding to states generated a schism between political appointees, like Azar and Mango, who argued states didn't need more funding, and doctors on the coronavirus task force, like Adams, White House coronavirus coordinator Deborah Birx and Anthony Fauci, director of the National Institute of Allergy and Infectious Diseases.

"The political people very much believed that it wasn't their responsibility and it should be left up to the states," the former adviser said. "The majority of the people running the Trump response at a high political level had zero medical experience or response experience and there was a disconnect between saying, 'I've already given them supplies, it shouldn't cost anything after that,' versus understanding that there are costs that have to do with the planning, with the spaces, with all of the PPE, with the training, security."

State public health officials weren't the only ones sounding the alarm over the lack of funding.

The National Governors Association had also directly warned the Trump administration that additional funding was needed.

"Without additional state and local funding to implement COVID-19 vaccine plans, we will be hampered in what we can accomplish. When can we expect more definitive information about resources related to this response?" NGA wrote to HHS on Oct 18.

HHS' response: The agency reiterated that $200 million had already been allocated to states and that "states should recognize that most of the major costs of a vaccine campaign are already being covered."

Congress eventually did allocate $4.5 billion to state governments, but the money only began to flow to states earlier this month. In the meantime, the Trump administration administered dramatically fewer vaccines than it had originally promised.

It's impossible to say definitively how the Trump administration's full-throated advocacy for state funding would have changed the course of the early vaccine rollout.

Mango told STAT that the early hiccups with the vaccine rollout were caused by states too closely following CDC recommendations for who to vaccinate first and by natural vaccine supply constraints, not lack of funding.

But independent public health officials weren't so sure.

"A lot of that could have been avoided or smoothed," said Amesh Adalja, a senior scholar at the Johns Hopkins Center for Health Security, regarding the scramble from states to begin vaccinating in December. "Having more money would have allowed them to devote more resources to planning for the vaccine, making sure they had enough vaccinators ... and get in place venues to do mass vaccinations."

About the Author

Nicholas Florko

Washington correspondent

Nicholas Florko is a Washington correspondent for STAT, reporting on the the intersection of politics and health policy. He is the author the newsletter "D.C. Diagnosis."

Administration Leaves Testing Responsibility to States in Report to Congress

By Amy Goldstein

May 24, 2020 at 10:08 p.m. EDT

In a report to Congress, the Trump administration is pledging to buy 100 million swabs by the year's end and distribute them to states to help expand the nation's capacity to test for the novel coronavirus.

The report, delivered on the Sunday deadline lawmakers had set for federal health officials to submit a national testing strategy, doubles down on the administration's stance that individual states, not the federal government, should bear primary responsibility for carrying out diagnostic tests to help curb the pandemic.

The Washington Post obtained the 81-page document, called Covid-19 Strategic Testing Plan, from an individual on Capitol Hill who was not authorized to disclose it. Federal health officials did not release it publicly, submitting it to four congressional committees as required by law.

The plan, sought by public health experts and congressional Democrats since the virus began circulating in the United States in late February, arrived as the nation's covid-19 cases exceeded 1.6 million and deaths closed in on 100,000 — both the highest in the world.

Public health authorities emphasize that diagnostic testing to identify who is infected, along with antibody testing to determine who might have immunity, are crucial tools to slow the spread of the highly infectious virus and to develop strategies to make it safe for states and communities to reopen. Without a nationwide strategy, states have developed their own approaches, creating a patchwork, with some parts of the country doing far more testing than others.

The administration's testing plan says every state should aim to test at least 2 percent of its population in May and June. The document, however, lists the testing targets each state reported to federal officials for May, totaling 12.9 million tests nationwide, rather than laying out goals the federal government is calling on each state to meet.

"With support from the federal government to ensure states are meeting goals, the state plans for testing will advance the safe opening of America," the plan says.

And in keeping with the portrayal by Trump and others in his administration that the pandemic is under control, the document says that epidemiologists and public health organizations have said that if 10 percent of tests are positive for the virus over the course of a week, that is "enough to assure broad coverage of the population." It says that 41 states already have achieved that goal.

Congress's Democratic leaders were expected to issue a reaction to the plan within hours of receiving it, but had not done so by Sunday evening.

The availability of tests and test kits has been a critical problem with the administration's pandemic response since the beginning. Testing began late because of problems in the central lab at the Centers for Disease Control and Prevention, which was at first the only source of a diagnostic test. Even when academic and commercial labs began developing their tests, government bureaucracy delayed their approval. And the supply of testing materials has been a recurrent problem, though the White House consistently says there are ample tests.

The number of tests nationwide has hovered lately around 400,000 a day, according to the Covid Tracking Project, which compiles and publishes state testing data. That is hundreds of thousands a day fewer than various research models say is necessary.

The new report, prepared by the Department of Health and Human Services, elaborates on a blueprint the White House released last month for increasing the nation's capacity for coronavirus testing. That 11-page document, released April 27, also placed responsibility primarily on states, saying the federal government's role would be to "provide strategic direction and technical assistance," while regulating tests and testing equipment. The government would "act as supplier of last resort," it said.

The blueprint said, for instance, that it was up to each state to devise a testing plan; determine where people could get tested; and monitor and seek to contain outbreaks. The private sector also had a role, developing new tests, getting them approved by federal regulators, and speeding up production of the tests and needed materials — all features of the strategy HHS submitted to Congress Sunday, as well.

Upon its release, the blueprint was immediately derided as inadequate by leading public health officials and other experts. The president issued it hours after a bipartisan group of 16 prominent former federal officials and academics — all with health-care expertise — sent a letter to lawmakers urging them to devote significantly more money to expand testing, as well as do more public health tracing to identity the contacts of infected people and then isolate them.

Congressional Democrats lambasted the blueprint as flawed. House Energy and Commerce Committee Chairman Frank Pallone Jr. (D-N.J.) called it "totally lacking in credibility," saying that it fell short of a national plan, was not enforceable, and was not accompanied by federal funding.

Under a $484 billion coronavirus relief package Congress adopted in late April — and that Trump signed into law — lawmakers devoted $25 billion for testing. The law says that each state must submit to HHS a detailed coronavirus testing plan for the rest of this year. It also requires the department to submit a national testing strategy to the four congressional committees — including plans to increase the amount of testing available and to curb disparities among different communities. The deadline for both was Sunday.

Some of the new testing plan borrows from advice federal health officials have given before. It says, for instance, that they will assist states if they need help in developing testing and surveillance efforts targeted to workers in 16 "critical infrastructure sectors" the CDC previously has addressed, including those in health care and food and agriculture.

It also includes an assertion made recently by Brett Giroir, an assistant HHS secretary in charge of testing, that the nation will have the capacity to perform 40 million to 50 million diagnostic tests a month by the end of the summer.

The document mentions actions the White House has taken already. They include collaborating with companies to operate drive-though testing sites, though fewer have been established than the president indicated when the idea was first announced.

The document also reiterates that the White House's plan for reopening the country calls for government officials to work with private companies on researching and developing new testing approaches.

Coronavirus: What you need to read

The Washington Post is providing some coronavirus coverage free, including:

Coronavirus maps: Cases and deaths in the U.S. | Cases and deaths worldwide

Coronavirus variants: What you need to know

Vaccine tracker: See how many doses will be available in your state

What you need to know: Vaccines FAQ | Covid-19 symptoms guide | Coronavirus etiquette | Your life at home | Personal finance guide | Make your own fabric mask | Follow all of our coverage and sign up for our free newsletter

Got a pandemic question? We answer one every day in our coronavirus newsletter

How to help: Your community | Seniors | Restaurants | Keep at-risk people in mind

It's Just Everywhere Already': How Delays in Testing Set Back the U.S. Coronavirus Response

A series of missed chances by the federal government to ensure more widespread testing came during the early days of the outbreak, when containment would have been easier.

By Sheri Fink and Mike Baker

March 10, 2020

Dr. Helen Y. Chu, an infectious disease expert in Seattle, knew that the United States did not have much time.

In late January, the first confirmed American case of the coronavirus had landed in her area. Critical questions needed answers: Had the man infected anyone else? Was the deadly virus already lurking in other communities and spreading?

As luck would have it, Dr. Chu had a way to monitor the region. For months, as part of a research project into the flu, she and a team of researchers had been collecting nasal swabs from residents experiencing symptoms throughout the Puget Sound region.

To repurpose the tests for monitoring the coronavirus, they would need the support of state and federal officials. But nearly everywhere Dr. Chu turned, officials repeatedly rejected the idea, interviews and emails show, even as weeks crawled by and outbreaks emerged in countries outside of China, where the infection began.

By Feb. 25, Dr. Chu and her colleagues could not bear to wait any longer. They began performing coronavirus tests, without government approval.

What came back confirmed their worst fear. They quickly had a positive test from a local teenager with no recent travel history. The coronavirus had already established itself on American soil without anybody realizing it.

"It must have been here this entire time," Dr. Chu recalled thinking with dread. "It's just everywhere already."

In fact, officials would later discover through testing, the virus had already contributed to the deaths of two people, and it would go on to kill 20 more in the Seattle region over the following days.

Federal and state officials said the flu study could not be repurposed because it did not have explicit permission from research subjects; the labs were also not certified for clinical work. While acknowledging the ethical questions, Dr. Chu and others argued there should be more flexibility in an emergency during which so many lives could be lost. On Monday night, state regulators told them to stop testing altogether.

The failure to tap into the flu study, detailed here for the first time, was just one in a series of missed chances by the federal government to ensure more widespread testing during the early days of the outbreak, when containment would have been easier. Instead, local officials across the country were left to work in the dark as the crisis grew undetected and exponentially.

Even now, after weeks of mounting frustration toward federal agencies over flawed test kits and burdensome rules, states with growing cases such as New York and California are struggling to test widely for the coronavirus. The continued delays have made it impossible for officials to get a true picture of the scale of the growing outbreak, which has now spread to at least 36 states and Washington, D.C.

Dr. Robert R. Redfield, director of the Centers for Disease Control and Prevention, said in an interview on Friday that acting quickly was critical for combating an outbreak. "Time matters," he said.

He insisted that despite the rocky start, there was still time to beat back the coronavirus in the United States. "It's going to take rigorous, aggressive public health — what I like to say, block and tackle, block and tackle, block and tackle, block and tackle," he said. "That means if you find a new case, you isolate it."

But the Seattle Flu Study illustrates how existing regulations and red tape — sometimes designed to protect privacy and health — have impeded the rapid rollout of testing nationally, while other countries ramped up much earlier and faster. Faced with a public health emergency on a scale potentially not seen in a century, the United States has not responded nimbly.

The C.D.C.'s own effort to create a system for monitoring the virus around the country, using established government surveillance networks for the flu, has not yet built steam. And as late as last week, after expanding authorizations for commercial and academic institutions to make tests, administration officials provided conflicting accounts of when a significant increase in tests would be available.

In states like Maine, Missouri and Michigan, where there are few or no known infections, state public health officials say they have more than enough tests to meet demand.

But it remains unclear how many Americans have been tested for the coronavirus. The C.D.C. says approximately 8,500 specimens or nose swabs have been taken since the beginning of the outbreak — a figure that is almost certainly larger than the number of people tested since one person can have multiple swabs. By comparison, South Korea, which discovered its first case around the same time as the United States, has reported having the capacity to test roughly 10,000 people a day since late February.

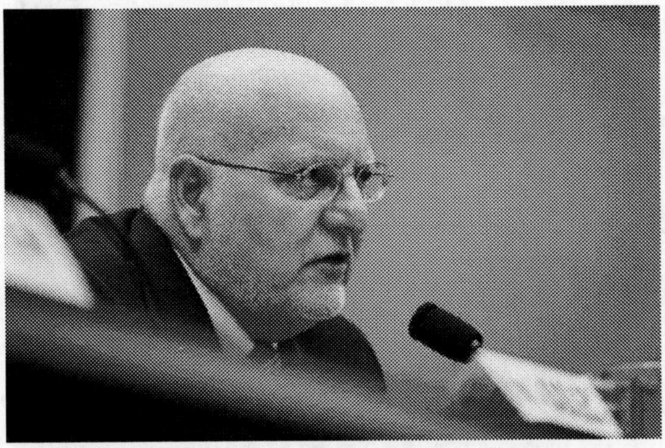

Dr. Robert Redfield, director of the Centers for Disease Control and Prevention, insisted that despite the rocky start, there was still time to beat back the coronavirus in the United States. T.J. Kirkpatrick for The New York Times.

A Prime Mission

As soon as the genetic sequence of the coronavirus was published in January, the C.D.C.'s first job was to develop a diagnostic test. "That's our prime mission," Dr. Redfield said, "to get eyes on this thing."

The agency also released criteria for deciding which individuals should be tested for the virus — at first only those who had a fever and respiratory issues and had traveled from the outbreak's origin in Wuhan, China.

The criteria were so strict that the sick man in the Seattle area who had visited Wuhan did not meet it. Still, worried state health officials pushed to get him checked, and the C.D.C. agreed. Local officials sent a sample to Atlanta and the results came back positive.

Officials monitored 70 people who were in contact with the man, including 50 who consented to getting nose swabs, and none tested positive for the coronavirus. But there was still the possibility that someone had been missed, said Dr. Scott Lindquist, the state epidemiologist for communicable diseases.

Around this time, the Washington State Department of Health began discussions with the Seattle Flu Study already going on in the state.

But there was a hitch: The flu project primarily used research laboratories, not clinical ones, and its coronavirus test was not approved by the Food and Drug Administration. And so the group was not certified to provide test results to anyone outside of their own investigators. They began discussions with state, C.D.C. and F.D.A. officials to figure out a solution, according to emails and interviews.

Dr. Scott F. Dowell, a former high-ranking C.D.C. official and a current deputy director at the Bill & Melinda Gates Foundation, which funds the Seattle Flu Study, asked for help from the leaders of the C.D.C.'s coronavirus response. "Hoping there is a solution," he wrote on Feb. 10.

The Coronavirus Outbreak

Latest Updates ›
Updated 36 minutes ago

- Iran will receive a shipment of the Russian coronavirus vaccine, the Islamic Republic's first. The Covid Tracking Project, a trusted source of data, will end on March 7.
- California prison authorities created a 'public health disaster' at San Quentin, a watchdog report says.

Later, Dr. Lindquist, the state epidemiologist in Washington, wrote an email to Dr. Alicia Fry, the chief of the C.D.C.'s epidemiology and prevention branch, requesting the study be used to test for the coronavirus.

C.D.C. officials repeatedly said it would not be possible. "If you want to use your test as a screening tool, you would have to check with F.D.A.," Gayle Langley, an officer at the C.D.C.'s National Center for Immunization and Respiratory Disease, wrote back in an email on Feb. 16. But the F.D.A. could not offer the approval because the lab was not certified as a clinical laboratory under regulations established by the Centers for Medicare & Medicaid Services, a process that could take months.

Dr. Chu and Dr. Lindquist tried repeatedly to wrangle approval to use the Seattle Flu Study. The answers were always no.

"We felt like we were sitting, waiting for the pandemic to emerge," Dr. Chu said. "We could help. We couldn't do anything."

Sense of Exasperation

As Washington State debated with the federal officials over what to do, the C.D.C. confronted the daunting task of testing more widely for the coronavirus.

The C.D.C. had designed its own test as it typically does during an outbreak. Several other countries also developed their own tests.

But when the C.D.C. shipped test kits to public labs across the country, some local health officials began reporting that the test was producing invalid results.

The C.D.C. promised that replacement kits would be distributed within days, but the problem stretched on for over two weeks. Only five state laboratories were able to test in that period. Washington and New York were not among them.

By Feb. 24, as new cases of the virus began popping up in the United States, the state labs were growing frantic.

The Association of Public Health Laboratories made what it called an "extraordinary and rare request" of Dr. Stephen Hahn, the commissioner of the F.D.A., asking him to use his discretion to allow state and local public health laboratories to create their own tests for the virus.

The Coronavirus Outbreak

Let Us Help You Better Understand the Coronavirus

- Are coronavirus case counts rising in your region? Our maps will help you determine how your state, county or country is fairing.
- Vaccines are rolling out and will reach many of us by spring. We've answered some common questions about the vaccines.
- Now that we are all getting used to living in a pandemic, you may have new questions about how to go about your routine safely, how your children will be impacted, how to travel and more. We're answering those questions as well.
- So far, the coronavirus outbreak has sickened more than 95 million people globally. More than 2 million people have died. A timeline of the events that led to these numbers may help you understand how we got here.

"We are now many weeks into the response with still no diagnostic or surveillance test available outside of C.D.C. for the vast majority of our member laboratories," Scott Becker, the chief executive of the association, wrote in a letter to Dr. Hahn.

Dr. Hahn responded two days later, saying in a letter that "false diagnostic test results can lead to significant adverse public health consequences" and that the laboratories were welcome to submit their own tests for emergency authorization.

But the approval process for laboratory-developed tests was proving onerous. Private and university clinical laboratories, which typically have the latitude to develop their own tests, were frustrated about the speed of the F.D.A. as they prepared applications for emergency approvals from the agency for their coronavirus tests.

Dr. Alex Greninger, an assistant professor at the University of Washington Medical Center in Seattle, said he became exasperated in mid-February as he communicated with the F.D.A. over getting his application ready to begin testing. "This virus is faster than the F.D.A.," he said, adding that at one point the agency required him to submit materials through the mail in addition to over email.

New tests typically require validation — running the test on known positive samples from a patient or a copy of the virus genome. The F.D.A.'s process called for five. Obtaining such samples has been hard because most hospital labs have not seen coronavirus cases yet, said Dr. Karen Kaul, chair of the department of pathology and laboratory medicine at NorthShore University HealthSystem in Illinois.

She said she had to scramble to obtain virus RNA from a laboratory in Europe. "Everyone is trying to figure out what we can get to help us gather the data that we need," she said.

The F.D.A. has disputed that it moved too slowly, saying that it provided emergency authorization for two laboratory-developed tests within 24 hours of a completed submission — one was the C.D.C.'s test and the other a test developed by New York's Wadsworth laboratory after it had trouble verifying the C.D.C.'s test.

'What Do We Do?'

On the other side of the country in Seattle, Dr. Chu and her flu study colleagues, unwilling to wait any longer, decided to begin running samples.

A technician in the laboratory of Dr. Lea Starita who was testing samples soon got a hit.

"I'm like, 'Oh my God,'" Dr. Starita said. "I just took off running" to the office of the study's program managers. "We got one," she told them. "What do we do?"

Members of the research group discussed the ethics of what to do next.

"What we were allowed to do was to keep it to ourselves," Dr. Chu said. "But what we felt like we needed to do was to tell public health." They decided the right thing to do was to inform local health officials.

The case was a teenager, in the same county where the first coronavirus case had surfaced, who had a flu swab just a few days before but had no travel history and no link to any known case.

The state laboratory, finally able to begin testing, confirmed the result the next morning. The teenager, who had recovered from his illness, was located and informed just after he entered his school building. He was sent home and the school was later closed as a precaution.

Later that day, the investigators and Seattle health officials gathered with representatives of the C.D.C. and the F.D.A. to discuss what happened. The message from the federal government was blunt. "What they said on that phone call very clearly was cease and desist to Helen Chu," Dr. Lindquist remembered. "Stop testing."

A Silent Spread

Still, the troubling finding reshaped how officials understood the outbreak. Seattle Flu Study scientists quickly sequenced the genome of the virus, finding a genetic variation also present in the country's first coronavirus case.

The implications were unnerving. There was a good chance that the virus had been circulating silently in the community for around six weeks, infecting potentially hundreds of people.

On a phone call the day after the C.D.C. and F.D.A. had told Dr. Chu to stop, officials relented, but only partially, the researchers recalled. They would allow the study's laboratories to test cases and report the results only in future samples. They would need to use a new consent form that explicitly mentioned that results of the coronavirus tests might be shared with the local health department.

They were not to test the thousands of samples that had already been collected.

The same day, the F.D.A. said it would relax its rules and allow clinical labs to begin using their own coronavirus tests as long as they submitted evidence that they worked to the agency. Under that new policy, according to an agency representative on Tuesday, it had heard from 14 labs, with 10 already beginning patient testing.

On March 2, the Seattle Flu Study's institutional review board at the University of Washington determined that it would be unethical for the researchers not to test and report the results in a public health emergency, Dr. Starita said. Since then, her laboratory has found and reported numerous additional cases, all of which have been confirmed.

As new samples came in, Dr. Starita's laboratory also worked their way backward through some older samples that had been sitting in the freezers for weeks, finding cases that date back to at least Feb. 20 — seven days before public health officials had any idea the virus was in the community.

The scientists said they believe that they will find evidence that the virus was infecting people even earlier, and that they could have alerted authorities sooner if they had been allowed to test.

But on Monday night, state regulators, enforcing Medicare rules, stepped in and again told them to stop until they could finish getting certified as a clinical laboratory, a process that could take many weeks.

In the days since the teenager's test, the Seattle region has spun into crisis, with dozens of people testing positive and at least 22 dying — many of them infected in a nursing home that had unknowingly been suffering casualties since Feb. 19.

The availability of testing for coronavirus remains uneven, with some people able to easily obtain tests in certain parts of the country while others have been turned away. Some state officials fear that the virus is spreading far faster than the capacity for testing is increasing.

Looking back, Dr. Chu said she understood why the regulations that stymied the flu study's efforts for weeks existed. "Those protections are in place for a reason," she said. "You want to protect human subjects. You want to do things in an ethical way."

The frustration, she said, was how long it took to cut through red tape to try to save lives in an outbreak that had the potential to explode in Washington State and spread in many other regions. "I don't think people knew that back then," she said. "We know it now."

Reporting was contributed by Nicholas Bogel-Burroughs, Joseph Goldstein, Sheila Kaplan, Michael D. Shear, Knvul Sheikh, Katie Thomas and Noah Weiland.

Months into Virus Crisis, U.S. Cities Still Lack Testing Capacity

With cases surging, some cities are seeing long testing lines and slow results.

By Sarah Mervosh and Manny Fernandez
Published July 6, 2020 Updated July 15, 2020

Lines for coronavirus tests have stretched around city blocks and tests ran out altogether in at least one site on Monday, new evidence that the country is still struggling to create a sufficient testing system months into its battle with Covid-19.

At a testing site in New Orleans, a line formed at dawn. But city officials ran out of tests five minutes after the doors opened at 8 a.m., and many people had to be turned away.

In Phoenix, where temperatures have topped 100 degrees, residents have waited in cars for as long as eight hours to get tested.

And in San Antonio and other large cities with mounting caseloads of the virus, officials have reluctantly announced new limits to testing: The demand has grown too great, they say, so only people showing symptoms may now be tested — a return to restrictions that were in place in many parts of the country during earlier days of the virus.

"It's terrifying, and clearly an evidence of a failure of the system," said Dr. Morgan Katz, an infectious disease expert at Johns Hopkins Hospital.

In the early months of the nation's outbreak, testing posed a significant problem, as supplies fell far short and officials raced to understand how to best handle the virus. Since then, the

United States has vastly ramped up its testing capability, conducting nearly 15 million tests in June, about three times as many as it had in April. But in recent weeks, as cases have surged in many states, the demand for testing has soared, surpassing capacity and creating a new testing crisis.

In many cities, officials said a combination of factors was now fueling the problem: a shortage of certain supplies, backlogs at laboratories that process the tests, and skyrocketing growth of the virus as cases climb in almost 40 states and the nation approaches a grim new milestone of three million total cases.

Fast, widely available testing is crucial to controlling the virus over the long term in the United States, experts say, particularly as the country reopens. With a virus that can spread through asymptomatic people, screening large numbers of people is seen as essential to identifying those who are carrying the virus and helping stop them from spreading it to others.

But the images of long lines at testing sites and complaints from mayors about the lack of a coordinated, overarching federal testing system have placed the White House on the defensive.

President Trump tweeted on Monday that "our great testing program continues to lead the World, by FAR!" Vice President Mike Pence said last week that the country had so improved its testing capacity that "we will literally test anyone who comes into a testing site or comes to their local pharmacy."

A spokeswoman for the Department of Health and Human Services said federal officials had been working closely with states to develop and meet testing goals since early April. So far, she said, the federal government has distributed about 26 million swabs nationwide, among other equipment, and was on track to "meet all the needs for July."

But testing in the United States has not kept pace with other countries, notably in Asia, which have been more aggressive. Chinese officials who were monitoring infections in Wuhan, where the pandemic began, tested 6.5 million people in a matter of days in May.

In Arizona, where reported cases have grown to more than 100,000, a shortage of testing has alarmed local officials, who say they feel ill-equipped to help residents on their own.

"The United States of America needs a more robust national testing strategy," Mayor Kate Gallego of Phoenix said in an interview.

Ms. Gallego, a Democrat, said she had been scrambling to lobby for help from anyone she could think of — the federal government, private companies like Walgreens, even a middle school friend who works at a European testing company. As the crisis has intensified in her state in recent weeks, she suggested that testing resources could be shifted from states with decreasing needs to those struggling like hers.

Arizona once had a stockpile of supplies, state officials say, but the surge in cases since Memorial Day has drained even basic items for testing, like swabs.

"That really speaks to the national and global supply chain issues," said Daniel Ruiz, Arizona's chief operating officer. "It's not that these things are in a warehouse ready to be delivered."

All along, the United States has struggled with issues tied to testing. In February, the federal government shipped a tainted testing kit to states, delaying a broader testing strategy and leaving states blind to a virus that was already beginning to circulate. Later, testing supplies became a choke point, and states called on the federal government to use the Defense Production Act to force additional production.

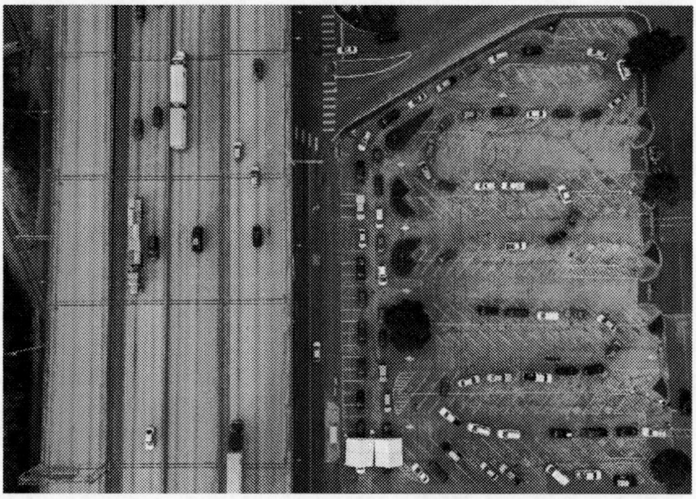

Vehicles snaked through a drive-through coronavirus testing site last week in Austin, Texas. Tamir Kalifa for The New York Times.

The Coronavirus Outbreak

Latest Updates
Updated 3 hours ago

- Some states in the U.S. are pulling back vaccine doses from the federal program for nursing homes.
- New data on the AstraZeneca-Oxford vaccine lend support for delaying its second doses.
- Cuomo expands vaccine eligibility in New York to include restaurant workers.

Many places have been able to overcome some of the supply constraints that defined the earlier days of the outbreak, in part with their own resources. New York City, once faced with severe shortages as an epicenter of the virus, is now testing 30,000 people a day, officials say, an expansion that included the city building its own testing kits and partnering with private labs.

But even as Gov. Andrew M. Cuomo announced last week that anyone in New York State who wanted a test could get one, officials in other states have been left seeking a more robust testing system, and setting new limits on who can take one.

"We are too fragmented," said Dr. Michael Mina, an assistant professor of epidemiology at Harvard's T.H. Chan School of Public Health. "We don't have a good way to load-balance the system."

Testing delays and shortages have increasingly become a problem in Texas, where cases are surging.

Cities like San Antonio and Austin have reverted to testing only those who are showing symptoms as a way to manage the demand and a backlog of tests.

"We're now focused on the highest priorities," Mayor Steve Adler of Austin said on Monday.

Mr. Adler, a Democrat, said the testing crunch was the result of the demand for tests statewide, brought on by the uptick in coronavirus cases after Texas reopened in fast-moving phases starting on May 1. He attributed the problem in large part to a backlog at laboratories; in some cases, test results take four to six days, far longer than the 24 hours health experts recommend to most effectively isolate the ill and track people they have had contact with.

Local officials in Austin had not relied on the state when it came to testing for the most part, the mayor said. And without a national testing program, he said, city and county officials had to fend for themselves in the private market.

"Maybe in retrospect if we had thought about this a half-year ago, we would have set up our own testing capacity," Mr. Adler said. "I don't know what else we'd do. We were out competing for tests. We were blocking up as many tests as we could block up on the market."

Mr. Adler said the testing system needed to be federalized, so that Austin and other cities would not have to compete for testing labs and supplies with other cities and other states.

The Coronavirus Outbreak

Let Us Help You Better Understand the Coronavirus

- Are coronavirus case counts rising in your region? Our maps will help you determine how your state, county or country is fairing.
- Vaccines are rolling out and will reach many of us by spring. We've answered some common questions about the vaccines.
- Now that we are all getting used to living in a pandemic, you may have new questions about how to go about your routine safely, how your children will be impacted, how to travel and more. We're answering those questions as well.
- So far, the coronavirus outbreak has sickened more than 95 million people globally. More than 2 million people have died. A timeline of the events that led to these numbers may help you understand how we got here.

The problem extends far beyond Texas and Arizona, among the hot spots that have led the country in rising cases in recent weeks.

In Idaho, where cases were also climbing, the state lab was so inundated that state officials sent a memo to nursing homes and long-term care facilities, saying the state could no longer meet all their testing needs. That has left the facilities in a crisis, desperate to find other labs to process tests for a particularly vulnerable population.

"Everyone is scrambling," said Robert Vande Merwe, the executive director of the Idaho Health Care Association.

Louisiana has also seen testing delays.

Dr. Jennifer Avegno, the director of the New Orleans Health Department, said the problem her agency was seeing now was different than the one it experienced in March, when states competed over swabs and test tubes. Now the problem is a shortage of reagents, she said, which are the chemical ingredients needed to detect whether the coronavirus is present in a sample.

The supply chain issues have led officials in New Orleans to reduce the tests they carry out: At one site on Monday, officials handed out just 150 tickets for testing, which were gone in minutes.

"We are telling everyone to do all the things you are supposed to do, and if they have any concerns about exposure or close contact or are feeling sick, there will be a test for you," Dr. Avegno said.

"And yet we're starting to have to turn them away," she said. "That is not what we want to do."

A locked testing site at Dillard University in New Orleans on Monday afternoon. All tests available were reserved before 8:15 a.m. Emily Kask for The New York Times

The urgent demand for tests also was affecting regions outside of those hardest hit.

In Omaha, a drive-through testing site in the parking lot of a former grocery store abruptly closed on Saturday.

Lab supplies fell short in the city, partly because they were needed in communities with bigger outbreaks than in Nebraska, where cases are prevalent but remain steady.

"We're getting put down on the priority list," said Dr. Anne O'Keefe, senior epidemiologist with the Douglas County Health Department in Omaha, citing a decision by the manufacturers of high-volume testing machines to prioritize supplies for those machines for other states before Nebraska.

The site in Omaha had tested nearly 3,500 people since it opened on June 17. Officials said they did not know when it would reopen.

"We really wanted to provide that extra capacity, to give people better options," Dr. O'Keefe said. "We're very, very disappointed that we can't do it."

Reporting was contributed by Mike Baker, Kimiko de Freytas-Tamura, Sheryl Gay Stolberg, Zolan Kanno-Youngs, Katie Rogers, Mark Walker and Elizabeth Williamson.

Health Workers Still Face Shortages of Critical Medical Supplies

January 26, 2021, 5:10 AM ET
Heard on Morning Edition
Yuki Noguchi

Since the start of the coronavirus pandemic, personal protective equipment, or PPE, has been in short supply. Exam gloves currently top the ever-changing list. What's holding up the supply?

Sarah Mccammon, Host

First, it was medical masks, then oxygen tanks and plastic pipette tips. Pandemic shortages have sent the country's hospitals, workers, labs and consumers scouring for critical medical supplies, and that does not include the shortage of vaccine. Many of those supplies are made overseas, and manufacturers are scrambling, too. NPR consumer health correspondent Yuki Noguchi joins us now to talk about why we're still facing shortages all these months later. Hi, Yuki.

YUKI NOGUCHI, BYLINE: Good morning.

MCCAMMON: So which supplies are the hardest to come by right now?

NOGUCHI: Well, you know, that list keeps evolving. But right now I'm hearing most about exam gloves. Also, sterilized water and portable oxygen cylinders are hard to find, particularly where COVID is sending a lot of people to the hospital because those are items that are used for respiratory treatment, and those supplies, you know, obviously become stressed when there's a lot of people in the hospital. But there's also stuff used in labs, like plastic pipette tips. You wouldn't normally think of that. So sometimes it's just the piece parts that are in short supply, but that affects a lot of other things. So now that mass vaccinations are about to get underway, that could also lead to different shortages of other items.

MCCAMMON: OK, President Biden invoked the Defense Production Act to compel companies to make more of these medical supplies. Is that going to solve this?

NOGUCHI: Well, you know, that prioritizes U.S. production of supplies, and government agencies have been using that since March, but it's just not a fast fix for a lot of things. Companies are already trying to boost production, and they have been; it's just that the crush of demand is global and sustained, and it's just very hard to meet that kind of demand. You need access to raw materials, and sometimes in order to make more, you need to make a factory first. So the situation with gloves, for example, the rubber components are running low, plus the machines to make them can take two years to build.

So David Hargraves is an executive at Premier, which buys medical products for, like, 40% of the country's hospitals, and he told me this.

DAVID HARGRAVES: There'll be new capacity that'll come online in 2022. Prices then should start to fall. But for this year, we've been urging our members to conserve the gloves they have.

MCCAMMON: So more factories have to be built to make the things that need to be made. Will any of those be here in the U.S.?

NOGUCHI: I think there's, you know, definitely domestic ramp-up here, and that may continue. But, you know, that's reversing a very long trend where we've come to rely on cheaper Asian medical supplies. And when that became unreliable, you know, to start the pandemic, everyone in America went looking for local suppliers. But there just aren't a lot of them.

And I talked to one of them, Prestige Ameritech. It has a factory in Texas making N95 respirators. Those are those molded medical masks that filter the virus. I think this company story's, especially over the last year, is really instructive. And I first talked to the co-owner, Mike Bowen, in February of last year. At the time, of course, supply of N95s were critically low, and the U.S. at the time only had 17 COVID cases. But nearly 3,000 Chinese people had died, and China stopped exporting N95s.

(SOUNDBITE OF ARCHIVED NPR BROADCAST)

MIKE BOWEN: We got a request for maybe a billion and a half masks, if you added up all the requests that I've got.

NOGUCHI: A billion and a half - wow. BOWEN: Yeah.

NOGUCHI: Hospitals, clinics and average people were begging him for supply.

BOWEN: Scared Americans and moms and old people and people saying, help me.

NOGUCHI: This might sound like a huge business windfall, but in fact, the overwhelming demand put Bowen in a tough spot. In order to make more masks, he needed to build more custom machines, each costing as much as a million dollars. But he couldn't justify spending that if American hospitals simply went back to buying much cheaper Chinese masks after the pandemic. Bowen had learned that lesson the hard way. A decade earlier, during the H1N1 flu pandemic, he boosted capacity. Afterward, business dried up as abruptly as it spiked, and Prestige nearly folded. So I recently reached back out to Bowen to see where things stood. Turns out his frantic pace hasn't abated.

BOWEN: Sorry, I'm out of breath.

NOGUCHI: Prestige since tripled its staff. It struck multiyear deals with U.S. hospitals. That helped fund nine new mask machines, and it now makes 80 times as many N95s, all earmarked for U.S. hospital workers.

BOWEN: We were selling 75,000 respirators a month. We're now selling 6 million, and we have another 4 million coming on board.

NOGUCHI: The last year, he says, has felt like five.

BOWEN: It's been the craziest year of my life. I mean, I'm in a movie. How weird is that?

NOGUCHI: We'll get to his Hollywood turn in a minute. Meanwhile, his business has seen lots of plot twists and villains. Fraudulent mask upstarts, Bowen says, sprouted everywhere.

BOWEN: For the last year, everybody's been able to sell anything that looks like a mask.

NOGUCHI: And not just copycat masks. Bowen himself had a fake replica. BOWEN: There's a Mike Bowen LinkedIn right now. It's not me.

NOGUCHI: Fighting fakes sucked up precious time.

BOWEN: Our website was copied by somebody in India. Several months ago, I was getting calls from people saying, we're about to wire you $1.6 million. Can you make sure it's you? And I said, it's not me - you're being scammed.

NOGUCHI: What irks Bowen most is that he predicted this crisis. Over 13 years, he wrote dozens of letters to presidents and federal officials warning of vulnerabilities in the U.S. supply chain. A pandemic, he told them, would put health workers and the public at risk. As recently as January a year ago, as COVID raged in China, Bowen frantically warned the Trump administration of a coming mask shortage. He says he was ignored. Now, of course, everyone's paying attention. Congress called Bowen to testify in May. He's even featured in the documentary "Totally under Control," about the Trump administration's pandemic response.

(SOUNDBITE OF DOCUMENTARY, "TOTALLY UNDER CONTROL")

BOWEN: I thought, you know, if I contact enough people in the administration, somebody, one of these people, are going to look at this and go, hey, this is a problem - maybe we ought to call this guy. And no, I couldn't get any - I didn't get any response there.

NOGUCHI: And the drama isn't over. Bowen worries the last year still hasn't changed how hospitals and government think about medical supply.

BOWEN: The entire supply could fail catastrophically if they continue to buy most of their products from outside the United States because when there's a pandemic, countries take care of themselves.

MCCAMMON: OK, Yuki, that raises an interesting question. What would the U.S. government need to change in order to avoid a situation like this in the future?

NOGUCHI: Well, it needs to start with mapping the supply chain, you know, detailed accounting of where and how our medical supplies are made. Right now there's no arm of government that really tracks that. And when you know that, then you can take steps to diversify the sources so the country's less susceptible to major disruptions like these.

MCCAMMON: That's NPR consumer health correspondent Yuki Noguchi. Thanks so much.

NOGUCHI: Thank you, Sarah.

(SOUNDBITE OF HELIOS' "ISOSTACY")

NPR transcripts are created on a rush deadline by Verb8tm, Inc., an NPR contractor, and produced using a proprietary transcription process developed with NPR. Accuracy and availability may vary. The authoritative record of NPR's programming is the audio record.

Oxygen Supply Shortages Bedevil Hospitals Already Overwhelmed by COVID-19 Patients

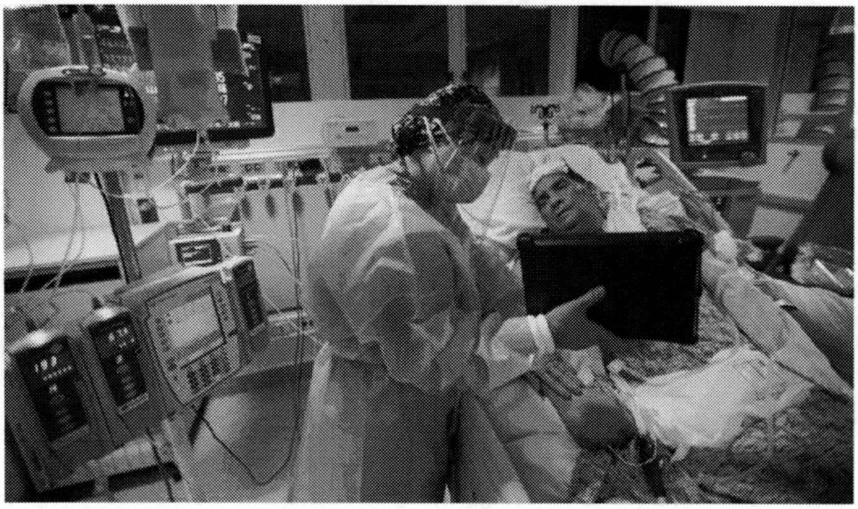

Nurse Kat Yi holds an iPad up to Eduardo Rojas, 50, so that his wife can talk to him at Providence St. Jude Medical Center in Fullerton on Christmas Day. (Francine Orr/Los Angeles Times).

By Rong-Gong Lin Ii, Luke Money, Hayley Smith
Dec. 29, 2020 4 AM PT

One of the myriad challenges facing Southern California's medical system, which is overwhelmed by COVID-19 patients, involves one of the most basic staples of any hospital.

Oxygen

Officials are having problems getting the amount of oxygen needed by critically ill COVID-19 patients who are struggling to breathe as their inflamed lungs are being damaged or destroyed.

Problems on Sunday caused at least five hospitals in L.A. County to declare an internal disaster, which closed the facilities to all ambulance traffic — not just certain types of ambulance patients, as is more typical.

It's not simply a shortage of oxygen itself, county and hospital officials say. There's a shortage of canisters, which patients need to return home, and aging hospital pipes are breaking down due to the huge amounts of oxygen needed to be distributed around the hospital.

There are two problems with the distribution of oxygen at aging hospitals.

First, there are so many patients needing a high rate of oxygen that the system cannot maintain the sufficient pressure needed in the pipes.

The second is that there is such high flow through the pipes that they freeze, "and obviously, if it freezes, then you can't have good flow of oxygen," said Dr. Christina Ghaly, L.A. County health services director.

Some hospitals are forced to move patients to lower floors, because it's easier to deliver oxygen there without needing the pressure to push it up to higher floors, Ghaly said.

California Coronavirus Hospitalizations

The number of hospital patients with a confirmed case

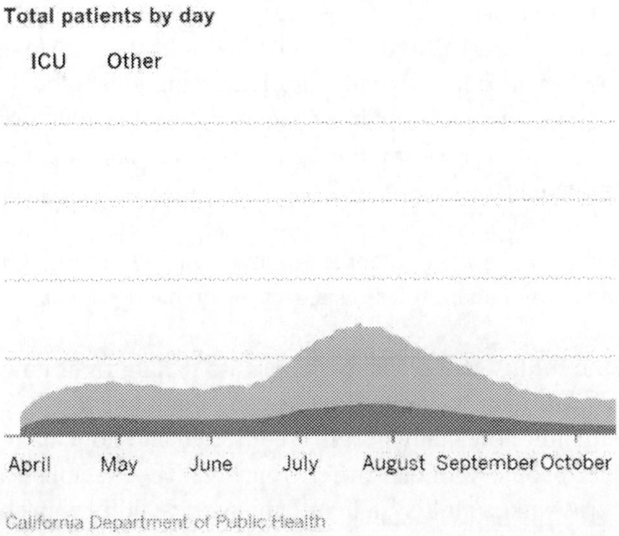

Memorial Hospital of Gardena is one of the centers facing oxygen issues. Chief Executive Kevan Metcalfe said the hospital has run low on oxygen.

If it runs out, the hospital would be in "deep, deep trouble," he said.

Doctors and nurses have learned since the early days of the pandemic to, as much as possible, avoid placing patients on ventilators, which involves sticking a breathing tube down the throat.

Many patients instead receive a high-flow oxygen treatment, in which oxygen is sent through plastic tubes placed in the nose.

While a non-COVID patient may receive six liters of oxygen per minute, COVID-19 patients need 60 to 80 liters a minute. So now, hospitals need far more oxygen than they did before.

One of the biggest concerns facing hospitals is that more patients are on the way.

The COVID-19 patients in the hospital now reflect coronavirus cases diagnosed two weeks earlier — a time at which L.A. County was averaging 11,000 new cases a day. That number has swelled since then — up to nearly 14,800 new cases a day for the seven-day period that ended Dec. 22 — before declining slightly to 14,000 cases a day as of Monday night.

That means hospitals are still expecting to see increasing demand into the new year because of infections that took place before Christmas. About 10% of people who test positive for the coronavirus in L.A. County end up needing hospital treatment.

Barbara Ferrer, L.A. County's public health director, said "all indicators tell us that our situation may only get worse as we begin 2021. The rate of community transmission remains extraordinarily high.... As cases continue to remain at these alarmingly high levels, hundreds more people are likely to die."

She added: "We all need to give our hospitals a fighting chance to handle the flood of COVID-19 patients that are arriving every single day."

The pace of the fall and winter surge has been staggering. On Nov. 1, L.A. County was averaging about 1,300 coronavirus cases a day on a weekly basis; L.A. County is now averaging 14,000 cases a day. The daily rate at which coronavirus test results are coming back positive is now 17% in L.A. County, more than quadruple the comparable figure Nov. 1, when the positivity rate was less than 4%.

L.A. County is now averaging about 90 COVID-19 deaths a day over the last week, one of the highest such numbers during the pandemic. The county death toll as of Monday night was 9,564, according to an independent Times count of local health jurisdictions; Ferrer said Monday that her agency is still sorting through a reporting backlog and it expects to add 432 deaths, pushing the death toll closer to 10,000.

County Supervisor Hilda Solis urged people against thinking that nothing could be done about the pandemic, and she asked people to stay home. A coronavirus test that shows up negative can easily become meaningless as a person can be infected and contagious by the time the results come back.

"I understand the futility that so many people are feeling right now — the idea that some people just want to throw their hands up. But we can't think like that," Solis said. "It's squarely within our control to limit how many people are infected and how many people can die.

It isn't just older people who can suffer from COVID-19, Solis said; a child this month died of the coronavirus-linked multisystem inflammatory syndrome in children, known as MIS-C, in L.A. County. There have been at least 51 cases of MIS-C in the county — all requiring hospitalization, with half treated in intensive care units. Latino children accounted for nearly three-quarters of those cases.

Ferrer said L.A. County has run 29 coronavirus samples for a genetic analysis, and none have been positive for the potentially more contagious variant of the coronavirus identified in Britain. Although there's a high probability the variant is here, she said, it doesn't appear to be dominant.

"Whether the variant is here or isn't here, the steps we need to take are exactly the same," Ferrer said.

The Stories Shaping California

Rong-Gong Lin II is a metro reporter based in San Francisco who specializes in covering statewide earthquake safety issues and the COVID-19 pandemic. The Bay Area native is a graduate of UC Berkeley and started at the Los Angeles Times in 2004.

Luke Money is a Metro reporter covering breaking news at the Los Angeles Times. He previously was a reporter and assistant city editor for the Daily Pilot, a Times Community News publication in Orange County, and before that wrote for the Santa Clarita Valley Signal. He earned his bachelor's degree in journalism from the University of Arizona.

Hayley Smith is a Metro reporter covering breaking news for the Los Angeles Times. Previously she was an intern on The Times' COVID-19 team who contributed to "The

Pandemic's Toll: Lives Lost in California" in partnership with the Pulitzer Center and USC. She holds a master's degree in journalism from USC.

Coronavirus and Pandemic

- Got a COVID-19 vaccine? You still need a mask to visit Downtown Disneyland
- Capt. Tom Moore, WWII vet whose walk cheered U.K., dies at 100
- L.A. City Council backs $5-an-hour 'hero pay' raise for grocery, drugstore workers
- When your chance for a COVID-19 shot comes, don't worry which one it is
- Tracking ICU capacity in California

Warning of Shortages, Researchers Look to Stretch Vaccine Supply

The N.I.H. and Moderna are examining whether doses of Moderna's coronavirus vaccine can be halved to double the supply, while scientists look for other ways to extend availability.

By Sheryl Gay Stolberg and Sharon LaFraniere
Published Jan. 5, 2021 Updated Jan. 21, 2021

WASHINGTON — Federal officials and drugmakers, faced with a slower-than-expected rollout of the coronavirus vaccine, are racing to find ways to expand the supply, looking at lowering the required dosage and extracting more doses from the supplies they have.

Just weeks into the vaccine program, scientists at the National Institutes of Health and the drugmaker Moderna are analyzing data to see if they can double the supply of the company's coronavirus vaccine by cutting doses in half. The study, though long planned, is increasingly urgent in the face of looming shortages as the country tries to fight off a surging pandemic.

Officials are also rushing to find supplies of more efficient syringes that could extract an additional dose from vials of the Pfizer-BioNTech vaccine. That could bolster the Pfizer supply by 20 percent.

With more than 355,000 Americans already dead of Covid-19, nearly 21 million cases reported in the United States and hospitals overflowing, the need to inoculate people grows more urgent every day. The nation is facing twin problems. At the moment, it has only enough vaccine on order to cover 185 million Americans by the end of June. At the same time, doses that vaccine makers rushed out of their factories are sitting unused and are in danger of expiring.

The Trump administration has shipped more than 15 million vaccine doses, and millions more are already in the federal government's hands. Yet only 4.5 million people have received them so far. State and local public health officials, already overwhelmed with rising infections, are struggling to administer the vaccine to hospital workers and at-risk older Americans while most people remain in the dark about when they might be protected.

Countries in Europe are grappling with their own rocky vaccine rollouts, only adding to a sense of panic as a new, more contagious variant of the novel coronavirus spreads across the globe.

"The total supply of vaccine has always been a concern," said Dr. John R. Mascola, director of the N.I.H.'s Vaccine Research Center, adding, "It's important to do these analyses that we're doing, and have all that data in our pocket in the event that there's a need to use it."

The Moderna dosage research, which also involves scientists from Operation Warp Speed, the government's vaccine initiative, could take two months, said Dr. Mascola, who described the work in an interview Tuesday. Any dosing changes would have to be approved by the Food and Drug Administration.

For the moment, the biggest problem is not a shortage of vaccine, but the difficulties that state and local governments face in distributing the doses they have. But in interviews, both Dr. Mascola and Dr. Anthony S. Fauci, the government's top infectious disease expert, warned of possible shortages to come.

"To me, what appears to be the imminent problem that's right in front of us is getting people vaccinated with the doses that we have," Dr. Fauci said. "That could change."

Those struggles will be global. Already, Italy, Greece and other countries are reporting shortages of needles. Spain has not trained enough nurses. France has only managed to vaccinate around 7,000 people. Poland's program was rocked by scandal after it was revealed that celebrities were given preferential treatment. There are calls in Germany to take control over vaccine purchases from the European Union authorities. Nearly every country in Europe has complained about burdensome paperwork.

In Washington, congressional Democrats are demanding an explanation for vaccination delays. Senator Patty Murray of Washington, the top Democrat on the Senate Health Committee, said in an interview on Tuesday that states needed more support and guidance from the federal government — an issue she said she raised on Monday with Gen. Gustave F. Perna, the chief operating officer of Operation Warp Speed.

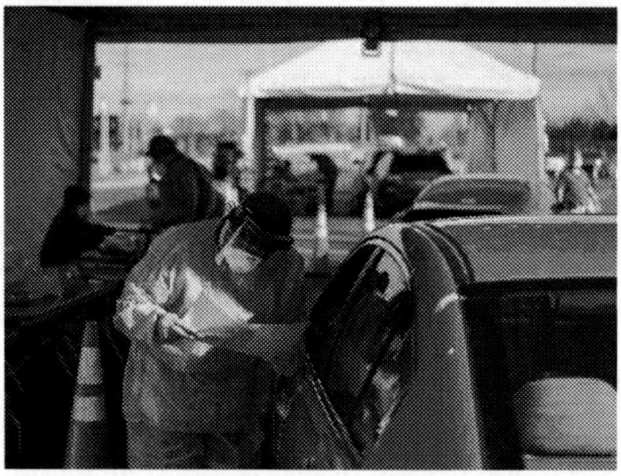

A testing site in Nashville in December. With more than 355,000 Americans already dead of Covid-19, and nearly 21 million cases reported in the United States, the need to inoculate people is becoming more urgent. William DeShazer for The New York Times.

President Trump "wants us all to just give him a lot of credit for having a vaccine this fast," Ms. Murray said. "But as the Trump administration has done with testing and everything else, it's, 'We did this — now it's up to the states.' Well, the states don't have capacity, and there isn't stability in the supply chain."

Dr. Jerome Adams, the surgeon general, conceded on Tuesday that the vaccine rollout was going slowly, and urged states not to stick rigidly to the Centers for Disease Control and Prevention guidelines about whom to vaccinate first. If fewer health care workers are willing to be vaccinated, he said, states should "move quickly to other priority groups," such as people older than 75 and essential workers.

"Your headline today really should be, 'Surgeon General Tells States and Governors to Move Quickly to Other Priority Groups,'" Dr. Adams said on NBC's "Today" show. "If the demand isn't there in 1a, go to 1b and continue on down. If the demand isn't there in one location, move those vaccines to another location."

Some states, like Texas and Florida, have already begun offering shots to people 65 and older who are not nursing home residents, and to those of any age with medical conditions that raise their risk of dying if they contract Covid-19. That has led to a desperate scramble among those eager to get vaccinated.

Covid-19 Vaccines: Answers to Your Vaccine Questions

Am I eligible for the Covid vaccine in my state?

Currently more than 150 million people — almost half the population — are eligible to be vaccinated. But each state makes the final decision about who goes first. The nation's 21 million health care workers and three million residents of long-term care facilities were the first to qualify. In mid-January, federal officials urged all states to open up eligibility to everyone 65 and older and to adults of any age with medical conditions that put them at high risk of becoming seriously ill or dying from Covid-19. Adults in the general population are at the back of the line. If federal and state health officials can clear up bottlenecks in vaccine distribution, everyone 16 and older will become eligible as early as this spring or early summer. The vaccine hasn't been approved in children, although studies are underway. It may be months before a vaccine is available for anyone under the age of 16. Go to your state health website for up-to-date information on vaccination policies in your area

- Is the vaccine free?
- Can I choose which vaccine I get?
- How long will the vaccine last? Will I need another one next year?
- Will my employer require vaccinations?
- Where can I find out more?

"People want to know: When is my turn? Is this happening? Where do I go?" Ms. Murray said.

Even if distribution kinks smooth out, a vaccine shortage looms in coming months because only two products so far — one developed by Moderna and the other by Pfizer-BioNTech — have been authorized for emergency use. Both vaccine makers have committed all their doses until midyear. That still leaves uncovered about 60 million of adult Americans eligible to be vaccinated.

Officials also have high hopes for a third, single-dose vaccine from Johnson & Johnson. The company is finishing its clinical trial this month and its vaccine could be authorized for emergency use in February. But even if it passes those tests, it is unclear how many more doses will be ready for distribution and by when.

With the proper syringes, federal officials hope to extract an extra dose from Pfizer's vials that were initially believed to contain only five doses, stretching Pfizer's vaccine further. But the government has yet to sign contracts to supply enough of those syringes, according to two experts familiar with the vaccine distribution system.

That has made the prospect of doubling the supply of Moderna doses that much more tantalizing. Dr. Moncef Slaoui, the head of Operation Warp Speed, said Sunday on the CBS program "Face the Nation" that data from Moderna's clinical trials demonstrated that people ages 18 to 55 who received two 50-microgram doses showed an "identical immune response" to the standard of two 100-microgram doses.

Both Dr. Mascola and Dr. Fauci confirmed that research.

But Dr. Slaoui went a step further, saying that the F.D.A. and Moderna were already discussing the possibility. The F.D.A. issued a statement on Monday that called the proposal "premature and not rooted solidly in the available science," although worthy of clinical research.

The finding Dr. Slaoui cited came from an early Phase 2 clinical trial, which involved 600 people and was meant to test only for immune response, and not for the effectiveness of the vaccine, according to Dr. Fauci and others. It compared the immune response in people given 50 micrograms with those given 100 micrograms.

The larger Phase 3 trial that found the vaccine was 94 percent effective involved 30,000 people, half of whom were given the 100-microgram dose and half of whom were given a placebo.

To provide the F.D.A. with the kind of data it would need to approve a change in dosing, scientists must first study blood samples from patients who participated in the Phase 3 trial to determine precisely what immune response correlates with protection against Covid-19.

Then, Dr. Mascola said, researchers would have to either look back at patients from the Phase 2 trial, or conduct a new one, to demonstrate that patients who received the 50-microgram dose developed the threshold immune response. If the results looked promising, he said, "all this then needs to be put together as a data package for review and discussion with F.D.A."

Because the vaccine was developed in a climate of intense partisan polarization, any effort to shift the dosing schedule must proceed cautiously and be balanced against the risk that it could scare those who have been hesitant to to be vaccinated, experts said.

"There would need to be a very strong rationale to shift off of the dose that was used in the study, and my concern would be that it would confuse people just as acceptance is increasing for a vaccine that's 95 percent effective," said Dr. Joshua M. Sharfstein, a former deputy commissioner of the F.D.A. who now teaches at the Johns Hopkins Bloomberg School of Public Health.

Dr. Richard E. Besser, a former acting director of the Centers for Disease Control and Prevention, said rigorous scientific research, clear communications about the findings and a public discussion by outside experts would be essential to making changes.

"Public trust is in short supply right now with these vaccines to begin with," he said, "and the more that there can be transparency around any changes to the approach to vaccination, the more you will be able to maintain and expand on that trust."

President Biden Announces American Rescue Plan

January 20, 2021

Legislation

Emergency Legislative Package to Fund Vaccinations, Provide Immediate, Direct Relief to Families Bearing the Brunt of the COVID-19 Crisis, and Support Struggling Communities

The COVID-19 pandemic and the corresponding economic crisis are devastating families across the country. More than 20 million Americans have contracted COVID-19, and at least

370,000 have died. From big cities to small towns, too many Americans are barely scraping by, or not scraping by at all. And the pandemic has shined a light on the persistence of racial injustice in our healthcare system and our economy. The need to act is clear in the lines at food banks, the small businesses that are closed or closing, and the growing number of Americans experiencing housing insecurity. After nearly a year of the public health crisis, our nation remains in this dark winter of the pandemic and facing a deep economic crisis.

President Biden is laying out the first step of an aggressive, two-step plan for rescue, from the depths of this crisis, and recovery, by investing in America, creating millions of additional good-paying jobs, combatting the climate crisis, advancing racial equity, and building back better than before.

While Congress's bipartisan action in December was a step in the right direction, it was only a down payment. It fell far short of the resources needed to tackle the immediate crisis. We are in a race against time, and absent additional government assistance, the economic and public health crises could worsen in the months ahead; schools will not be able to safely reopen; and vaccinations will remain far too slow.

As last month's jobs report underscored, the virus and our economy are intertwined. We cannot rescue our economy without containing this virus.

Today, President Biden is announcing the American Rescue Plan to change the course of the pandemic, build a bridge towards economic recovery, and invest in racial justice. The American Rescue Plan will address the stark, intergenerational inequities that have worsened in the wake of COVID-19. Researchers at Columbia University estimate that these proposals will cut child poverty in half.

Specifically, President Biden's American Rescue Plan will:

- Mount a national vaccination program, contain COVID-19, and safely reopen schools, including by setting up community vaccination sites nationwide, scaling up testing and tracing, eliminating supply shortage problems, investing in high-quality treatments, providing paid sick leave to contain spread of the virus, addressing health disparities, and making the necessary investments to meet the president's goal of safely reopening a majority of K-8 schools in the first 100 days.
- Deliver immediate relief to working families bearing the brunt of this crisis bysending $1,400 per-person checks to households across America, providing direct housing and nutrition assistance, expanding access to safe and reliable childcare and affordable healthcare, increasing the minimum wage, extending unemployment insurance, and giving families with kids and childless workers an emergency boost this year.
- Support communities that are struggling in the wake of COVID-19 by providing support for the hardest-hit small businesses, especially small businesses owned by entrepreneurs of color, and protecting the jobs of the first responders, transit workers, and other essential workers we depend on.

In addition to addressing the public health and economic crises head on, the President's plan will provide emergency funding to upgrade federal information technology infrastructure and address the recent breaches of federal government data systems. This is an urgent national security issue that cannot wait.

President Biden's $1.9 trillion American Rescue Plan is ambitious, but achievable, and will rescue the American economy and start beating the virus. Congress should act expeditiously to help working families, communities, and small businesses persevere through the pandemic.

This legislative package is needed now to address the immediate crises. In the coming weeks, President Biden will lay out his economic recovery plan to invest in America, create millions of additional good-paying jobs, combat the climate crisis, and build back better than before.

Mount a National Vaccination Program, Contain COVID-19, and Safely Reopen Schools

The pandemic is raging, with record high infection and death rates. A new strain of the virus that is even more contagious is appearing in communities across the country. Meanwhile, Americans are waiting to get their vaccines, even while doses are sitting on shelves. More than ten months into the pandemic, we still lack necessary testing capacity and are suffering from shortages of supplies like basic protective equipment for those on the front lines. Americans of color are being infected and are dying from COVID-19 at greater rates because of lasting systemic racism in our health care system. And, older Americans continue to suffer at disproportionate rates.

We can't wait to slow the spread of this virus. And, we can't fight this pandemic in fits and starts. President Biden is putting forward a comprehensive plan to deal with this crisis and launch a whole-of-government COVID-19 response plan that will change the course of the pandemic by ensuring we have necessary supplies and protective gear, increasing testing to mitigate spread, vaccinating the US population, safely reopening schools, and addressing COVID-19 health disparities.

To support this plan, President Biden is calling on Congress to provide the $160 billion in funding necessary to save American lives and execute on his plan to mount a national vaccination program, expand testing, mobilize a public health jobs program, and take other necessary steps to build capacity to fight the virus. He is also calling on Congress to ensure our schools have everything they need to safely reopen and to provide emergency paid leave so people can stay home when needed to help contain the spread of the virus. Altogether, this would put over $400 billion toward these critical measures for addressing COVID-19.

President Biden's rescue proposal will:

Mount a National Vaccination Program

Current vaccination efforts are not sufficient to quickly and equitably vaccinate the vast majority of the U.S. population. We must ensure that those on the ground have what they need to get vaccinations into people's arms. The president's proposal will invest $20 billion in a national vaccination program in partnership with states, localities, Tribes and territories. This will include launching community vaccination centers around the country and deploying mobile vaccination units to hard-to-reach areas. The Biden Administration will take action to ensure all people in the United States–regardless of their immigration status–can access the vaccine free-of-charge and without cost-sharing. To help states ensure that all Medicaid enrollees will be vaccinated, President Biden will also work with Congress to expand the Federal Medicaid Assistance Percentage (FMAP) to 100% for the administration of vaccines.

Scale up Testing to Stop the Spread of COVID, Safely Reopen Schools, and Protect at-Risk Populations

While we are working to vaccinate the population, we need to focus on what we know works. Testing is a critical strategy for controlling the spread of COVID-19, yet the U.S. is still not using it effectively. Despite innovations to improve testing, tests are still not widely available. The president's plan invests $50 billion in a massive expansion of testing, providing funds for the purchase of rapid tests, investments to expand lab capacity, and support to help schools and local governments implement regular testing protocols. Expanded testing will ensure that schools can implement regular testing to support safe reopening; that vulnerable settings like prisons and long-term care facilities can regularly test their populations; and that any American can get a test for free when they need one.

Mobilize a Public Health Jobs Program to Support COVID-19 Response

The president's plan includes an historic investment in expanding the public health workforce. This proposal will fund 100,000 public health workers, nearly tripling the country's community health roles. These individuals will be hired to work in their local communities to perform vital tasks like vaccine outreach and contact tracing in the near term, and to transition into community health roles to build our long-term public health capacity that will help improve quality of care and reduce hospitalization for low-income and underserved communities.

Address Health Disparities and COVID-19

While COVID-19 has devastated the entire country, it has hit some groups and communities of color much harder than others. President Biden is committed to addressing the disparities evident in the pandemic at every step, from ensuring equitable distribution of vaccines and supplies to expanding health care services for underserved communities. His proposal includes funding to provide health services for underserved populations, including expanding Community Health Centers and investing in health services on tribal lands. These funds will support the expansion of COVID treatment and care, as well as our ability to provide vaccination to underserved populations.

Protect Vulnerable Populations in Congregate Settings

Long-term care residents and workers account for almost 40% of all U.S. COVID-19 deaths. Further, African-American and Latina women, who have borne the brunt of the pandemic, are overrepresented among long-term care workers. The president's proposal provides critical funding for states to deploy strike teams to long-term care facilities experiencing COVID-19 outbreaks–which may impede vaccination of residents and workers–and to conduct better infection control oversight.

1 in 5 state and federal prisoners in the U.S. has had COVID-19, and African Americans and Latinos are overrepresented among incarcerated individuals. The proposal also supports COVID-19 safety in federal, state, and local prisons, jails, and detention centers by providing funding for COVID-19 mitigation strategies, including supplies and physical distancing; safe re-entry for the formerly incarcerated; and the vaccination of both incarcerated people and staff

.

Identify and Address Emerging Strains of COVID-19

The identification of new strains of SARS-CoV-2 in the United Kingdom and South Africa highlight a key vulnerability in our nation's COVID response: we simply do not have the kind of robust surveillance capabilities that we need to track outbreaks and mutations. Tracking the way the virus is changing and moving through the population is essential to understanding outbreaks, generating treatments and vaccines, and controlling the pandemic. The president's proposal includes funding to dramatically increase our country's sequencing, surveillance, and outbreak analytics capacity at the levels demanded by the crisis.

Provide Emergency Relief and Purchase Critical Supplies and Deploy National Guard

Persistent supply shortages – from gloves and masks to glass vials and test reagents – are inhibiting our ability to provide testing and vaccination and putting frontline workers at risk. The president's plan will invest $30 billion into the Disaster Relief Fund to ensure sufficient supplies and protective gear, and to provide 100% federal reimbursement for critical emergency response resources to states, local governments, and Tribes, including deployment of the National Guard. The president will call for an additional $10 billion investment in expanding domestic manufacturing for pandemic supplies. These funds will support President Biden in fulfilling his commitment to fully use the Defense Production Act and to safeguard the country by producing more pandemic supplies in the U.S.

Invest in Treatments for COVID-19

Months into this pandemic, we still do not have reliable and accessible treatments. The federal government urgently needs to invest to support development, manufacturing, and purchase of therapies to ensure wide availability and affordability of effective treatments, as well as invest in studies of the long-term health impacts of COVID-19 and potential therapies to address them.

Protect Workers against COVID-19

Millions of Americans, many of whom are people of color, immigrants, and low-wage workers, continue to put their lives on the line to keep the country functioning through the pandemic. They should not have to lie awake at night wondering if they'll make it home from work safely the next day, or if they'll bring home the virus to their loved ones and communities. The president is calling on Congress to authorize the Occupational Safety and Health Administration to issue a COVID-19 Protection Standard that covers a broad set of workers, so that workers not typically covered by OSHA, like many public workers on the frontlines, also receive protection from unsafe working conditions and retaliation. And, President Biden is calling on Congress to provide additional funding for OSHA enforcement and grant funding, including for the Susan Harwood grant program, for organizations to help keep vulnerable workers healthy and safe from COVID-19. These steps will help keep more workers healthy, reopen more businesses safely, and beat the virus.

Restore U.S. Leadership Globally and Build Better Preparedness

Protecting the United States from COVID-19 requires a global response, and the pandemic is a grave reminder that biological threats can pose catastrophic consequences to the United States and the world. The president's plan will provide $11 billion including to support to the international health and humanitarian response; mitigate the pandemic's devastating impact on global health, food security, and gender-based violence; support international efforts to develop and distribute medical countermeasures for COVID-19; and build the capacity required to fight COVID-19, its variants, and emerging biological threats.

Provide Schools the Resources They Need to Reopen Safely

A critical plank of President Biden's COVID-19 plan is to safely reopen schools as soon as possible – so kids and educators can get back in class and parents can go back to work. This will require immediate, urgent action by Congress. The COVID-19 pandemic created unprecedented challenges for K-12 schools and institutions of higher education, and the students and parents they serve. School closures have disproportionately impacted the learning of Black and Hispanic students, as well as students with disabilities and English language learners. While the December down payment for schools and higher education institutions was a start, it is not sufficient to address the crisis. President Biden is calling on Congress to provide $170 billion — supplemented by additional state and local relief resources — for K-12 schools and institutions of higher education. These resources will help schools serve all students, no matter where they are learning, and help achieve President Biden's goal to open the majority of K-8 schools within the first 100 days of his Administration.

- Provide $130 billion to help schools to safely reopen. Schools need flexible resources to safely reopen and operate and/or facilitate remote learning. The president's plan will provide $130 billion to support schools in safely reopening. These funds can be used to reduce class sizes and modify spaces so students and teachers can socially distance; improve ventilation; hire more janitors and implement mitigation measures; provide personal protective equipment; ensure every school has access to a nurse; increase transportation capacity to facilitate social distancing on the bus; hire counselors to support students as they transition back to the classroom; close the digital divide that is exacerbating inequities during the pandemic; provide summer school or other support for students that will help make up lost learning time this year; create and expand community schools; and cover other costs needed to support safely reopening and support students. These funds will also include provisions to ensure states adequately fund education and protect students in low-income communities that have been hardest hit by COVID-19. Districts must ensure that funds are used to not only reopen schools, but also to meet students' academic, mental health and social, and emotional needs in response to COVID-19, (e.g., through extended learning time, tutoring, and counselors), wherever they are learning. Funding can be used to prevent cuts to state pre-k programs. A portion of funding will be reserved for a COVID-19 Educational Equity Challenge Grant, which will support state, local and tribal governments in partnering with teachers, parents, and other stakeholders to advance equity- and evidence-based policies to respond to COVID-related educational challenges and give all students the support they need to succeed. In addition to this funding, schools will be able to access FEMA Disaster Relief Fund resources to get reimbursed for certain COVID-19 related expenses and will receive support to implement regular testing protocols.
- Expand the Higher Education Emergency Relief Fund. The president's plan will ensure colleges have critical resources to implement public health protocols, execute distance learning plans, and provide emergency grants to students in need. This $35

billion in funding will be directed to public institutions, including community colleges, as well as, public and private Historically Black Colleges and Universities and other Minority Serving Institutions. This funding will provide millions of students up to an additional $1,700 in financial assistance from their college.

- Hardest Hit Education Fund. Provide $5 billion in funds for governors to use to support educational programs and the learning needs of students significantly impacted by COVID-19, whether K-12, higher education, or early childhood education programs.

Provide Emergency Paid Leave to 106 Million More Americans to Reduce the Spread of the Virus

No American should have to choose between putting food on the table and quarantining to prevent further spread of COVID-19. And yet, nearly 1 in 4 workers and close to half of low-income workers lack access to paid sick leave, disproportionately burdening Americans of color. Lack of paid leave is threatening the financial security of working families and increasing the risk of COVID-19 infections, hospitalizations, and deaths. Congress did the right thing last year when it created an emergency paid leave program through the Families First Coronavirus Response Act. That action decreased daily infections by 400 cases per state per day in states that previously had no paid sick leave requirement. While the December down payment extended the Families First employer tax credits through March 2021, it did not renew the requirement that employers provide leave. President Biden is calling on Congress to:

- Put the requirement back in place and eliminate exemptions for employers with more than 500 and less than 50 employees. He will also make it clear that healthcare workers and first responders get these benefits, too. Closing these loopholes in the Families First Coronavirus Response Act will extend emergency paid leave to up to 106 million additional workers.
- Provide expanded paid sick and family and medical leave. The president will provide over 14 weeks of paid sick and family and medical leave to help parents with additional caregiving responsibilities when a child or loved one's school or care center is closed; for people who have or are caring for people with COVID-19 symptoms, or who are quarantining due to exposure; and for people needing to take time to get the vaccine.
- Expand emergency paid leave to include federal workers. This measure will provide paid leave protections to approximately 2 million Americans who work for the federal government.
- Provide a maximum paid leave benefit of $1,400 per-week for eligible workers. This will provide full wage replacement to workers earning up to $73,000 annually, more than three-quarters of all workers.
- Reimburse employers with less than 500 employees for the cost of this leave. Extending the refundable tax credit will reimburse employers for 100 percent of the cost of this leave.
- Reimburse state and local government for the cost of this leave.
- Extend emergency paid leave measures until September 30, 2021. With so much uncertainty surrounding the pandemic, extending paid leave until the end of September will help to limit the spread of COVID-19 and provide economic security to millions of working families.

Deliver Immediate, Direct Relief to Families Bearing the Brunt of the Crisis

As a result of the COVID-19 crisis, millions of Americans are hurting through no fault of their own. More than 10 million Americans are unemployed, and 4 million have been out of work for half a year or longer. The jobs crisis is particularly severe in communities of color, where 1 in 10 Black workers and 1 in 11 Latino workers are unemployed. Large numbers of families are struggling to pay rent or their mortgages and put food on the table. And, last month, it only got worse: we lost 140,000 jobs in December, including 20,000 public educators, and nearly 400,000 jobs at restaurants and bars.

President Biden is calling on Congress to take urgent action to deliver immediate, direct relief to Americans bearing the brunt of this crisis. Altogether, this would devote about $1 trillion towards building a bridge to economic recovery for working families and, according to researchers at Columbia University, cut child poverty in half.

President Biden's plan will:

Give working families a $1,400 per-person check to help pay their bills, bringing their total relief payment from this and the December down payment to $2,000. More than 1 in 3 households — and half of Black and Latino households — are struggling to pay for usual household expenses like rent and groceries during the pandemic. In this crisis, working families need more than the $600 per person that Congress passed last year. President Biden is calling on Congress to increase that direct financial assistance to $2,000. An additional $1,400 per person in direct checks will help hard-hit households cover expenses, spend money at local businesses in their communities, and stimulate the economy. President Biden's plan will also expand eligibility to adult dependents who have been left out of previous rounds of relief and all mixed status households. And, his plan will ensure that the Treasury Department has the flexibility and resources it needs to deliver stimulus checks to the families that need them most, including the millions of families that still haven't received the $1,200 checks they are entitled to under the CARES Act.

Extend and Expand Unemployment Insurance Benefits so American Workers Can Pay Their Bills

Around 18 million Americans rely on the unemployment insurance program. Congress did the right thing by continuing expanded eligibility and extending the number of weeks unemployed workers can receive benefits. One study estimates that extending pandemic unemployment insurance programs through 2021 could create or save over five million jobs. But these benefits are set to expire in weeks — even as the COVID-19 pandemic worsens. Millions of Americans are receiving benefits through unemployment insurance programs that will no longer serve new beneficiaries starting in mid-March.

President Biden is calling on Congress to extend these and other programs, providing millions of hard-hit workers with the financial security and peace of mind they need and deserve. And, he believes Congress should provide a $400 per-week unemployment insurance supplement to help hard-hit workers cover household expenses. The president is committed to providing these emergency supports to families for as long as the COVID-19 crisis continues and employment opportunities remain limited. The president is proposing to extend these emergency unemployment insurance programs through September 2021, and will work with Congress on ways to automatically adjust the length and amount of relief depending on health and economic conditions so future legislative delay doesn't undermine the recovery and families' access to benefits they need.

President Biden's plan will:

- Extend financial assistance for workers who have exhausted their regular unemployment compensation benefits. Extending and increasing the additional weeks provided under the emergency unemployment insurance program will ensure that approximately 5 million Americans continue to receive assistance in the months ahead.
- Extend financial assistance for unemployed workers who do not typically qualify for unemployment compensation benefits. The president believes Congress should extend unemployment support for self-employed workers, like ride-share drivers and many grocery delivery workers, who do not typically qualify for regular unemployment compensation. And, he supports increasing the number of weeks these workers can receive the benefit to provide long-term financial security to the program's approximately 8 million beneficiaries.
- Fully fund states' short-time compensation programs and additional weeks of benefits. Short-time compensation programs, also known as work sharing, help small businesses stay afloat and economically vulnerable workers make ends meet by enabling workers to stay on the job at reduced hours, while making up the difference in pay. These programs avoid layoffs and pave the way for rapid rehiring and an accelerated recovery.

Help Struggling Households Keep a Roof over Their Heads

The economic fallout of COVID-19 has made it more difficult for working families, especially families of color, to cover their housing expenses. Across the country, 1 in 5 renters and 1 in 10 homeowners with a mortgage are behind on payments. Congress took an important step in the right direction by securing $25 billion in rental assistance and extending the federal eviction moratorium until January 31. However, American families already owe $25 billion in back rent, and the threat of widespread evictions will still exist at the end of January. Further, more than 10 million homeowners have fallen behind on mortgage payments. Failing to take additional action will lead to a wave of evictions and foreclosures in the coming months, overwhelming emergency shelter capacity and increasing the likelihood of COVID-19 infections. And Americans of color, who have on average a fraction of the wealth available to white families, face higher risks of eviction and housing loss without critical assistance.

President Biden is calling on Congress to take immediate action to forestall a coming wave of COVID-related evictions and foreclosures.

- *Ensure that families hit hard by the economic crisis won't face eviction or foreclosure.* The president is calling on Congress to extend the eviction and foreclosure moratoriums and continue applications for forbearance on federally-guaranteed mortgages until September 30, 2021. These measures will prevent untold economic hardship for homeowners, while limiting the spread of COVID-19 in our communities. The president is also calling on Congress to provide funds for legal assistance for households facing eviction or foreclosure.

- *Help renters and small landlords make ends meet by providing an additional $30 billion in rental and critical energy and water assistance for hard-hit individuals and families.* While the $25 billion allocated by Congress was an important down payment on the back rent accrued during this crisis, it is insufficient to meet the scale of the need. That's why President Biden is proposing an additional $25 billion in rental assistance to provide much-needed rental relief, especially for low- and moderate-income households who have lost jobs or are out of the labor market. The president is also proposing $5 billion to cover home energy and water costs and arrears through programs like the Low Income Home Energy Assistance Program, for struggling renters. These funds will ensure that the hardest-hit renters and small landlords, including those in disadvantaged communities that have suffered disproportionately in terms of pollution and other environmental harms, aren't put in the position where they can't cover their own housing expenses. This program includes a competitive set-aside of funding for states to invest in clean energy and energy efficiency projects that reduce electricity bills for families in disadvantaged communities.
- *Deliver $5 billion in emergency assistance to help secure housing for people experiencing or at risk of homelessness.* This funding will allow states and localities to help approximately 200,000 individuals and families obtain stable housing, while providing a downpayment on the president's comprehensive approach to ending homelesness and making housing a right for all Americans. Specifically, these funds will provide flexibility for both congregate and non-congregate housing options, help jurisdictions purchase and convert hotels and motels into permanent housing, and give homeless services providers the resources they need to hire and retain staff, maintain outreach programs, and provide essential services.

Address the Growing Hunger Crisis in America

About 1 in 7 households nationwide, including more than 1 in 5 Black and Latino households and many Asian American and Pacific Islander households, are struggling to secure the food they need. While the December down payment provided $13 billion to strengthen and expand federal nutrition programs, it will not solve the hunger crisis in America. President Biden is calling on Congress to ensure all Americans, regardless of background, have access to healthy, affordable groceries. The president's plan will:

- *Extend the 15 percent Supplemental Nutrition Assistance Program (SNAP) benefit increase.* Maintaining the increase through the summer – when childhood hunger spikes due to a lack of school meals – is a critical backstop against rising food insecurity. This change will help keep hunger at bay for around 40 million Americans. The president is calling for this to be extended through September 2021. He is also committed to providing this boost for as long as the COVID-19 crisis continues, and will work with Congress on ways to automatically adjust the length and amount of relief depending on health and economic conditions so future legislative delay doesn't undermine the recovery and families' access to benefits they need.
- *Invest $3 billion to help women, infants and children get the food they need.* This multi-year investment in the Special Supplemental Nutrition Program for Women, Infants, and Children (WIC) is needed to account for increased enrollment due to growing

hunger and to increase outreach to ensure that low-income families have access to high-quality nutritious food and nutrition education.

- *Partner with restaurants to feed American families and keep restaurant workers on the job at the same time.* The FEMA Empowering Essential Deliveries (FEED) Actwill leverage the resources and expertise of the restaurant industry to help get food to families who need it, and help get laid-off restaurant workers across the country back on the job.
- *Support SNAP by temporarily cutting the state match.* The president is calling for a one time emergency infusion of administrative support for state anti-hunger and nutrition programs to ensure that benefits get to the kids and families that need it most.
- *Provide U.S. Territories with $1 billion in additional nutrition assistance for their residents.* Bolstering the Nutrition Assistance Program block grant will help thousands of working families in Puerto Rico, American Samoa, and the Commonwealth of the Northern Mariana Islands put food on the table for the duration of the pandemic.

Raise the Minimum Wage to $15 per Hour

Throughout the pandemic, millions of American workers have put their lives on the line to keep their communities and country functioning, including the 40 percent of frontline workers who are people of color. As President Biden has said, let's not just praise them, let's pay them. Hard working Americans deserve sufficient wages to put food on the table and keep a roof over their heads, without having to keep multiple jobs. But millions of working families are struggling to get by. This is why the president is calling on Congress to raise the minimum wage to $15 per hour, and end the tipped minimum wage and sub-minimum wage for people with disabilities so that workers across the country can live a middle class life and provide opportunity for their families.

Call on Employers to Meet Their Obligations to Frontline Essential Workers and Provide Back Hazard Pay

Essential workers — who are disproportionately Black, Latino, and Asian American and Pacific Islander– have risked their lives to stock shelves, harvest crops, and care for the sick during this crisis. They have kept the country running even during the darkest days of the pandemic. A number of large employers, especially in the retail and grocery sectors, have seen bumper profitability in 2020 and yet done little or nothing at all to compensate their workers for the risks they took. The president believes these employers have a duty to do right by their frontline essential workers and acknowledge their sacrifices with generous back hazard pay for the risks they took across 2020 and up to today. He and the Vice President will call on CEOs and other business leaders to take action to meet these obligations.

Expand Access to High-Quality, Affordable Child Care

We are facing an acute, immediate child care crisis in America, which is exacerbating our economic crisis. Due to increased costs and lower enrollment, a recent survey of child care providers showed that most child care providers expect that they will close within a few months without relief or are uncertain how long they can stay open. If left unaddressed, many child care providers will close — some permanently — and millions of children could go without necessary care, and millions of parents could be left to make devastating choices this winter between caring for their children and working to put food on the table. Early childcare providers are almost entirely women, among whom 40 percent are people of color, and so these closures could devastate engines of opportunity for minority- and women-owned businesses. President Biden is calling on Congress to take immediate actions to address this crisis by helping child care centers reopen and remain open safely, and by making that care affordable to families who need it.

In addition, too many families are unable to afford child care, while early educators earn wages so low that they can't support their own families. This challenge existed before COVID-19, and the pandemic has exacerbated it. President Biden is calling on Congress to ease the financial burden of care for families, expand financial support for child care providers so that this critical sector can stay afloat during the pandemic and beyond, and make critical investments to improve wages and benefits for the essential child care sector. President Biden's plan will:

- Help hard-hit child care providers, including family child care homes, cover their costs and operate safely by creating a $25 billion emergency stabilization fund. This Emergency Stabilization Fund will help hard-hit child care providers that are in danger of closing and provide support to nearly half of all child care providers. It will also assist those that have had to shut down meet their financial obligations during the pandemic, so that they can reopen. It will help providers pay for rent, utilities, and payroll, as well as increased costs associated with the pandemic including personal protective equipment, ventilation supplies, smaller group sizes, and modifications to make the physical environment safer for children and workers.
- Expand child care assistance to help millions of families and help parents return to work. Millions of parents are risking their lives as essential workers, while at the same time struggling to obtain care for their children. Others have become 24/7 caregivers while simultaneously working remotely. Still more are unemployed, caring for their children full-time, and worrying about how they will make ends meet or afford child care when they do find a job. And, the limited access to child care during the pandemic has caused more women to leave the workforce. While the December down payment provides $10 billion in funding through the Child Care and Development Block Grant program, the president's proposal expands this investment with an additional $15 billion in funding, including for those who experienced a job interruption during the COVID-19 pandemic and are struggling to afford child care. This additional assistance with child care costs will help the disproportionate number of women who left the labor force to take on caregiving duties reenter the workforce. And, this expanded investment will also help rebuild the supply of child care providers, and encourage states to take meaningful steps towards increasing the pay and benefits of child care workers.
- Increase tax credits to help cover the cost of childcare. To help address the childcare affordability crisis, President Biden is calling on Congress to expand child care tax credits on an emergency basis for one year to help working families cover the cost of childcare. Families will get back as a tax credit as much as half of their spending on child care for children under age 13, so that they can receive a total of up to $4,000 for one child or $8,000 for two or more children. The tax credit will be refundable,

meaning that families who don't owe a lot in taxes will still benefit. The full 50 percent reimbursement will be available to families making less than $125,000 a year. And, all families making between $125,000 and $400,000 will receive a partial credit so they receive benefits at least as generous as those they can receive today.

Bolster financial Security for Families and Essential Workers in the Midst of the Pandemic

The lowest income families are particularly vulnerable in the midst of the pandemic, and President Biden is calling for one year expansions of key supports for families on an emergency basis. The Child Tax Credit should be made fully refundable for the year. Currently, 27 million children live in families with household incomes low enough that they didn't qualify for the full value of the Child Tax Credit, and this measure would give these children and their families additional needed resources. The president is also calling to increase the credit to $3,000 per child ($3,600 for a child under age 6) and make 17 year-olds qualifying children for the year.

He is also calling for an expansion of the Earned Income Tax Credit for the year to ensure that the lowest income workers get critical support including millions of essential workers. He is proposing to raise the maximum Earned Income Tax Credit for childless adults from roughly $530 to close to $1,500, raise the income limit for the credit from about $16,000 to about $21,000, and expand the age range that is eligible including by eliminating the age cap for older workers and expanding eligibility for younger workers so that they can claim the credit they deserve. Expanding the Earned Income Tax Credit for childless adults would give a needed boost to the earnings of several million workers, including cashiers, home health aides, delivery people, and other people working in essential occupations. The president also is committed to making sure that Americans who see their earnings fall in 2021 due to the pandemic don't see the Earned Income Tax Credit reduced as a result.

Lastly, the president is calling for an additional $1 billion for states to cover the additional cash assistance that Temporary Assistance to Needy Families (TANF) recipients needed as a result of the pandemic crisis. The pandemic has led to increased TANF caseloads, generated higher costs for many TANF recipients – from higher utility costs to the need for internet access for remote schooling – and longer periods of joblessness given high unemployment. These funds will provide sorely needed relief.

Preserving and Expanding Health Coverage

Roughly two to three million people lost employer sponsored health insurance between March and September, and even families who have maintained coverage may struggle to pay premiums and afford care. Further, going into this crisis, 30 million people were without coverage, limiting their access to the health care system in the middle of a pandemic. To ensure access to health coverage, President Biden is calling on Congress to subsidize continuation health coverage (COBRA) through the end of September. He is also asking Congress to expand and increase the value of the Premium Tax Credit to lower or eliminate health insurance premiums and ensure enrollees – including those who never had coverage through their jobs – will not pay more than 8.5 percent of their income for coverage. Together, these policies would reduce premiums for more than ten million people and reduce the ranks of the uninsured by millions more.

Expanding Access to Behavioral Health Services

The pandemic has made access to mental health and substance use disorder services more essential than ever. The president is calling on Congress to appropriate $4 billion to enable the Substance Abuse and Mental Health Services Administration and the Health Resources and Services Administration to expand access to these vital services.

Ensure Adequate Funding for Veterans' Health

COVID-19 has put enormous pressure on America's veterans and on the Veterans Health Administration that is charged with providing and facilitating top-notch care for them. The president is committed to ensuring America delivers on its promise to the people who have served our country. To account for increased usage as many veterans have lost access to private health insurance, higher overall costs, and other pandemic-related impacts, the president is immediately requesting an additional $20 billion to make sure that veterans' health care needs can be met through this crisis.

Combat Increased Risk of Gender-Based Violence

The COVID-19 pandemic has exacerbated domestic violence and sexual assault, creating a "shadow pandemic " for many women and girls who are largely confined to their home with their abuser and facing economic insecurity that makes escape more difficult. President Biden is calling for at least $800 million in supplemental funding for key federal programs that protect survivors.

Provide Critical Support to Struggling Communities

COVID-19 and the resulting economic crisis has devastated communities across the country. Schools remain closed, with students struggling with remote learning and parents – 1.6 million mothers this fall – leaving the workforce. Small businesses, the backbones of their communities that employ nearly half of American workers, are unable to keep their doors open. And, some state and local essential workers are seeing their wages reduced or their jobs disappear. President Biden is calling on Congress to send a lifeline to small businesses; protect educators, public transit workers, and first responders from lay-offs; and keep critical services running at full strength. Altogether, his plan would provide approximately $440 billion in critical support to struggling communities. This is in addition to funds that President Biden is requesting for safely reopening schools throughout the country.

President Biden's plan will:

Provide Small Businesses with the Funding They Need to Reopen and Rebuild

Small businesses sustain half of the private sector jobs in America, and they have struggled in the wake of COVID-19. Black- and Brown-owned small businesses, and those in hard-hit industries like restaurants, hotels, and the arts, have suffered disproportionately. Nationally, small business revenue is down 32 percent, and at least 400,000 firms have permanently closed. To help hard-hit firms survive the pandemic and fully recover, President Biden is calling on Congress to:

- Provide grants to more than 1 million of the hardest hit small businesses. This $15 billion in flexible, equitably distributed grants will help small businesses get back on their feet, put the current disaster behind them, and build back better.
- Leverage $35 billion in government funds into $175 billion in additional small business lending and investment. With a $35 billion investment in successful state, local, tribal, and non-profit small business financing programs, Congress can generate as much as $175 billion in low-interest loans and venture capital to help entrepreneurs — including those in the clean energy sector — innovate, create and maintain jobs, build wealth, and provide the essential goods and services that communities depend on.

In addition, the president wants to work with Congress to make sure that restaurants, bars, and other businesses that have suffered disproportionately have sufficient support to bridge to the recovery, including through the Community Credit Corporation at the U.S. Department of Agriculture (USDA).

Provide Support for first Responders and Other Essential Workers

Throughout the COVID-19 pandemic, first responders, frontline public health workers, and countless other essential workers have risked their lives to keep our communities safe and functioning. Educators have worked tirelessly to keep our children learning and growing, coming up with new ways to reach and engage their students, often while balancing caring for their own children. Without these front line workers, we will not be able to effectively respond to the pandemic, administer the vaccine, or safely reopen our schools. President Biden is calling on Congress to provide $350 billion in emergency funding for state, local, and territorial governments to ensure that they are in a position to keep front line public workers on the job and paid, while also effectively distributing the vaccine, scaling testing, reopening schools, and maintaining other vital services. The president is also calling on Congress to allocate $3 billion of this funding to the Economic Development Administration (EDA). Grants from EDA provide resources directly to state and local government entities, tribal institutions, institutions of higher education, and non-profits to fund initiatives that support bottom's up economic development and enable good-paying jobs. This funding – double the amount provided by the CARES Act – will support communities nationwide with a broad range of financial needs as they respond to and recover from COVID-19.

Protect the Future of Public Transit

Safe and dependable public transit systems are critical for a robust and equitable economy recovery. The president is calling for $20 billion in relief for the hardest hit public transit agencies. This relief will keep agencies from laying off transit workers and cutting the routes that essential workers rely on every day while making these transit systems more resilient and ensuring that communities of color maintain the access to opportunity that public transportation provides.

Support Tribal Governments' Response to COVID-19

COVID-19 has exacted an especially high toll in Indian Country. People living on reservations are four times more likely to have COVID-19 and American Indian and Alaska Natives are nearly twice as likely to die from COVID-19 than white Americans. While the December down payment had many beneficial provisions, it included little direct funding to help Tribal governments respond to COVID-19. President Biden is calling on Congress to give Tribes the resources they need to obtain sufficient personal protective equipment, increase access to clean water and electricity, and expand internet access so that children can learn remotely and more families can obtain basic health care through telemedicine. President Biden's plan would invest $20 billion in Indian Country to support Tribal governments' response to the pandemic.These resources will help to reduce stark and persistent inequities in COVID-19 transmission, hospitalization, and death, while improving economic conditions and opportunity.

Modernize Federal Information Technology to Protect against Future Cyber Attacks

In addition to the COVID-19 crisis, we also face a crisis when it comes to the nation's cybersecurity. The recent cybersecurity breaches of federal government data systems underscore the importance and urgency of strengthening U.S. cybersecurity capabilities.

President Biden is calling on Congress to launch the most ambitious effort ever to modernize and secure federal IT and networks. To remediate the SolarWinds breach and boost U.S. defenses, including of the COVID-19 vaccine process, President Biden is calling on Congress to:

- Expand and improve the Technology Modernization Fund. A $9 billion investment will help the U.S. launch major new IT and cybersecurity shared services at the Cyber Security and Information Security Agency (CISA) and the General Services Administration and complete modernization projects at federal agencies. In addition, the president is calling on Congress to change the fund's reimbursement structure in order to fund more innovative and impactful projects.
- Surge cybersecurity technology and engineering expert hiring. Providing the Information Technology Oversight and Reform fund with $200 million will allow for the rapid hiring of hundreds of experts to support the federal Chief Information Security Officer and U.S. Digital Service.
- Build shared, secure services to drive transformational projects. Investing $300 million in no-year funding for Technology Transformation Services in the General Services Administration will drive secure IT projects forward without the need of reimbursement from agencies.
- Improving security monitoring and incident response activities. An additional $690M for CISA will bolster cybersecurity across federal civilian networks, and support the piloting of new shared security and cloud computing services.

Executive Order on Ensuring a Data-Driven Response to COVID-19 and Future High-Consequence Public Health Threats

January 21, 2021
Presidential Actions

By the authority vested in me as President by the Constitution and the laws of the United States of America, it is hereby ordered as follows:

Section 1. Policy

It is the policy of my Administration to respond to the coronavirus disease 2019 (COVID-19) pandemic through effective approaches guided by the best available science and data, including by building back a better public health infrastructure. This stronger public health infrastructure must help the Nation effectively prevent, detect, and respond to future biological threats, both domestically and internationally.

Consistent with this policy, the heads of all executive departments and agencies (agencies) shall facilitate the gathering, sharing, and publication of COVID-19-related data, in coordination with the Coordinator of the COVID-19 Response and Counselor to the President (COVID-19 Response Coordinator), to the extent permitted by law, and with appropriate protections for confidentiality, privacy, law enforcement, and national security. These efforts shall assist Federal, State, local, Tribal, and territorial authorities in developing and implementing policies to facilitate informed community decision-making, to further public understanding of the pandemic and the response, and to deter the spread of misinformation and disinformation.

Sec. 2. Enhancing Data Collection and Collaboration Capabilities for High-Consequence Public Health Threats, Such as the COVID-19 Pandemic

a) The Secretary of Defense, the Attorney General, the Secretary of Commerce, the Secretary of Labor, the Secretary of Health and Human Services (HHS), the Secretary of Education, the Director of the Office of Management and Budget (OMB), the Director of National Intelligence, the Director of the Office of Science and Technology Policy (OSTP), and the Director of the National Science Foundation shall each promptly designate a senior official to serve as their agency's lead to work on COVID-19- and pandemic-related data issues. This official, in consultation with the COVID-19 Response Coordinator, shall take steps to make data relevant to high-consequence public health threats, such as the COVID-19 pandemic, publicly available and accessible.

b) The COVID-19 Response Coordinator shall, as necessary, convene appropriate representatives from relevant agencies to coordinate the agencies' collection, provision, and analysis of data, including key equity indicators, regarding the COVID-19 response, as well as their sharing of such data with State, local, Tribal, and territorial authorities.

c) The Director of OMB, in consultation with the Director of OSTP, the United States Chief Technology Officer, and the COVID-19 Response Coordinator, shall promptly review the Federal Government's existing approaches to open data, and shall issue supplemental guidance, as appropriate and consistent with applicable law, concerning how to de-identify COVID-19-related data; how to make data open to the public in human- and machine-readable formats as rapidly as possible; and any other topic the Director of OMB concludes would appropriately advance the policy of this order. Any guidance shall include appropriate protections for the information described in section 5 of this order.

d) The Director of the Office of Personnel Management, in consultation with the Director of OMB, shall promptly:

   (i) review the ability of agencies to hire personnel expeditiously into roles related to information technology and the collection, provision, analysis, or other use of data to address high-consequence public health threats, such as the COVID-19 pandemic; and
   (ii) take action, as appropriate and consistent with applicable law, to support agencies in such efforts.

Sec. 3. Public Health Data Systems

The Secretary of HHS, in consultation with the COVID-19 Response Coordinator and the heads of relevant agencies, shall promptly:

a) review the effectiveness, interoperability, and connectivity of public health data systems supporting the detection of and response to high-consequence public health threats, such as the COVID-19 pandemic;

b) review the collection of morbidity and mortality data by State, local, Tribal, and territorial governments during high-consequence public health threats, such as the COVID-19 pandemic; and

c) issue a report summarizing the findings of the reviews detailed in subsections (a) and (b) of this section and any recommendations for addressing areas for improvement identified in the reviews.

Sec. 4. Advancing Innovation in Public Health Data and Analytics

The Director of OSTP, in coordination with the National Science and Technology Council, as appropriate, shall develop a plan for advancing innovation in public health data and analytics in the United States.

Sec. 5. Privileged Information

Nothing in this order shall compel or authorize the disclosure of privileged information, law-enforcement information, national-security information, personal information, or information the disclosure of which is prohibited by law.

Sec. 6. General Provisions

a) Nothing in this order shall be construed to impair or otherwise affect:

   i) the authority granted by law to an executive department or agency, or the head thereof; or

   ii) the functions of the Director of the Office of Management and Budget relating to budgetary, administrative, or legislative proposals.

b) This order shall be implemented consistent with applicable law and subject to the availability of appropriations.

c) This order is not intended to, and does not, create any right or benefit, substantive or procedural, enforceable at law or in equity by any party against the United States, its departments, agencies, or entities, its officers, employees, or agents, or any other person.

JOSEPH R. BIDEN JR.
THE WHITE HOUSE, January 21, 2021.

Executive Order on a Sustainable Public Health Supply Chain

January 21, 2021
Presidential Actions

By the authority vested in me as President by the Constitution and the laws of the United States of America, including the Defense Production Act of 1950, as amended (50 U.S.C. 4501 *et seq.*), sections 319 and 361 of the Public Health Service Act (42 U.S.C. 247d and 264), sections 306 and 307 of the Robert T. Stafford Disaster Relief and Emergency Assistance Act (42 U.S.C. 5149 and 5150), and section 301 of title 3, United States Code, it is hereby ordered as follows:

Section 1. Purpose

The Federal Government must act urgently and effectively to combat the coronavirus disease 2019 (COVID-19) pandemic. To that end, this order directs immediate actions to secure supplies necessary for responding to the pandemic, so that those supplies are available, and remain available, to the Federal Government and State, local, Tribal, and territorial authorities, as well as to America's health care workers, health systems, and patients. These supplies are vital to the Nation's ability to reopen its schools and economy as soon and safely as possible.

Sec. 2. Immediate Inventory of Response Supplies and Identification of Emergency Needs

a) The Secretary of State, the Secretary of Defense, the Secretary of Health and Human Services, the Secretary of Homeland Security, and the heads of appropriate executive departments and agencies (agencies), in coordination with the COVID-19 Response Coordinator, shall:

  I) immediately review the availability of critical materials, treatments, and supplies needed to combat COVID-19 (pandemic response supplies), including personal protective equipment (PPE) and the resources necessary to effectively produce and distribute tests and vaccines at scale; and

  II) assess, including by reviewing prior such assessments, whether United States industry can be reasonably expected to provide such supplies in a timely manner.

b) Where a review and assessment described in section 2(a)(i) of this order identifies shortfalls in the provision of pandemic response supplies, the head of the relevant agency shall:

  I) promptly revise its operational assumptions and planning factors being used to determine the scope and prioritization, acquisition, and distribution of such supplies; and

  II) take appropriate action using all available legal authorities, including the Defense Production Act, to fill those shortfalls as soon as practicable by acquiring additional stockpiles, improving distribution systems, building market capacity, or expanding the industrial base.

c) Upon completing the review and assessment described in section 2(a)(i) of this order, the Secretary of Health and Human Services shall provide to the President, through the COVID-19 Response Coordinator, a report on the status and inventory of the Strategic National Stockpile.

d) The Secretary of State, the Secretary of Defense, the Secretary of Health and Human Services, the Secretary of Homeland Security, and the heads of any other agencies relevant to inventorying pandemic response supplies shall, as soon as practicable, provide to the President, through the COVID-19 Response Coordinator, a report consisting of:

  I) an assessment of the need for, and an inventory of current supplies of, key pandemic response supplies;

  II) an analysis of their agency's capacity to produce, provide, and distribute pandemic response supplies;

III) an assessment of their agency's procurement of pandemic response supplies on the availability of such supplies on the open market;

IV) an account of all existing or ongoing agency actions, contracts, and investment agreements regarding pandemic response supplies;

V) a list of any gaps between the needs identified in section 2(a)(i) of this order and supply chain delivery, and recommendations on how to close such gaps; and

VI) a compilation and summary of their agency's existing distribution and prioritization plans for pandemic response supplies, which shall include any assumptions or planning factors used to determine such needs and any recommendations for changes to such assumptions or factors.

e) The COVID-19 Response Coordinator, in coordination with the heads of appropriate agencies, shall review the report described in section 2(d) of this order and submit recommendations to the President that address:

I) whether additional use of the Defense Production Act, by the President or agencies exercising delegated authority under the Act, would be helpful; and

II) the extent to which liability risk, regulatory requirements, or other factors impede the development, production, and procurement of pandemic response supplies, and any actions that can be taken, consistent with law, to remove those impediments.

f) The heads of agencies responsible for completing the requirements of this section, as appropriate and in coordination with the COVID-19 Response Coordinator, shall consult with State, local, Tribal, and territorial authorities, as well as with other entities critical to assessing the availability of and need for pandemic response supplies.

Sec. 3. Pricing

To take steps to address the pricing of pandemic response supplies:

a) The Secretary of Health and Human Services shall promptly recommend to the President, through the COVID-19 Response Coordinator, whether any changes should be made to the authorities delegated to the Secretary by Executive Order 13910 of March 23, 2020 (Preventing Hoarding of Health and Medical Resources To Respond to the Spread of COVID-19), with respect to scarce materials or materials the supply of which would be threatened by accumulation for the purpose of hoarding or price gouging.

b) The Secretary of Defense, the Secretary of Health and Human Services, and the Secretary of Homeland Security shall promptly review and provide to the President, through the COVID-19 Response Coordinator, recommendations for how to address the pricing of pandemic response supplies, including whether and how to direct the use of reasonable pricing clauses in Federal contracts and investment agreements, or other related vehicles, and whether to use General Services Administration Schedules to facilitate State, local, Tribal, and territorial government buyers and compacts in purchasing pandemic response supplies using Federal supply schedules.

Sec. 4. Pandemic Supply Chain Resilience Strategy

Within 180 days of the date of this order, the Secretary of Defense, the Secretary of Health and Human Services, and the Secretary of Homeland Security, in coordination with the Assistant to the President for National Security Affairs (APNSA), the Assistant to the President for Domestic Policy, the COVID-19 Response Coordinator, and the heads of any agencies or entities selected by the APNSA and COVID-19 Response Coordinator, shall provide to the President a strategy to design, build, and sustain a long-term capability in the United States to manufacture supplies for future pandemics and biological threats. This strategy shall include:

(a) mechanisms to respond to emergency supply needs of State, local, Tribal, and territorial authorities, which should include standards and processes to prioritize requests and delivery and to ensure equitable distribution based on public health criteria;

(b) an analysis of the role of foreign supply chains in America's pandemic supply chain, America's role in the international public health supply chain, and options for strengthening and better coordinating global supply chain systems in future pandemics;

(c) mechanisms to address points of failure in the supply chains and to ensure necessary redundancies;

(d) the roles of the Strategic National Stockpile and other Federal and military stockpiles in providing pandemic supplies on an ongoing or emergency basis, including their roles in allocating supplies across States, localities, tribes, and territories, sustaining supplies during a pandemic, and in contingency planning to ensure adequate preparedness for future pandemics and public health emergencies;

(e) approaches to assess and maximize the value and efficacy of public/private partnerships and the value of Federal investments in latent manufacturing capacity; and

(f) an approach to develop a multi-year implementation plan for domestic production of pandemic supplies.

Sec. 5. Access to Strategic National Stockpile

The Secretary of Health and Human Services shall consult with Tribal authorities and take steps, as appropriate and consistent with applicable law, to facilitate access to the Strategic National Stockpile for federally recognized Tribal governments, Indian Health Service healthcare providers, Tribal health authorities, and Urban Indian Organizations.

Sec. 6. General Provisions

(a) Nothing in this order shall be construed to impair or otherwise affect:

(i) the authority granted by law to an executive department or agency, or the head thereof; or

(ii) the functions of the Director of the Office of Management and Budget relating to budgetary, administrative, or legislative proposals.

(b) This order shall be implemented consistent with applicable law and subject to the availability of appropriations.

(c) This order is not intended to, and does not, create any right or benefit, substantive or procedural, enforceable at law or in equity by any party against the United States, its departments, agencies, or entities, its officers, employees, or agents, or any other person.

JOSEPH R. BIDEN JR.

THE WHITE HOUSE,
January 21, 2021.

Executive Order on Establishing the COVID-19 Pandemic Testing Board and Ensuring a Sustainable Public Health Workforce for COVID-19 and Other Biological Threats

January 21, 2021
Presidential Actions

By the authority vested in me as President by the Constitution and the laws of the United States of America, including section 301 of title 3, United States Code, it is hereby ordered as follows:

Section 1. Policy

It is the policy of my Administration to control coronavirus disease 2019 (COVID-19) by using a Government-wide, unified approach that includes: establishing a national COVID-19 testing and public health workforce strategy; working to expand the supply of tests; working to bring test manufacturing to the United States, where possible; working to enhance laboratory testing capacity; working to expand the public health workforce; supporting screening testing for schools and priority populations; and ensuring a clarity of messaging about the use of tests and insurance coverage.

Sec. 2. COVID-19 Pandemic Testing Board

a) Establishment and Membership. There is established a COVID-19 Pandemic Testing Board (Testing Board), chaired by the Coordinator of the COVID-19 Response and Counselor to the President (COVID-19 Response Coordinator) or his designee. The Testing Board shall include representatives from executive departments and agencies (agencies) that are designated by the President. The heads of agencies so designated shall designate officials from their respective agencies to represent them on the Testing Board.

b) Mission and Functions. To support the implementation and oversight of the policy laid out in section 1 of this order, the Testing Board shall:

   i) coordinate Federal Government efforts to promote COVID-19 diagnostic, screening, and surveillance testing;

   ii) make recommendations to the President with respect to prioritizing the Federal Government's assistance to State, local, Tribal, and territorial authorities, in order to expand testing and reduce disparities in access to testing;

   iii) identify barriers to access and use of testing in, and coordinate Federal Government efforts to increase testing for:

      A) priority populations, including healthcare workers and other essential workers;

      B) communities with major shortages in testing availability and use;

      C) at-risk settings, including long-term care facilities, correctional facilities, immigration custodial settings, detention facilities, schools, child care settings, and food processing and manufacturing facilities; and

      D) high-risk groups, including people experiencing homelessness, migrants, and seasonal workers;

   iv) identify methods to expand State, local, Tribal, and territorial capacity to conduct testing, contact tracing, and isolation and quarantine, in order for schools, businesses, and travel to be conducted safely;

   v) provide guidance on how to enhance the clarity, consistency, and transparency of Federal Government communication with the public about the goals and purposes of testing;

   vi) identify options for the Federal Government to maximize testing capacity of commercial labs and academic labs; and

   vii) propose short- and long-term reforms for the Federal Government to: increase State, local, Tribal, and territorial capacity to conduct testing; expand genomic sequencing; and improve the effectiveness and speed of the Federal Government's response to future pandemics and other biological emergencies.

c) The Chair of the Testing Board shall coordinate with the Secretary of Health and Human Services (HHS) and the heads of other relevant agencies or their designees, as necessary, to ensure that the Testing Board's work is coordinated with the Public Health Emergency Countermeasures Enterprise within HHS.

Sec. 3. Actions to Address the Cost of COVID-19 Testing

a) The Secretary of the Treasury, the Secretary of HHS, and the Secretary of Labor, in coordination with the COVID-19 Response Coordinator, shall promptly, and as appropriate and consistent with applicable law:

  i) facilitate the provision of COVID-19 testing free of charge to those who lack comprehensive health insurance; and

  ii) clarify group health plans' and health insurance issuers' obligations to provide coverage for COVID-19 testing.

b) The Secretary of HHS, the Secretary of Education, and the Secretary of Homeland Security, through the Administrator of the Federal Emergency Management Agency (FEMA), in coordination with the COVID-19 Response Coordinator, shall promptly, and as appropriate and consistent with applicable law:

  i) provide support for surveillance tests for settings such as schools; and

  ii) expand equitable access to COVID-19 testing.

Sec. 4. Establishing a Public Health Workforce Program

a) The Secretary of HHS and the Secretary of Labor shall promptly consult with State, local, Tribal, and territorial leaders to understand the challenges they face in pandemic response efforts, including challenges recruiting and training sufficient personnel to ensure adequate and equitable community-based testing, and testing in schools and high-risk settings.

b) The Secretary of HHS shall, as appropriate and consistent with applicable law, as soon as practicable:

  i) provide technical support to State, local, Tribal, and territorial public health agencies with respect to testing and contact-tracing efforts; and

  ii) assist such authorities in the training of public health workers. This may include technical assistance to non-Federal public health workforces in connection with testing, contact tracing, and mass vaccinations, as well as other urgent public health workforce needs, such as combating opioid use.

b) The Secretary of HHS shall submit to the President, through the COVID-19 Response Coordinator, the Assistant to the President for Domestic Policy (APDP), and the Assistant to the President for National Security Affairs (APNSA), a plan detailing:

i) how the Secretary of HHS would deploy personnel in response to future high-consequence public health threats; and

ii) five-year targets and budget requirements for achieving a sustainable public health workforce, as well as options for expanding HHS capacity, such as by expanding the U.S. Public Health Service Commissioned Corps and Epidemic Intelligence Service, so that the Department can better respond to future pandemics and other biological threats.

c) The Secretary of HHS, the Secretary of Homeland Security, the Secretary of Labor, the Secretary of Education, and the Chief Executive Officer of the Corporation for National and Community Service, in coordination with the COVID-19 Response Coordinator, the APDP, and the APNSA, shall submit a plan to the President for establishing a national contact tracing and COVID-19 public health workforce program, to be known as the U.S. Public Health Job Corps, which shall be modeled on or developed as a component of the FEMA Corps program. Such plan shall include means by which the U.S. Public Health Job Corps can be part of the National Civilian Community Corps program, as well as recommendations about whether it would be appropriate for the U.S. Public Health Job Corps to immediately assign personnel from any of the agencies involved in the creation of the plan, including existing AmeriCorps members, to join or aid the U.S. Public Health Job Corps. The U.S. Public Health Job Corps will:

i) conduct and train individuals in contact tracing related to the COVID-19 pandemic;

ii) assist in outreach for vaccination efforts, including by administering vaccination clinics;

iii) assist with training programs for State, local, Tribal, and territorial governments to provide testing, including in schools; and

iv) provide other necessary services to Americans affected by the COVID-19 pandemic.

Sec. 5. General Provisions

a) Nothing in this order shall be construed to impair or otherwise affect:

i) the authority granted by law to an executive department or agency, or the head thereof; or

ii) the functions of the Director of the Office of Management and Budget relating to budgetary, administrative, or legislative proposals.

b) This order shall be implemented consistent with applicable law and subject to the availability of appropriations.

c) This order is not intended to, and does not, create any right or benefit, substantive or procedural, enforceable at law or in equity by any party against the United States, its departments, agencies, or entities, its officers, employees, or agents, or any other person.

JOSEPH R. BIDEN JR.
THE WHITE HOUSE,

January 21, 2021.

Biden Covid Team Derides Trump Plan While Borrowing Playbook

By Josh Wingrove and Riley Griffin
January 29, 2021, 2:00 AM EST; Updated on January 29, 2021, 9:00 AM EST

Biden inherited system already meeting target pace of shots
Biden to use DPA, like Trump, and order doses from old deals

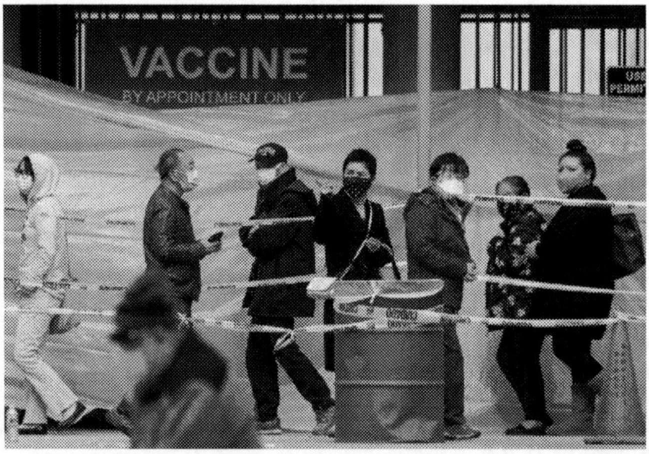

People wait in line at a vaccination site at Lincoln Park in Los Angeles, California, on Jan. 28. *Photographer: Mario Tama/Getty Images.*

President Joe Biden and his top advisers have derided the Trump administration's playbook for distributing coronavirus vaccines, but so far have made only modest changes to the plan that's meeting their target pace of more than one million shots a day.

Biden has said vaccine distribution was in "worse shape than we anticipated." White House Chief of Staff Ron Klain said a Trump administration plan "did not really exist." Adviser Cedric Richmond said they "didn't leave a plan." Xavier Becerra, Biden's choice for health secretary, said it was like taking over a plane in a nosedive.

But while Biden's approach to the virus – frank warnings about the pandemic, mask mandates on federal property – is a reversal from Trump's policies, his administration's distribution of vaccines so far looks little different from that of its predecessor. Before Biden was sworn in, vaccines already were being delivered at a pace to meet his goal of 100 million doses in his first 100 days as president.

The Biden administration has said they'll order new doses, but will do so by exercising options in contracts negotiated by the previous administration, which thought it premature to do so.

They say they'll use the Defense Production Act, which Trump used repeatedly. Rather than a total overhaul, they have otherwise made course corrections and modest shifts. Data released Friday by Johnson & Johnson will fuel hopes that a third vaccine soon could hit the U.S. market.

J&J Single-Dose Vaccine Provides Strong Shield against Covid

Still, Biden's ability to sharply change direction is inherently limited. The sheer magnitude of the distribution efforts would make any major changes costly and risk backsliding, even if temporarily. Some aspects of the program don't offer much wiggle room to begin with, while the trickiest parts are yet to come – and entirely on Biden's shoulders.

Any efforts by Biden to shape the program also were undercut by Trump, who delayed the transition as he disputed the results of the election and refused to concede. Trump's team said more than 300 transition briefings were held with health officials, though Biden officials have said the information exchange was limited until just days before the inauguration.

Partisan Rhetoric

Some officials who led Trump's efforts have objected to what they see as partisan sniping from Biden's team, warning that it's hurting morale among career staff who are working on the vaccine rollout.

"The transition is happening less well than I, and my team, had been hoping," said Moncef Slaoui, chief scientific adviser to Operation Warp Speed, the joint effort between the Department of Health and Human Services and the Department of Defense to develop and distribute vaccines in record time. Biden's team dropped the name, in hopes of boosting confidence in the shots, and forced out Slaoui.

"The team doesn't understand why the Operation is being criticized as it is. It is so unfair and unjustified," Slaoui said. "If it wasn't for this Operation, we may not have as many vaccines as we will now."

Among those who've pumped the brakes on claims that Biden was handed nothing is Anthony Fauci, the nation's top infectious disease expert who was sidelined by Trump and now serves as an adviser to Biden.

"We certainly are not starting from scratch," Fauci said last week. "It's taking what's gone on, but amplifying it in a big way." Biden, too, has given credit to scientists and the Trump administration for getting the vaccine program off the ground. "And that credit is absolutely due," he said.

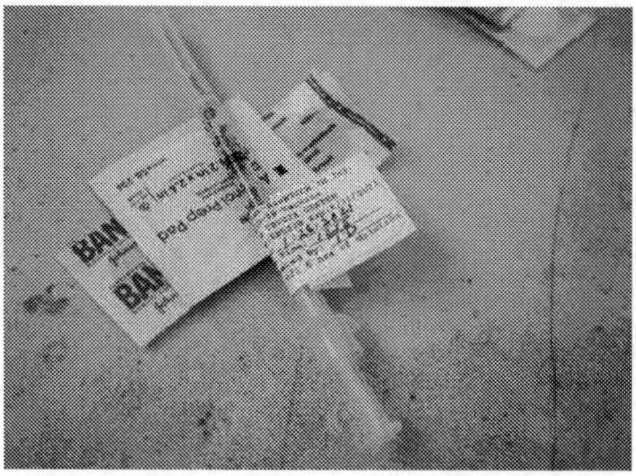

Producers can't make vaccines fast enough and supplies are scarce. *Photographer: David Ryder/Getty Images.*

Biden's Approach

There are differences. Biden is endorsing federally run community vaccination centers and mobile clinics, and is aiming to provide states with a three-week supply preview. They have moved to boost the number of people available to administer it, although Trump officials said the shortage is in vaccines, not vaccinators. Biden has pledged to let science lead the way and made briefings public, in stark contrast to Trump, who sidelined health advisers in favor of those who reinforced his own view.

Biden has also pressed to address equity – saying that communities of color have been disproportionately hurt by the virus and can't be left out in the response. Vaccinations could get more complicated as months stretch on, supply grows and the easier groups to access – including health care workers and long-term care residents – are fully vaccinated.

But the biggest pieces of the distribution effort remain unchanged, undercutting claims from some Biden advisers that they inherited no plan. Many of the most stubborn bottlenecks don't stem from the federal government's decisions: Companies simply can't produce vaccines fast enough and supplies are scarce; even if distribution goes smoothly, the administration of doses gets backed up at the local level.

"What we're seeing here is them marching through the playbook of Operation Warp Speed," added Michael Pratt, a former Health and Human Services official under Trump. "Something cannot simultaneously be a dismal failure and have already accomplished the 'ambitious goal' you set."

Nearly every industrialized nation has been beset by vaccine delays. The European Union has moved to restrict vaccine exports. The U.S. has administered 8.3 doses per 100 people, trailing the U.K. and Israel yet outpacing Germany, Canada, France and the EU overall, according to Bloomberg's Vaccine Tracker.

The war of words has ramped up since inauguration day. Slaoui said he'd been told by the Biden administration that he would remain as a consultant, only to later read in news reports that he had been asked to resign. He said he asked Zients about the reports and was told that he should resign.

"I accepted to do it that way at their request," Slaoui said in an interview. "There's two ways to look good, you either look good because you do great things, or you look good because you make others look bad. I hope that the new administration doesn't get into that game."

Biden has kept other key Trump personnel in place, including General Gustave Perna, who co-lead Operation Warp Speed alongside Slaoui, focusing on distribution.

100-Day Pledge

Biden has bristled at questions about whether 100 million doses in 100 days – a target he set before vaccinations began – is too modest a goal. The U.S. reported more than one million daily doses for the first time on Jan. 13, and the rolling daily average topped one million on Jan. 23, Biden's third full day in office. Two days later, Biden revised his goal, saying he thinks 1.5 million daily doses was achievable in the first 100 days. The U.S. has only so far hit that mark once: inauguration day.

"It is really incorrect to say there was no plan – because we're already achieving 1.3 million doses in arms per day, which exceeds the first goal President Biden had," said Brett Giroir, who led the previous administration's efforts to ramp up testing.

A key unknown remains – when another vaccine will hit the market. Johnson & Johnson's vaccine generated strong protection against Covid-19 in a large, late-stage trial, the company announced Friday. Its single-dose vaccine is more easily stored, and is expected to be quickly brought to market without the missed delivery timelines of the P fizer Inc.-BioNTech SE shots. If the J&J vaccine is authorized, Biden's team could quickly hit 2 million total doses a day, a former Trump official said.

Biden on Tuesday announced the U.S. would exercise options for an additional 100 million doses each from Pfizer and Moderna Inc., a move that puzzled Trump officials. The doses will cost roughly $3.6 billion and won't be ready until summer.

"I would have waited to see what the J&J vaccine does before talking about deals for additional doses," Slaoui said.

Biden said that doesn't bother him.

"I hope you're all asking me by the end of the summer that: You have too much vaccine left over. You have too much equipment left over. That's not my worry," he said this week. "I hope that becomes the problem"

Biden announced that shipments to states would rise for the next three weeks – to 10 million doses from about 8.6 million. The administration hasn't said where the extra doses are coming from, but Trump officials said Moderna had been scheduled to bring more production online under agreements made before Biden took office.

One pillar of the Biden response is use of the Defense Production Act to prioritize certain materials and supplies. Trump's administration used it regularly, but there's always a tradeoff – pushing something to the front of the line can displace other crucial production. Biden administration officials have declined to detail how they're using DPA.

Slaoui said the DPA was used 18 times to support vaccine manufacturing. "There's nothing new about that," he said.

(Updates with Johnson & Johnson data in fourth, 22nd paragraphs)

No Good Vaccine Deed

The Biden team shows no gratitude to the man who sped up the Covid shots.

By The Editorial Board
Jan. 29, 2021 6:31 pm ET

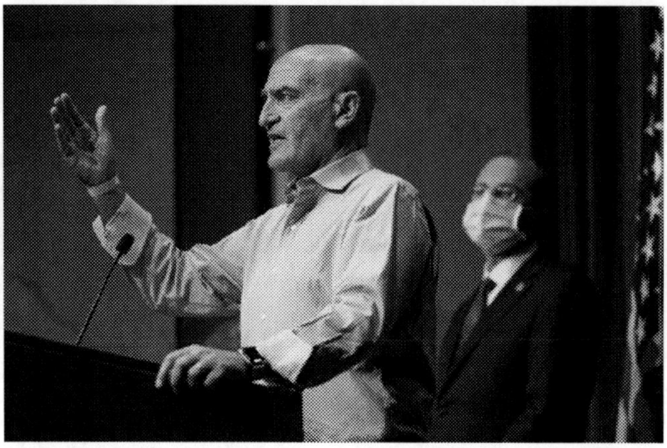

Dr. Moncef Slaoui, chief science adviser to Operation Warp Speed, speaks during a news conference on Operation Warp Speed and COVID-19 vaccine distribution, Tuesday, Jan. 12, 2021, in Washington. Photo: Patrick Semansky/Press Pool.

Johnson & Johnson and Novavax this week reported that their vaccines were effective in clinical trials, and what fortunate timing. The U.S. urgently needs a supply boost. But at this juncture it's also worth noting how former Operation Warp Speed chief Moncef Slaoui positioned the Biden Administration for a vaccine triumph.

Covid, Kids and Teachers Unions

One of Mr. Slaoui's inspired ideas was to diversify the federal government's vaccine bets with six manufacturers when nobody knew which, if any, would work. The vaccine candidates used different technologies—Moderna and Pfizer -BioNTech (mRNA), J&J and AstraZeneca (adenovirus), and Novavax and Sanofi -GSK (recombinant protein).

The J&J and AstraZeneca vaccines were hobbled by trial delays in the fall. But J&J reported Friday that its vaccine was 66% effective at protecting people from moderate to severe disease in a global trial, and 85% against severe illness. Early trial data from AstraZeneca suggests similar efficacy. Novavax reported Thursday its shot appears to be nearly 90% effective.

The Moderna and Pfizer-BioNTech vaccines are about 95% effective, so it's fortuitous that their trial results came first so their shots could inoculate the elderly and others most at highest risk. But even if somewhat less effective, the other vaccines may be good candidates for young people and boost supply this spring.

Operation Warp Speed removed the financial risk for drug makers by financing trials and manufacturing in advance so vaccines could roll out as soon as they are approved. This is the reason some 20 million Americans have already been inoculated. President Biden this week ordered another 200 million doses from Pfizer and Moderna to be delivered this summer.

These extra doses may or may not be needed if other vaccines are approved—J&J could add 100 million this spring—but the reason they will be available is contracts that Operation Warp Speed negotiated with drug makers that gave the feds the option to order more. We point this out because White House officials have been griping that they are "starting from scratch."

That's false. Operation Warp Speed created the incentives for vaccine development, and assisted with rapid approvals and distribution infrastructure, which Mr. Biden will undoubtedly claim credit for as the rollout gains speed and breadth. The Biden team showed its gratitude by deposing Mr. Slaoui via a nasty news leak that criticized his good work.

Mr. Slaoui graciously agreed to remain on the job for a few weeks as a consultant. He deserves praise for his excellent public service, all the more because the Biden Administration so ungraciously won't acknowledge it.

Why Operation Warp Speed Worked

The successful vaccine program followed the model of U.S. mobilization in World War II.

By Arthur Herman
Feb. 1, 2021 6:28 pm ET

Every day new questions and criticisms arise about Operation Warp Speed, the public-private vaccine development initiative launched by presidential order in May 2020. Most of that criticism focuses on the distribution bottlenecks that have developed in different states, as Americans are impatient with the slow pace of the rollout. Jen Psaki, President Biden's press secretary, has claimed to see an "urgent need to address failures of the Trump team approach to vaccine distribution." Some in the new administration even want to rename the program.

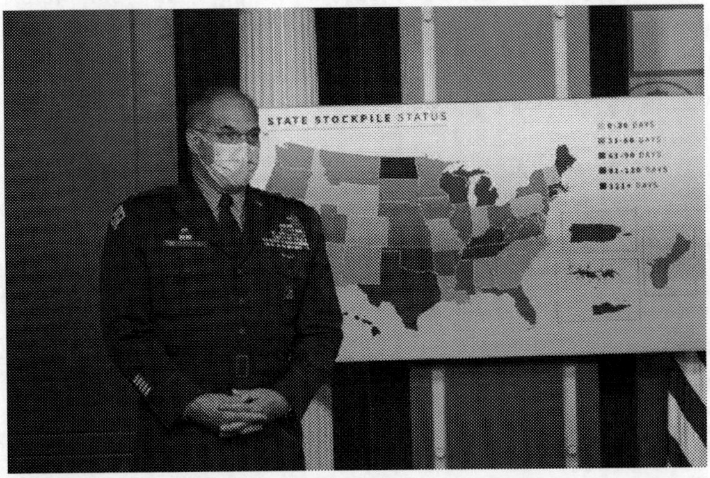

Gen. Gustave F. Perna during am Operation Warp Speed press briefing in Washington, Nov. 19, 2020. Photo: Chris Kleponis/Zuma Press.

Nearly all these claims rest on a misunderstanding both of Operation Warp Speed's mission and its nature as a government program. While President Trump's Health and Human Services Secretary Alex Azar and others dubbed the original project MP2, or Manhattan Project 2, after the crash effort to build an atomic bomb, Operation Warp Speed's leadership borrowed a more practical model: the industrial mobilization during World War II that produced the so-called Arsenal of Democracy.

Will Biden Cut a Covid Deal with Republicans?

That model can still push the vaccine rollout over the finish line. Governors and other state officials in particular need to realize the federal government is operating in the wake of a health-care version of Pearl Harbor, and adjust their operations accordingly.

From the beginning the principal mission of Operation Warp Speed was the development, manufacturing, and distribution—i.e., shipping—of coronavirus vaccines. To date, the program has managed to produce and deliver about 50 million vaccine doses—all made in the U.S.—with hundreds of millions more on the way. It also had 97,000 certified receivers distributing the vaccine across the U.S.

It is the most remarkable achievement in modern medicine, made possible by following the model of the World War II mobilization effort. That model rests on three principles.

First, set a clear target and a firm deadline. Operation Warp Speed's goal was 20 million vaccine doses by December 2020. Aiming at that target enabled the program's leaders, Gen. Gustave Perna and Dr. Moncef Slaoui (who resigned last month at the Biden administration's request but will stay on as a consultant), to focus everyone in Operation Warp Speed on achieving a single result.

Second, mobilize the best pharmaceutical and drug manufacturing companies to hit the target, so that private industry invests its energy and productivity in the plan. During World War II, the big automotive and electrical companies became the driving engine of the mobilization effort, though many had never before produced arms or weapons.

In Operation Warp Speed's case, the vaccine effort went from a single manufacturing facility in the U.S. to a network of facilities where the country's drug companies could pool efforts to develop and manufacture vaccines. What traditional health-care experts thought of as a laboratory process became an industrial process—with prodigious results. Companies like FedEx and UPS were pressed into service to deliver the finished product.

Third, maintain government oversight from start to finish. The Commerce, Defense, and Health and Human Services departments invoked the Defense Production Act 18 times to prioritize materials and supplies for Operation Warp Speed, and get government contracts for vaccine development and manufacturing to the head of the line. The use of federal authority to guide but not micromanage the private economy's efforts was key to producing victory in World War II and to creating the Covid vaccine in record time.

In the U.S. federal system, however, state governments can't be steamrolled by Washington. The Arsenal of Democracy was able to ship its goods to two all-powerful federal agencies, the War and Navy departments, which knew how to get those weapons to the soldiers, sailors and airmen who would use them. There's no corresponding federal agency in this case.

About 50 million vaccination doses have been made and shipped, but only half have been administered, while fewer than six million people have received second doses. While some states have dealt with the crisis well, many have found the process of getting shots into arms overwhelming.

It isn't too late to turn things around, if governors start using the World War II model. One step would be appointing their National Guard adjutants general as vaccine czars with clear authority to override state agency procedures and coordinate with federal leadership.

A second step would be to set a statewide target for inoculation aimed at twice the number of inoculations in half the time recommended by state health-care bureaucrats and experts. An urgent deadline can focus minds and trigger innovative thinking in ways that can transform the effort.

Another step would be to turn major businesses with large distribution networks into links in a logistical chain that can put as much vaccine as Operation Warp Speed can supply into as many arms as need it. With some 97,000 approved distribution centers already on the books there are plenty of opportunities for speeding up dispersal as part of an all-state government effort.

Some states are doing so. West Virginia has distributed nearly 90% of its first vaccine shot supply. But much more can be done in every state by combining planning with authority and imagination—and relying on guidance from the Arsenal of Democracy model.

There's still plenty to be done on manufacturing. The Novavax and Johnson & Johnson vaccines look promising and could be available this spring. One could argue that Moderna and Pfizer should focus now on making booster shots for the South African strain. The original architects of the World War II mobilization model would see all these issues as opportunities not obstacles. Thanks to Operation Warp Speed, America has established clear leadership in vaccine manufacturing. It is now poised to do the same for getting that vaccine to every American, starting with those who need it most.

Mr. Herman is a senior fellow at the Hudson Institute and author of "Freedom's Forge: How American Business Produced Victory in World War II."

Appeared in the February 2, 2021, print edition.

December 18, 2020
Governor Andrew Cuomo, Chair
Governor Asa Hutchinson, Vice Chair
National Governors Association

Re: Prioritizing hotel employees for inclusion in phase 1b distribution of the COVID-19 vaccine

Dear Chair Cuomo and Vice Chair Hutchinson,

We greatly appreciate your ongoing leadership and efforts to protect the public as we continue to face this unprecedented public health crisis.

As the rollout of the COVID-19 vaccine begins across the nation, we are now one step closer to ending the pandemic. And as you are likely aware, the Centers for Disease Control and Prevention's (CDC) Advisory Committee on Immunization Practices (ACIP) shared recommendations for allocation of the vaccine. Phase 1 of the CDC's proposed rollout, split into three stages, prioritizes health care providers and long-term care residents (phase 1a), essential workers (phase 1b) and adults with high-risk medical conditions and adults 65 and older (phase 1c). Now, as governors and state public health agencies begin to finalize COVID-19 vaccine distribution plans, we urge states to consider hotel employees for inclusion in phase "1b" of the vaccination rollout.

The Cybersecurity and Infrastructure Security Agency (CISA), a division of the Department of Homeland Security (DHS), classifies essential workers as "workers who conduct a range of operations and services that are typically essential to continued infrastructure viability." CISA identifies "management and staff at hotels and other temporary lodging facilities that provide for COVID-19 mitigation, containment, and treatment measures or provide accommodations for essential workers" as essential workers. Hotels have been utilized as places to quarantine for many during the pandemic and helped support all levels of government by opening our doors to first responders and medical professionals for a place to stay closer to their hospital or place work as they provide around-the-clock care to patients. Hotel employees also remain on the frontlines, and each day that they come to work, they welcome both global and domestic travelers increasing their likelihood of contracting the virus. While hotels have protocols in place to ensure limited contact between employees and guests, prioritizing employees with access to the vaccine would provide another layer of protection.

Since the onset of the pandemic, the hotel industry has worked diligently to support frontline healthcare workers and first responders through AHLA's "Hospitality for Hope Initiative." The initiative was launched in March and designed to match emergency and healthcare workers who require temporary housing with hotels during this unprecedented health crisis.

Established in partnership with AHLA's partner state associations, Hospitality for Hope identified more than 17,000 properties nationwide located in close proximity to healthcare facilities at the ready to assist government efforts. Hospitality for Hope partnered the hotel industry with the U.S. Department of Health and Human Services (HHS), in coordination with the US Army Corps of Engineers and local emergency management and public health agencies to provide access to hotel properties and room to support frontline workers in need of temporary housing while working on the front lines of the pandemic. And as the nation continues to battle the pandemic, the hotel industry remains committed to serving and housing the frontline medical staff and vulnerable populations across the nation.

The hotel industry has a longstanding commitment to cleanliness and safety for our employees and guests and rolled out our Safe Stay Guidelines to elevate our cleaning and disinfection efforts even further. However, our employees continue to be on the front lines for interstate travelers which increases exposure risk – another important reason why hotel workers should be included in the Phase 1b vaccine distribution. Additionally, given their often close proximity to hospitals and critical infrastructure such as airports and interstates, hotels could potentially be utilized during vaccine distribution, therefore increasing the need for vaccine distribution among hotel employees.

During the pandemic, we have continued and built upon this commitment to ensure hotels are cleaner and safer than ever before. In accordance with guidance issued by public health authorities, including the Centers for Disease Control and Prevention (CDC), AHLA launched "Safe Stay" – an industry-wide commitment to enhanced cleaning protocols and safety guidelines to meet and exceed the concerns created during the COVID-19 pandemic. Safe Stay has been endorsed by leading scientists, physicians and public health experts in epidemiology and infectious diseases.

Travel and tourism are critical drivers of the American economy, and while travel demand has hit record lows, ensuring hotel employees are prioritized during the vaccine rollout will help keep both employees and guests safe when it becomes safe to travel and resume meetings and events once again.

As an industry of people taking care of people, the hotel industry has taken steps to support and strengthen the community during this public health crisis. We ask that the employees who power our industry are prioritized during phase 1b of the vaccine roll out.

Once again, we thank you for your support, and we ask that you prioritize hotel employees as states finalize recommendations for COVID-19 vaccine distribution.

Sincerely, Chip Rogers
President and CEO of the American Hotel and Lodging Association
CC: Governors of the United States

January 14, 2021
Jeffrey Zients
Biden-Harris Transition Team

Dear Mr. Zients,

America's hotels stand ready to work alongside America's governors as states continue to move forward in administrating the COVID-19 vaccine. By quickly mobilizing an existing network of sites, hotels can help strengthen the delivery and distribution of the COVID-19 vaccine in communities across the country to better streamline and build on current state efforts.

As you know, administering the vaccine on a national level will be a significant undertaking requiring innovative solutions and collaboration. To aide in the distribution, the hotel industry is asking that hotels be considered as an option for vaccine administration sites in partnership with public health departments.

Hotels have existing infrastructure and operational capabilities to serve as vaccine administration sites and capacity to assist. The American Hotel & Lodging Association (AHLA) under its "Hospitality for Hope" initiative has the infrastructure in place to support public health agencies and private sector partners through a network of more than 20,000 hotels which could be quickly ready serve as locations to administer the COVID-19 vaccine. Through this program, the hotel industry has already successfully partnered with federal and local governments to provide assistance to those in need, including frontline and emergency workers as well as state and municipal public health departments.

The hotel industry is ready to step in and assist our community and alleviate the current burdens on our health systems in a time of national need and has the following capabilities:

- *Geographic reach:* With more than 50,000 hotels in every state, including properties located in cities, suburbs, and rural communities, hotels have the geographic reach to support a wide distribution of the vaccine.
- *Available Capacity and Operate 24/7:* Hotels have private rooms, meeting rooms, conference and ball rooms as well as outside areas, hotels are equipped for 24-hour operations to allow for round-the-clock vaccination administration. This will also ensure there is adequate space to maintain physical distancing, capacity limits and other safety protocols. Further, as hotels are currently running at less than 50 percent

occupancy rates, families or individuals who might be traveling to receive the vaccine will have access to comfortable and flexible lodging options should they need

- *Comprehensive cleanliness protocols:* The industry has also adopted AHLA's Safe Stay, an enhanced cleaning initiative that builds on the hotel industry's long-standing commitment and operations procedures to ensure the safety of guests during the ongoing public health crisis.
- *Infrastructure:* Hotels also offer ample parking and are often accessible from major transportation networks, including highways and public transportation routes. Hotels also have outdoor capabilities that can provide safe, weather-proof vaccination services where parking lots could be utilized for vaccination administration, similar to drive-thru testing sites.
- *Refrigeration Capabilities:* With many hotels being temperature controlled and the majority of hotels having refrigeration capabilities to store vaccines, issues concerning vaccine storage will be limited or can be quickly addressed to meet the requirements necessary for safe and effective vaccine storage.

Since the start of the pandemic, our industry has been on the frontlines to support national public health and safety priorities. AHLA launched the "Hospitality for Hope" initiative in early 2020, identifying more than 20,000 hotels willing to provide temporary housing for emergency and healthcare workers during the COVID-19 public health crisis. The initiative identified a total combined 2.3 million rooms located in close proximity to established healthcare facilities for frontline workers to use as they worked around the clock to save lives and provide lodging for those exposed to COVID to quarantine safely. Additionally, as part of this effort, hotels are supporting the national guard by providing lodging to those who Washington D.C. and surrounding region to provide additional security around the inauguration.

With the next phases of vaccination distribution underway, hotels have the unique capability to help provide additional locations to assist with the administration of the vaccine. As an industry, we have always stepped up to help our neighbors and communities in a time of need, including early-on in the pandemic through Hospitality for Hope. The industry looks forward to continuing this work in partnership with the public and private sector to support this next phase of recovery.

Sincerely, Chip Rogers
President and CEO
American Hotel & Lodging Association
Cc: Governor Andrew Cuomo, Chair, National Governors Association
Governor Asa Hutchinson, Vice Chair, National Governors Association
Moncef Slaoui, Operation Warp Speed
Dr. Robert R. Redfield, Centers for Disease Control and Prevention
The Honorable Alex Azar, U.S. Department of Health & Human Services
US Conference of Mayors

January 27, 2021

Dr. Jose R. Romero, MD, FAAP

Chair, Advisory Committee on Immunization Practices
U.S. Centers for Disease Control and Prevention
RE: Docket No. CDC–2021–0002, Advisory Committee on Immunization Practices, January 27

Dear Chair Jose Romero:

We greatly appreciate your ongoing leadership and efforts to protect the public as we continue to face this unprecedented public health crisis. As the rollout of the COVID-19 vaccine begins across the nation, we are now one step closer to ending the pandemic. The Centers for Disease Control and Prevention's (CDC) Advisory Committee on Immunization Practices (ACIP) plays a critical role in allocation of the vaccine and as you continue to provide recommendations, we urge you to consider the importance of prioritizing hotel employees in phase "1" of the vaccination rollout. Additionally, we request the Committee clarify "other essential workers" in the "1c" vaccination classification.

The Cybersecurity and Infrastructure Security Agency (CISA), a division of the Department of Homeland Security (DHS), classifies essential workers as "workers who conduct a range of operations and services that are typically essential to continued infrastructure viability." CISA identifies "management and staff at hotels and other temporary lodging facilities that provide for COVID-19 mitigation, containment, and treatment measures or provide accommodations for essential workers" as essential workers. Hotels have been utilized as places to quarantine for many during the pandemic and helped support all levels of government by opening our doors to first responders and medical professionals for a place to stay closer to their hospital or place work as they provide around-the-clock care to patients. Hotel employees also remain on the frontlines, and each day that they come to work, they welcome both global and domestic travelers increasing their likelihood of contracting the virus. While hotels have protocols in place to ensure limited contact between employees and guests, prioritizing employees with access to the vaccine would provide another layer of protection.

Since the onset of the pandemic, the hotel industry has worked diligently to support frontline healthcare workers and first responders through AHLA's "Hospitality for Hope Initiative." The initiative was launched in March and designed to match emergency and healthcare workers who require temporary housing with hotels during this unprecedented health crisis.

Established in partnership with AHLA's partner state associations, Hospitality for Hope identified more than 17,000 properties nationwide located in close proximity to healthcare facilities at the ready to assist government efforts. Hospitality for Hope partnered the hotel industry with the U.S. Department of Health and Human Services (HHS), in coordination with the US Army CORPS of Engineers and local emergency management and public health agencies to provide access to hotel properties and room to support frontline workers in need of temporary housing while working on the front lines of the pandemic. And as the nation continues to battle the pandemic, the hotel industry remains committed to serving and housing the frontline medical staff and vulnerable populations across the nation, including working with federal, state and local governments to serve as vaccinations sites.

The hotel industry has a longstanding commitment to cleanliness and safety for our employees and guests and rolled out our Safe Stay Guidelines to elevate our cleaning and disinfection efforts even further. However, our employees continue to be on the front lines for interstate travelers which increases risk exposure – another important reason why hotel workers should be included in the Phase 1c vaccine distribution. Additionally, given their often close proximity to hospitals and critical infrastructure such as airports and interstates, hotels could potentially be utilized during vaccine distribution, therefore increasing the need for vaccine distribution among hotel employees. Clarification of "other essential workers" to include hotel employees will also ensure that state and local municipalities are well equipped to provide vaccinations to those that need it most.

During the pandemic, we have continued and built upon this commitment to ensure hotels are cleaner and safer than ever before. In accordance with guidance issued by public health authorities, including the CDC, AHLA launched "Safe Stay" – an industry-wide commitment to enhanced cleaning protocols and safety guidelines to meet and exceed the concerns created during the COVID-19 pandemic. Safe Stay has been endorsed by leading scientists, physicians and public health experts in epidemiology and infectious diseases.

Travel and tourism are critical drivers of the American economy, and while travel demand has hit record lows, ensuring hotel employees are prioritized during the vaccine rollout will help keep both employees and guests safe when it becomes safe to travel and resume meetings and events once again.

As an industry of people taking care of people, the hotel industry has taken steps to support and strengthen the community during this public health crisis. We ask that the employees who power our industry are prioritized during phase 1 of the vaccine roll out and to provide clarity to municipalities that hotel workers are considered essential.

Once again, we thank you for your support, and we ask that you prioritize hotel employees as states finalize recommendations for COVID-19 vaccine distribution.

Sincerely,
Chip Rogers
President and CEO of the American Hotel and Lodging Association

American Pharmaceutical Resilience

By Scott Lincicome

Shortly after the COVID-19 outbreak began last year, numerous politicians and pundits proclaimed that the pandemic revealed massive vulnerabilities in global supply chains for essential medical goods - vulnerabilities that imperiled Americans' health and national security and therefore necessitated major government interventions (read: subsidies and protectionism) to bolster U.S. supply chain "resiliency." Pharmaceuticals, in particular, topped the list of medical goods that required government action, and the alleged threat to American pharmaceutical access - supposedly dependent on China and India - was so dire that the Trump administration fast-tracked hundreds of millions of dollars in federal support to domestic producers of drugs and raw materials in order to "reduce reliance on other countries for drugs."

At the time, I and others noted repeatedly that, while there were some gaps in the public data, the information we had on U.S. pharmaceutical production, R&D, and trade did not indicate a forthcoming pharmaceutical crisis. Now, the nonpartisan United States International Trade Commission has provided additional data in a massive new report on "U.S. industries producing COVID-19 related goods and the supply chain challenges and constraints that impacted the availability of such goods," which for the most part confirms that our skepticism was warranted.

The report overall reveals a far more complicated and benign picture of the medical goods situation in the United States - one characterized by unprecedented supply and demand shocks, as well as substantial domestic resources (especially for pharmaceuticals, medical devices, and N95 masks), quickly-adapting domestic and international supply chains, and beneficial global specialization and cooperat io n. It's a great resource for those interested in manufacturing issues, and should help to inform the broader debate in Washington about the pandemic, supply chain resiliency, and national security.

The report also should temper specific concerns about the pharmaceutical supply chain, which the USITC finds worked quite well during the once-in-a-generation pandemic due in part to its globalized business model (emphasis mine):

> The United States has a large, geographically diverse pharmaceutical industry with established supply chains that proved resilient during the first half of 2020. The flexibility and number of manufacturing sites inherent in the global footprint of the pharmaceutical sector allowed firms to respond relatively quickly to demand and deliver additional medicines to aid in the response to the pandemic ... The U.S. industry, which comprises companies ranging from large multinational firms to small and medium-sized firms (SMEs), was operating at almost full capacity in the second quarter of 2020 to meet demand. These supplies were delivered via the existing wholesale distribution network....

The Commission's report also details the immense size and scope of the U.S. pharmaceutical industry (which has supposedly shriveled due to globalization) - nearly 5,000 establishments spanning numerous states and all stages of production (upstream, downstream, and "fill and finish"); increasing shipments that reached $268.7 billion in 2019; and an expanding workforce that hit 310,000 workers in early 2020. The report further notes that U.S. manufacturers responded to the pandemic by substantially increasing pharmaceutical shipments (even while bringing new COVID-19 products to the market) because they maintained their own "emergency plans" to utilize significant available inventories, different production sites, or contract manufacturers. Finally, the USITC report shows that some of the industry's resilience has stemmed from its diverse foreign sourcing of raw materials and finished products, while noting that China and India are significant (but not dominant) suppliers - essentially confirming my analysis of the import data earlier this year.

For those (like me) who have been fascinated by the COVID-19 vaccine rollout in the United States, the USITC's conclusions about the pharmaceutical supply chain's resilience during the pandemic shouldn't come as much of a surprise: Pfizer, for example, utilized its existing U.S. manufacturing capacity, as well as other domestic and international resources (not to mention lots of immigrants), to test and produce millions of vaccine doses with unprecedented speed. Moderna, meanwhile, has relied on smaller in-house facilities and a partnership with a large Swiss pharmaceutical manufacturer, which has production sites in the United States and Switzerland. As a result of these and other multinational efforts, the vaccine bottlenecks we're now experiencing have been related to government distribution, not private sector production, of finished doses. (Lessons abound).

Still, the USITC report has a wealth of new data and is especially welcome given the incoming Biden administration's plans to "rebuild" American pharmaceutical supply chains through top-down mandates like the Defense Production Act. Surely, the pandemic has put real strains on Americans' access to essential medical goods as demand skyrocketed and supply raced to catch up, and it'd be good for the country to get a better handle on the virus and vaccine distribution. But the pharmaceutical supply chains themselves have fared pretty well so far, and there's little evidence that government could improve them.

Global Supply Chains and Economic "Resilience": (More) Evidence from the Pandemic

By Scott Lincicome

The last few months have provided several counterexamples to the trendy claim that "re-nationalizing" global supply chains for essential goods would have bolstered the United States' economic "resilience" during the pandemic (and thus is a necessity in the future). As I explain in a forthcoming paper on trade, manufacturing, and national security, these claims never made much sense: "greater trade and investment openness might make an economy more vulnerable to external supply or demand shocks, but it also helps reduce a nation's vulnerability to (and improve its recovery from) domestic shocks." New economic research confirms this intuition (and those anecdotes) with respect to COVID-19:

In a mid-2020 analysis of the pandemic's earliest days, economists Barthelemy Bonadio, Zhen Huo, Andrei A. Levchenko and Nitya Pandalai-Nayar-

> show that the average real GDP downturn due to the Covid-19 shock is expected to be - 29:6%, with one quarter of the total due to transmission through global supply chains. However, "renationalizat ion" of global supply chains does not in general make countries more resilient to pandemic-induced contractions in labor supply. The average GDP drop would have been - 30:2% in a world without trade in inputs and final goods. This is because eliminating reliance on foreign inputs increases reliance on the domestic inputs, which are also disrupted due to nationwide lockdowns. In fact, trade can insulate a country imposing a stringent lockdown from the pandemic- shock, as its foreign inputs are less disrupted than its domestic ones.

Their initial conclusions were subsequently confirmed in a new paper from World Bank economists Alvaro Espitia, Aaditya Mattoo, Nadia Rocha, Michele Ruta, Deborah Winkler, who summarized their findings in a recent VoxEU article:

> Econometric results for the first six months of the health crisis confirm a nuanced view of the roe of [global value chains] during a pandemic. GVCs have certainly acted as a transmitter of shocks. Exports of firms relying on upstream suppliers from countries in lockdown suffered more. So did exports of firms supplying inputs to countries severely hit by Covid-19. But exports of domestic producers participating in GVCs fared better during the pandemic, as diversification through trade turned out to be an asset. These findings suggest that thinking of better ways to improve GVC resilience in the face of a pandemic or other shocks is crucial. Nationalisation of production is not a solution - it would result in lower exposure to foreign shocks at the cost of higher exposure to domestic shocks.

The authors' conclusions are summarized in the following chart, which shows that exporters who utilized imported inputs fared worse when their supplier markets were hit by COVID-19 ("upstream supply shock") *but* fared better when their own home market was hit.

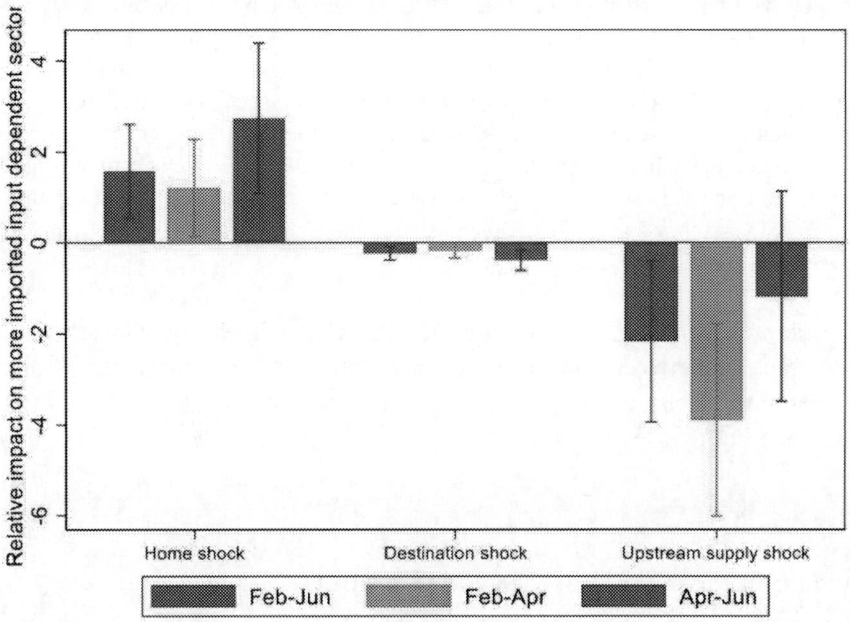

With respect to the latter scenario, they calculate that that the harm of a domestic shock for sectors with low value-chain participation has been 20 percentage points worse, on average, than for sectors with high participat ion. These findings are particularly important for the United States, which continues to struggle with a domestic COVID-19 shock (especially as compared to other key economies).

Finally, a November 2020 analysis from OECD economists Christine Arriola, Przemyslaw Kowalski, Frank van Tongeren finds that the economic costs of "localizing" global supply chains would significantly exceed any benefits from doing so and *still* wouldn't insulate countries from external shocks:

> [A] localised regime (where economies are less interconnected) has significantly lower levels of economic activity and lower incomes. A shift to the localised regime is estimated to decrease global real GDP by more than 5% relative to the post-Covid-19 baseline. Reductions in economic activity are significant across all regions and countries, and in some cases reach double digits. Increased localisation would thus add further GDP losses to the economic slowdown caused by the pandemic. Further, even with the support and protection offered to domestic producers under a localised regime, not all stages of production can be undertaken in the home country, and trade in intermediate inputs and raw materials continues to play an important role in domestic production. In that context, less international diversification of sourcing and sales means that most domestic markets are required to shoulder more of the adjustments to absorb shocks. This translates into larger price swings and large changes of production, ultimately leading to greater variability of incomes. In this sense, the more localised regime delivers neither greater efficiency nor greater security of supply.
>
> Recent analysis on the global value chain of face masks during the Covid-19 outbreak offers a concrete illustration. It shows that producing face masks requires a multitude of inputs

> along the value chain, from non-woven fabric made with polypropylene to specialised machinery for ultra-sonic welding. While the production itself does not require high-tech inputs, localising the production of just this one good would require high capital investments which would need to be supported during periods when demand shrinks, and localised production is not competitive. With current technologies it would therefore be excessively costly for every country to develop production capacity that matches crisis-induced surges in demand, and which encompasses the whole value chain from raw materials through distribution for a whole catalogue of essential goods to match any potential crisis, foreseen and otherwise.
>
> More localisation also means more reliance on fewer sources of (and often more expensive) inputs. In this regime, when a disruption occurs somewhere in the supply chain, it is harder and more costly to find ready substitutes, giving rise to greater risk of insecurity in supply. This is also the case for sectors that are often seen as strategic, such as food, basic pharmaceuticals, motor vehicles, and electronics.

All of these studies, along with the aforementioned anecdotes, show that the United States' openness to trade and investment is compatible with - and often bolsters - our ability to withstand economic shocks, even a once-in-a-generation global pandemic. Policymakers would be wise to remember that lesson before trying to rewire global supply chains in the name of "resilience."

Coronavirus: Operation Warp Speed Timeline

Using the resources of the Federal Government and the U.S. private sector, Operation Warp Speed (OWS) will accelerate the testing, supply, development, and distribution of safe and effective vaccines, diagnostics, and therapeutics to counter COVID-19 by January 2021.

Jan. 12, 2021

The Department of Health and Human Services (HHS) and the Department of Defense (DOD) announces the purchase of 1.25 million additional treatment courses of Regeneron's investigational monoclonal antibody therapeutic to be delivered in the first half of 2021 to treat non-hospitalized, high-risk COVID-19 patients

Army Gen. Gustave F. Perna, chief operating officer of Operation Warp Speed; Dr. Moncef Slaoui, chief advisor to Operation Warp Speed; Secretary of Health and Human Services Alex M. Azar II; and Dr. Robert R. Redfield, Director of the Centers for Disease Control and Prevention brief the news media on Operation Warp Speed.

Jan. 6, 2021

Army Gen. Gustave F. Perna, chief operating officer of Operation Warp Speed; Dr. Moncef Slaoui, chief advisor to Operation Warp Speed; and Health and Human Services Secretary Alex M. Azar II brief the media on the progress of Operation Warp Speed.

Dec. 30, 2020

Army Gen. Gustave F. Perna, chief operating officer of Operation Warp Speed, and Dr. Moncef Slaoui, chief advisor to Operation Warp Speed, brief the media on Operation Warp Speed and COVID-19 vaccine distribution.

Dec. 28, 2020

Novavax begins Phase 3 clinical trials.

Dec. 23, 2020

The U.S. Department of the Health and Human Services and DOD jointly announce an agreement with Merck to continue the development and large-scale manufacturing of investigational COVID-19 treatment MK-7110.

The Administration announces that it will purchase an additional 100 million doses of COVID-19 vaccine from Pfizer through the U.S. Department of Health and Human Services and DOD.

Army Gen. Gustave F. Perna, chief operating officer of Operation Warp Speed; Dr. Moncef Slaoui, chief advisor to Operation Warp Speed; and Health and Human Services Secretary Alex M. Azar II brief the media on the progress of Operation Warp Speed.

Dec. 21, 2020

Army Gen. Gustave F. Perna, chief operating officer of Operation Warp Speed; Dr. Moncef Slaoui, chief advisor to Operation Warp Speed; and Health and Human Services Secretary Alex M. Azar II brief the media on the progress of Operation Warp Speed.

Dec. 19, 2020

Army Gen. Gustave F. Perna, chief operating officer of Operation Warp Speed, briefs the media on Operation Warp Speed and COVID-19 vaccine distribution.

Dec. 18, 2020

U.S. Food and Drug Administration issues an Emergency Use Authorization for Moderna's COVID-19 vaccine.

Dec. 16, 2020

Army Gen. Gustave F. Perna, chief operating officer of Operation Warp Speed; Dr. Moncef Slaoui, chief advisor to Operation Warp Speed; and Health and Human Services Secretary Alex M. Azar II brief the media on Operation Warp Speed and COVID-19 vaccine distribution.

Dec. 14, 2020

Army Gen. Gustave F. Perna, chief operations officer for Operation Warp Speed; Health and Human Services Secretary Alex M. Azar II; and Dr. Moncef Slaoui, chief advisor for OWS, conduct a briefing on Operation Warp Speed beginning nationwide vaccine distribution.

Dec. 12, 2020

Army Gen. Gustave F. Perna, chief operations officer for Operation Warp Speed, conducts a briefing on Operation Warp Speed planning for nationwide vaccine distribution.

Dec. 11, 2020

DOD purchases an additional 100 million doses of Moderna's COVID-19 vaccine.

U.S. Food and Drug Administration issues an Emergency Use Authorization to Pfizer for its COVID-19 vaccine.

Nov. 24, 2020

Army Gen. Gustave F. Perna, chief operations officer for Operation Warp Speed, Health and Human Services Secretary Alex M. Azar II and Dr. Moncef Slaoui, chief advisor for OWS, conduct a briefing on Operation Warp Speed.

Nov. 23, 2020

Congressional/media engagement on Emergency Use Authorization of Regeneron's investigational monoclonal antibody therapeutic cocktail.

Nov. 21, 2020

U.S. Food and Drug Administration issues an Emergency Use Authorization for Regeneron's investigational monoclonal antibody therapeutic cocktail comprised of the drugs casirivimab and imdevimab for treatment of non-hospitalized patients with mild or moderate confirmed cases of COVID-19 at high risk of hospitalization.

Nov. 18, 2020

Army Gen. Gustave F. Perna, chief operations officer for Operation Warp Speed, Health and Human Services Secretary Alex M. Azar II and Dr. Moncef Slaoui, chief advisor for OWS, conduct a briefing on Operation Warp Speed.

Nov. 12, 2020

The U.S. government partnered with large chain pharmacies and networks covering approximately 60 percent of pharmacies throughout the United States, Puerto Rico, and the U.S. Virgin Islands to maximize access to COVID-19 vaccines.

Nov. 10, 2020

Congressional/media engagement on OWS vaccine distribution and therapeutics.

Nov. 9, 2020

U.S. Food and Drug Administration issues an Emergency Use Authorization for Eli Lilly's COVID-19 investigational antibody therapeutic.

Oct. 28, 2020

The Department of Health and Human Services and DOD announce an agreement with Eli Lilly and Company to purchase 300,000 doses of the company's COVID-19 investigational antibody therapeutic for $375 million. These doses will be available for patient care if the U.S. Food and Drug Administration authorizes use of the therapeutic, as outlined in agency guidance.

Oct. 23, 2020

AstraZeneca resumes COVID-19 Phase 3 vaccine clinical trials in the United States after the FDA and an independent safety review board completed an examination of all safety data from trials globally and concluded it was safe to resume.

Congressional/media engagement on OWS vaccine distribution and minority enrollment in clinical trials.

Oct. 19, 2020

All 64 jurisdictions have submitted initial COVID-19 vaccine distribution plans to the Centers for Disease Control and Prevention, a significant milestone in the ongoing collaboration between the federal government and jurisdictions to prepare for delivery of a safe, effective vaccine to the American people.

Oct. 16, 2020

The Department of Health and Human Services and DOD announce agreements with CVS and Walgreens to provide COVID-19 vaccine with no out-of-pocket costs to protect vulnerable Americans in long-term care facilities nationwide once vaccines are available and recommended for them.

Oct. 13, 2020

$31 million agreement with Cytiva to expand manufacturing capacity for products essential in producing COVID-19 vaccines, such as liquid and dry powder cell culture media, cell culture buffers, mixer bags, and XDR bioreactors.

Oct. 9, 2020

$486 million agreement with AstraZeneca for late-stage development and large-scale manufacturing of the company's COVID-19 investigational prophylaxis product, a cocktail of two monoclonal antibodies, that may help treat or prevent the coronavirus that causes COVID-19.

Congressional/media engagement on OWS vaccine distribution.

Sept. 23, 2020

Johnson & Johnson begins Phase 3 clinical trials.

Sept. 16, 2020

The Department of Health and Human Services and DOD release two documents outlining the Administration's strategy to deliver safe and effective COVID-19 vaccine doses to Americans as quickly and reliably as possible. The documents provide a strategic distribution overview along with an interim playbook for jurisdiction operations.

Congressional/media engagement on OWS vaccines.

Sept. 8, 2020

AstraZeneca pauses clinical trials due to an unexpected adverse event in a study participant in the Phase 2/3 trial in the UK. AstraZeneca is working with the FDA to facilitate review of the information and the agency will decide when the U.S. trial can resume.

Sept. 3, 2020

As part of the Operation Warp Speed goal to deliver safe and effective vaccines and therapeutics by January 2021, five DOD medical treatment facilities are identified for Phase 3 COVID-19 vaccine trials. The selected sites are located in the National Capital Region, San Antonio and San Diego.

Aug. 29, 2020

AstraZeneca begins Phase 3 clinical trials.

Aug. 28, 2020

Congressional/media engagement on OWS vaccine distribution.

Aug. 23, 2020

U.S. Food and Drug Administration issues an Emergency Use Authorization for convalescent plasma.

Aug. 17, 2020

$106 million contract with Ology Bioservices Inc. to reserve production capacity of more than 180 million doses of COVID-19 medical countermeasures.

Aug. 14, 2020

CDC selects McKesson Corporation to support distribution of COVID-19 vaccines and related supplies.

Aug. 13, 2020

Congressional/media engagement on OWS vaccine prioritization.

Aug. 11, 2020

$1.5 billion agreement with Moderna to support the large-scale manufacture and delivery of a vaccine candidate.

Aug. 5, 2020

$1.5 billion agreement with Moderna to support the large-scale manufacture and delivery of a vaccine candidate.

Aug. 4, 2020

$160 million awarded to Grand River Aseptic ManufacturingInc. for domestic aseptic fill and finish manufacturing capacity for critical vaccines and therapeutics.

July 31, 2020

$2 billion agreement with Sanofi and GlaxoSmithKline to support the advanced development, including clinical trials and large-scale manufacturing, of a vaccine candidate.

July 30, 2020

Congressional/media engagement on OWS vaccines.

July 27, 2020

Moderna and Pfizer begin Phase 3 clinical trials.

Texas A&M University and FUJIFILM announce a task order with Texas A&M University and FUJIFILM to advance domestic manufacturing capabilities and capacity for a potential COVID-19 vaccine.

July 22, 2020

$1.95 billion agreement with Pfizer for the large-scale manufacturing and nationwide distribution of 100 million doses of their vaccine candidate.

July 13, 2020

Congressional/media engagement on OWS vaccines.

July 7, 2020

$1.6 billion agreement to support the large-scale manufacturing of Novavax's vaccine candidate.

July 2, 2020

GEN Gustave Perna is Senate-confirmed to serve as chief operating officer.

June 18, 2020

GEN Gustave Perna confirmation hearing.

June 15, 2020

Congressional/media engagement on OWS vaccines.

June 11, 2020

$143 million agreement with SiO2 Materials Science to ramp up capacity to produce the company's glass-coated plastic container.

June 9, 2020

$204 million agreement with Corning to expand the domestic manufacturing capacity to produce approximately 164 million Valor Glass vials per year.

June 1, 2020

Emergent BioSolutions announces a task order to advance domestic manufacturing capabilities and capacity for a potential COVID-19 vaccine as well as therapeutics.

May 21, 2020

$1.2 billion agreement in support for AstraZeneca's candidate vaccine.

May 15, 2020

White House announces Operation Warp Speed, or OWS.

May 12, 2020

$138 million contract with ApiJect for more than 100 million prefilled syringes for distribution across the United States by year-end.

April 16, 2020

$483 million agreement in support available for Moderna's candidate vaccine, which began Phase 1 trials on March 16, 2020, and received a fast-track designation from the U.S. Food & Drug Administration.

March 30, 2020

$456 million for Johnson & Johnson's candidate vaccine.

FAQs

DOD is collaborating closely with public and private sector partners to provide an unprecedented response to the coronavirus outbreak. Our crucial support includes assistance for the accelerated development and rapid distribution of a safe, effective vaccine or vaccines and therapeutics for COVID-19. Below is information on this American vaccine effort.

Operation Warp Speed

Using the resources of the federal government and the U.S. private sector, Operation Warp Speed (OWS) will accelerate the testing, supply, development, and distribution of safe and effective vaccines, therapeutics, and diagnostics to counter COVID-19 by January 2021.

Coronavirus: DOD Response

The Defense Department is working closely with the Department of Health and Human Services and the State Department to provide support in dealing with the coronavirus outbreak.

Operation Warp Speed Staffers Refute Claim Biden Is Starting from Scratch on Vaccines

By Tobias Hoonhout and Ryan Mills
January 26, 2021 6:30 AM

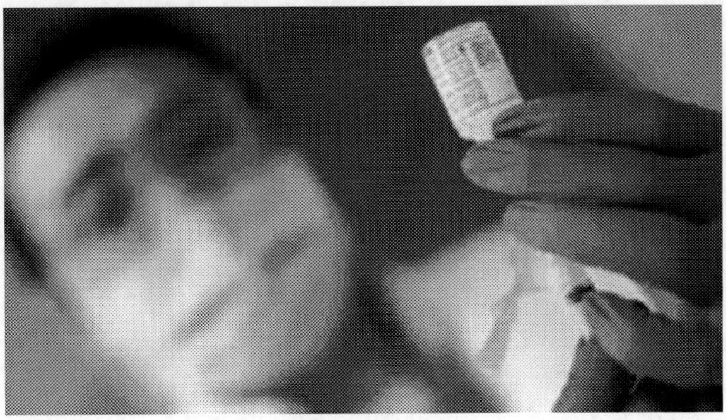

Pharmacist Danny Huynh fills a syringe with the Moderna coronavirus vaccine in Chula Vista, Calif., January 21, 2021. (Mike Blake/Reuters).

Current and Former Staffers Say They Helped Set Biden's Administration on a Glide Path to Its Vaccination Goal

Leaders of the Trump administration's Operation Warp Speed spent months working with states and cities to improve their coronavirus vaccine rollout plans, and helped set President Joe Biden's administration on a glide path to its goal of vaccinating 100 million people in 100 days, according to current and former operation officials who spoke with NATIONAL REvIEw.

Those officials pushed back on Biden administration members who have both publicly and privately bashed their predecessors for leaving "no coronavirus vaccine distribution plan to speak of." The Biden officials are simply "passing the buck" and trying to lower expectations, two Trump administration officials said.

Last week, CNN White House correspondent MJ Lee published a story titled "Biden inheriting nonexistent coronavirus vaccine distribution plan and must start 'from scratch,' sources say." It included quotes from anonymous Biden administration officials saying things like "there is nothing for us to rework" and that they were starting from "square one." Though Dr. Anthony Fauci has publicly refuted the claim, Biden officials have continued to imply it.

"The sad part is the last administration didn't leave anything. They didn't leave a plan," Biden senior adviser Cedric Richmond told CNN on Saturday. On *Meet the Press*, Biden chief of staff Ron Klain said "the process to distribute the vaccine, particularly outside of nursing homes and hospitals out into the community as a whole, did not really exist when we came into the White House."

The White House has set a goal of 100 million vaccinations in Biden's first 100 days, though CDC director Dr. Rochelle Walensky said Sunday that she didn't know "how much vaccine we have," a statement echoed by Biden press secretary Jen Psaki on Monday.

"The confusion around this issue — which, we acknowledge, there is some confusion — speaks to a larger problem, which is what we're inheriting from the prior administration," Psaki said. "Which is much worse than we could have imagined."

But per vaccination data from *Bloomberg*, the U.S. has now hit 1 million vaccinations for four days in a row, with a rolling seven-day average of 1.2 million. And on Monday, Biden himself said he hoped to raise the threshold to 1.5 million soon.

The new administration's ability to hit its daily target immediately after the benchmark was set is evidence that they inherited a workable plan from the Trump administration, according to current and former officials.

"We provided the Biden team over 300 transition meetings, including the very first one on Warp Speed which I kicked off myself," former Health and Human Services chief of staff Brian Harrison told NATIONAL REvIEw. "The idea that they're walking in, having no clue what was going on, is absolutely preposterous."

Another former senior administration official noted the difference between the distribution of vaccines – the logistical efforts to transport the vaccines to the proper locations – and the actual administration of the vaccines, or actually getting needles into arms.

The former official described the distribution plan, which is being managed by U.S. Army general Gustave Perna, as "extraordinarily detailed" and "comprehensive."

"It's gone flawlessly," the former official said. "Like, out of tens of thousands of deliveries under extreme cold storage conditions, I think three out of like 30,000 didn't make it to the right place at the right time. So, it's a 99.99 percent success rate of shipping to the right place at the right time in the right quantity, under the right conditions."

As for the actual administration of the vaccine, officials said that there were also plans in place for rollout, led by the U.S. Centers for Disease Control and Prevention.

"CDC was the one who volunteered — not volunteered, asserted — itself to the task, and said that they were going to be in charge of this because they were in charge of pandemic influenza distribution and allocation," one former senior HHS official said.

The former official added that the incoming administration's insistence on blaming the outgoing one for challenges associated with vaccine distribution amounts to "playing politics with public health."

"They're shifting blame. That's the most polite way I could describe it. But I'll tell you that the guys at Warp Speed were pushing the CDC really hard to basically demonstrate that the plans were more than just paper," the official said. "They pushed them as hard as they could, but again, CDC was strident in its view that they're the experts. They're the ones with the relationships with the states. They're the ones who could do this and that."

"It's disgraceful that the CDC is pointing its finger at Warp Speed, when CDC was the one that said that they were in charge and basically said they were the one responsible party," he continued. "It's passing the buck, and I just think that's disgraceful."

A disagreement over governing philosophy accounts for much of the division between the vaccine rollout plan implemented by the Trump administration and the one preferred by the Biden team. The Biden team believes in centralizing control of the rollout under the federal government, while the Trump team sought to empower the states and public health jurisdictions.

"There was this very big feeling in the Trump administration we need to leave this to the states," one senior administration official involved with Operation Warp Speed told NATIONAL REvIEw. "There was fear of we don't want to dictate to the states of how we do this, but we can get it there. If they tell us where to send it, we can deliver it."

Under the Trump administration, there wasn't one vaccine rollout plan, but rather 64 plans, one from each of the nation's public health jurisdictions. Those plans were crafted, starting in mid-September, based on a 60-page operating book provided by the CDC, which gave guidance to local officials about operations, logistics, information technology, and storage requirements, among other things. The jurisdictions turned in their vaccine administration plans in mid-October, one former official said.

"We actually created a rating system that has seven criteria for each one. And we rated them as red, yellow and green. And where we saw yellow and red, we worked with the states. We even sent strike teams out to the states and jurisdictions to help them get their plans well developed," the former official said.

The planning process wrapped up in early December, the former official said.

"They were all in good shape," the former official said. "I don't want to say all the reds turned to green, but they certainly all turned to yellow. And we felt pretty good about them. There was an immense amount of planning that went on over several months' time."

The states that have been most successful were those whose leaders were engaged from the beginning, and those who worked well with local community leaders, the former official explained.

"I can tell you the single biggest difference, and that is, was the governor engaged in the fall or wasn't he or she?" the former official said. "You had some of them front and center taking notes, asking questions. … Other governors didn't give a crap. Some didn't show up to a single governors call when we discussed all of this."

There were some hurdles and unexpected challenges, the former official acknowledged. For one, the CDC's Advisory Committee on Immunization Practices (ACIP) provided guidance over the winter, recommending that front-line workers and people who live in congregant settings be prioritized. Some jurisdictions applied those guidelines so rigidly, that when some of the intended vaccine recipients declined to take the vaccine, there was no backup plan for how to distribute the extra doses, the former official said.

"When ACIP came out with its recommendations, I would have had every doctor on television saying, 'Guys, these are just recommendations. You should do what's best for your states,'" the former official said.

The former official also said Pfizer's vaccine rollout was slower than expected, and the federal government received fewer doses than initially planned.

"We probably shouldn't have had as much confidence in that globally respected pharmaceutical company and its CEO who made promises to us that they didn't keep," the former official said.

As for the Biden administration's claims that there was no vaccine rollout plan, the Trump administration's rollout was already hitting the goal of distributing 1 million doses daily.

"It appears to me they are lowering expectations so they can look like they're heroes," the former official said, adding, "I think they're both naïve and a little bit arrogant about what they believe the federal government can do to make this any better than what it has."

One pharmaceutical adviser working with Operation Warp Speed said that what has been accomplished already has been "remarkable, and hopefully will continue to improve."

"I think that we have accomplished something that has never been accomplished before," said the adviser, who is still working with the project. "There are things that could have worked better, of course. When you do something like this, you can always point at something that could have been better."

Tobias Hoonhout is a media reporter for NATIONAL REvIEw ONLINE. *Ryan Mills is a media reporter for* NATIONAL REvIEw ONLINE *who previously worked as a breaking news reporter, investigative reporter, and editor at newspapers in Florida.*

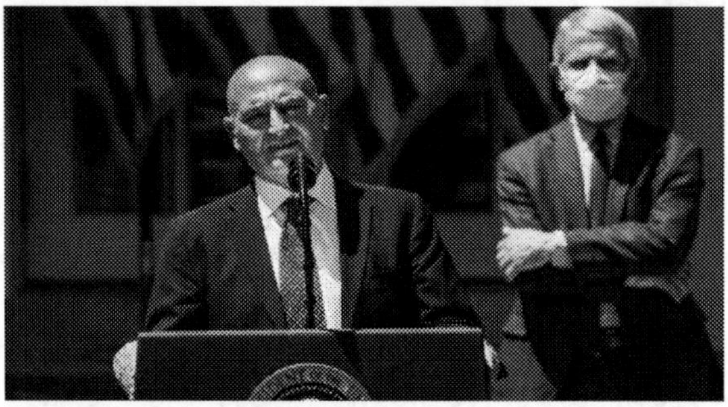

Moncef Slaoui last spring spoke at a White House ceremony that announced his appointment as scientific head of Operation Warp Speed.
Jabin Botsford/The *Washington Post* Via Getty Images.

Proud of Vaccine Success, Warp Speed's Ex-Science Head Talks Politics, Presidents, and Future Pandemics

By Jon Cohen
Jan. 25, 2021, 4:1O PM

When President Joe Biden took office last week, his administration swiftly announced it would be renaming Operation Warp Speed, the Trump administration's crash program to develop

COVID-19 vaccines. The decision puzzled immunologist Moncef Slaoui, scientific head of Warp Speed, but he attributes it to a word he says with disdain: politics.

Slaoui recently resigned from his post, but has agreed to help the Biden transition team into February. In a lengthy chat with Science from his home in Pennsylvania last week, he reflected on his time with Operation Warp Speed, discussing challenging interactions with former President Donald Trump and how to be better prepared for a future pandemic. Never a Trump supporter—he's a Democrat—Slaoui had reluctantly taken the Warp Speed job because, as the former head of vaccines at GlaxoSmithKline (GSK), he thought he could help solve one of the world's most urgent problems.

But long before COVID-19 surfaced, Slaoui had become frustrated that the vaccine industry had such a haphazard, ad hoc response to emerging infectious diseases. About 6 years ago at GSK, he began working with the company to create a nonprofit division they called a Biopreparedness Organization (BPO) that would exist solely to make vaccines to prevent pandemics. In 2016, after recent outbreaks of Ebola and Zika had made headlines, he explained why the project was sorely needed. "Unfortunately, one of these days, one of these agents is going to be global and very lethal. It's going to be catastrophic," he said on a TV show. "So we have to have a longer term commitment and solution that governments and a long-term institution should drive and fund."

The company ended up buying a defunct drug manufacturing plant in Rockville, Maryland, but it wanted financial help to launch the BPO. The U.S. government, which has sunk more than $11 billion into Warp Speed vaccine R&D, wasn't interested. GSK helped form the Coalition for Epidemic Preparedness Innovations in 2017, a nonprofit that would fund vaccine development, but it, too, ultimately didn't want to bankroll the BPO, and the idea died. The plant is now called GSK's Slaoui Center for Vaccines Research.

During his undergraduate years at the Free University of Brussels, Slaoui was a militant in a secret organization that wanted to spark a revolution in Morocco, his native country. "What I realized at the very end as I got in trouble with the regime was that, at least as far as I'm concerned, I want to participate in changing the world."

Deeply proud of what he and the Warp Speed team accomplished, Slaoui is chagrined that Biden has called the vaccine rollout a "dismal failure." He shares the dismay that there have been significant problems administering the vaccine doses Warp Speed has sent to the states—the troubles make him "sad" and "reflective" about what else he could have done. But he says most of the troubles stem from overwhelmed local public health systems, issues outside of Warp Speed's purview. "Hundreds of people worked 20-hour days for the last 8 months," he says. "I cannot wait to actually celebrate with all the people that worked together, someplace where we have a great dinner and we just take time to say, 'great job, everyone.'"

Earlier today, Slaoui received his first dose of a COVID-19 vaccine, from Moderna, on whose board he once sat. "I feel a joy I am sure every person that has been vaccinated has felt—a form of liberation," Slaoui told Science immediately afterward. The interview below has been edited for clarity and brevity.

Q: *We met 4 years ago to talk about your vision for a pandemic preparedness vaccine manufacturing plant. It didn't get off the ground. Would it have made a difference?*

A: Absolutely. The whole concept—after we went through the flu pandemic, the Ebola outbreak, the Zika outbreak—was to say, "Listen, the problem is always the same, which is there are no manufacturing facilities sitting there idle, waiting to be used. Even if we had one, we would have trouble because we would have to stop manufacturing other vaccines, which are essential for saving people's life." So we thought, "Why don't we take a dedicated facility and have them work on discovering vaccines against known potential outbreak agents, one after the other?" They would become incredibly skilled and trained at going fast, discovering vaccines. The company was prepared to make available the facility and ask just for the cost of running it. Unfortunately, it didn't fly. [For the COVID-19 vaccines,] the biggest challenge we've had to work on the hardest has been manufacturing.

Q: *So you think you would have been better prepared if the BPO was up and running?*

A: Yes. I have already started discussing this with my successor with the new administration, David Kessler [Biden's chief science officer for COVID-19 response]. This pandemic is costing $23 billion a day to the U.S. economy, every single day. Investing $300 million to $500 million a year into such a facility is peanuts and would save countless lives.

Q: *There must be some "I told you so."*

A: It's never my philosophy to say, "I told you so." I think it's a negative, it's not helpful. For me, it's more, OK, we learned more. Let's set ourselves an ambitious objective and try to now make this happen, capitalizing on everything we've learned. Clearly, we can develop vaccines within 8, 9 months against an unknown pathogen. That's just amazing.

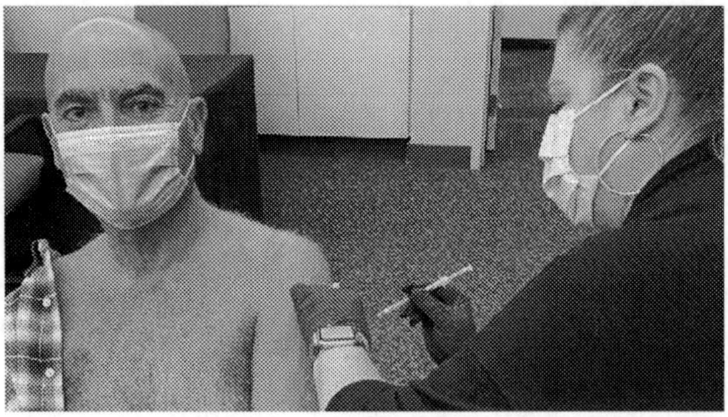

Moncef Slaoui receives his first dose of Moderna's COVID-19 vaccine.
MONCEF SLAOUI.

Q: *What did you think of Trump?*

A: I completely disagree with the values that he projects, as a person, in terms of respect, in terms of capacity to listen, accepting diversity. Many of the policy decisions that ended up politicizing this pandemic were wrong, particularly around wearing the mask. But at the same time, I do think that Warp Speed was absolutely visionary to put together science, government, the military, and the private sector and just give us full empowerment. It was the right thing to do.

My preference is even after the fact, not to politicize this. I worked so hard to stay out of any politics, because I was convinced it would derail it. Even now I think it could derail it when I see the headlines. It just kind of makes me sad.

Q: *What headlines are you referring to?*

A: That there's absolutely no plan for the vaccines. I saw that today on CNN. How can you have discovered two vaccines, developed them all the way to approval, manufacture, and distribute with 99.9% precision 14 million doses to 14,000 sites and it's labeled as there is no plan? We had to do everything from scratch. The biggest lesson for politicians in public health is: Never politicize. Just let people do the work, and if there are things that are wrong, let's fix them versus make a whole story out of that because it freaks out people.

Q: *Trump had a concern about a deep state, the worry that people in the government were working against him. Did he ever confront you and say, "You're a Democrat, you didn't vote for me, are you working behind my back?" Did he ever get in your face?*

A: Absolutely not. He never told me, "Why can't you make it happen sooner?" He asked me, "Can it happen sooner?" And I should say also, frankly, that Jared Kushner, with whom I had a lot of interactions, was absolutely straight, no interference, very rational, and very balanced.

Q: *Trump made an assertion that Pfizer delayed announcing its efficacy data until after the 3 November 2020 presidential election to hurt him. What was your reaction when you heard him say that?*

A: He asked me. And I said, "No, this is not how it works." There is a data safety monitoring board and they're independent. These companies have processes, they have tens of thousands of people in them. They can't do this. It would be the end of the company if they did that, and I've been on the board of a big pharma company and an executive in a big pharma company. I know how it works. The CEO will be fired in a second. I have frankly big respect for [Pfizer CEO] Albert Bourla for just having said it's going to be this day and then it was that day and that's what it is.

Q: *Where were you when you learned the Pfizer data?*

A: Albert Bourla emailed and then called me. I was in my hotel place in Washington, D.C., which is very close to the White House. I was expecting high efficacy, but it was an unbelievable joy. It may have been 5 a.m., and I remember telling myself, "I'm not going to scream." When I think about this now, it gets emotional. I just realized, "Oh my God, we're going to control this pandemic."

Q: *One of the problems you had from the very beginning was allegations of your own conflicts of interest and you were very upset by Senator Elizabeth Warren's (D–MA) attack on you and all the media accounts. What do you think of the way you were criticized? [Slaoui was on Moderna's board, which received substantial Warp Speed support, and also retained GSK stock, though offered to donate to research any increase in value it had turning his tenure.]*

A: I was proactive and decided to resign from the Moderna board and agreed I would sell my shares to make sure there is no conflict whatsoever. I don't complain about that, but if you look at the share price at the time I sold and the share price now, I left an enormous amount of money on the table.

Q: *How much approximately would you have made had you not taken this job?*

A: Maybe between 8 [million] and 12 million. But honestly, I'm not calculating, that's not what I stand for, believe it or not. I've dedicated all my professional life to make sure I help and support global health by being inside a big company and driving its policies. I was shocked by people saying, "You're corrupt, you're doing this for the money," by making an assertion that because you're a pharmaceutical executive, you have to be a person with no values and no principles. That crossed a line. Even now I'll ask, Elizabeth Warren, which vaccine did you take as a senator? The Pfizer vaccine maybe or the Moderna vaccine? Aren't you happy you had the vaccine? Did I make a penny? Was I helpful?

Q: *Warp Speed has been heavily criticized for not getting vaccines into more arms. What do you think about that? [To date, 41 million doses have been distributed to states and about half have been administered.]*

A: There has been a huge misunderstanding. Between May [2020] and now, we've moved five vaccines into phase III trials, two have been authorized, two are completing phase III—and one of those could be approved imminently. One other vaccine is in phase IIb. By all standards, this is absolutely exceptional.

Our mission in its second piece, with my co-leader Gen. [Gustave] Perna, was to distribute the vaccines, take them from point A to the point of immunization. That's how we designed it and worked it out with all the jurisdictions in the country. We went to the departments of health of various states, we explained that we're going to ship vaccine on a weekly basis as they are produced and quality controlled. We will proportionately give doses to each jurisdiction based on the population so that it's fair.

Indeed, the immunization definitely is not working appropriately. And as long as that is not working appropriately, we're failing. Overall, we're failing, because the objective is to immunize.

Q: *The Trump administration from the beginning of the pandemic response said, "We'll help, but this is up to the states and local jurisdictions." The Biden administration comes in and says, "No, the federal government can coordinate this."*

A: Frankly I've been caught in the middle of that. But if I am [a state or local official] who is deciding how many doses I need, I should at least say, "Hey guys, I don't have the resources to immunize." We have never been told that.

Q: *But the Trump administration told us there would be 300 million doses by January. We were not told in a transparent fashion how many doses are coming week by week—there's no dashboard that everyone can see. So there's confusion about how many doses really are available.*

A: What's really important is to truly understand how we can solve the problem. I have always said, "Listen, if there is a problem, please come and help us with a specific proposal and let's pull up our sleeves together and work it out." I did vaccines for a long time. Manufacturing is very difficult and very complex.

Q: *In addition to what the companies are producing, would you have the government build another manufacturing plant?*

A: Yes. My proposal would be for the government to have a license to these technologies for pandemic agents exclusively, not for commercial use.

Q: *The Trump administration has been criticized for not being helpful to the Biden administration during the transition. Was it bumpier than you had hoped it would be?*

A: I had interactions with David Kessler during the summer. I spoke to him regularly. Once the election happened, it was absolute silence—it was against the law for us, as federal employees or contractors, to talk to nonfederal people. I was surprised that nothing happened. We had no contact, no meeting, no nothing. And then somewhere in the second half of December [2020], we had a first meeting with Jeff Zients [coordinator of Biden's pandemic response] and David Kessler and others, where we just introduced each other and discussed what was involved.

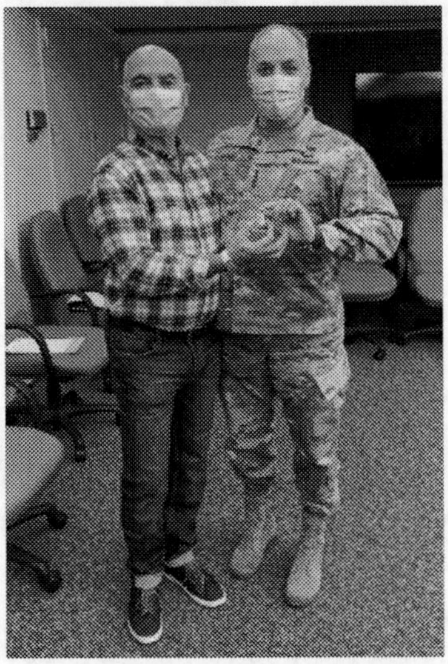

Moncef Slaoui (left) and Gen. Gustave Perna, co-leaders of Operation Warp Speed, hold a vial of COVID-19 vaccine on the day they both get vaccinated.
MONCEF SLAOUI.

Q: *Do you think Trump's failure to concede made it more difficult to transition the information to the next team?*

A: For sure. It was at least very, very unfortunate, to use a polite word.

Q: *When will you leave?*

A: I am very supportive of the new administration. I don't want to turn my back and leave. They proposed that we could have a notice period of 30 days after I resign, and that gives us time to cover the transition. So I did that on that on 12 January, and my last day will be 12 February.

I've since had many very good discussions with David Kessler over the phone that last more than an hour each to share everything I know. I'm totally committed to help 100%.

I'm surprised we got an email yesterday saying, "As of tomorrow, you cannot use the name Operation Warp Speed any more." I asked myself, why? What's the added value? This is probably why I'm not a politician. It just escapes rationality and understanding. Because in a way, everybody that works under Operation Warp Speed feels like, "What did we do wrong?"

I'm not married to that name. I don't care. Honestly, I feel so fortunate and happy to have served and hey, that's all that counts. I would redo it in the blink of an eye. But next pandemic virus, please, do not come during an election year.

Statement for the Record, Submitted by the Premier Inc. Healthcare Alliance, Road to Recovery: Ramping up COVID-19 Vaccines, Testing, and Medical Supply Chain, House Energy and Commerce Subcommittee on Health, February 3, 2021

The Premier healthcare alliance appreciates the opportunity to submit a statement for the record on the House Energy and Commerce Health Subcommittee's hearing titled "*Road to Recovery:*

Ramping Up COVID-19 Vaccines, Testing, and Medical Supply Chain," scheduled for February 3, 2021. We applaud the leadership of Chairs Pallone and Eshoo, Republican Leaders Rodgers and Guthrie and members of the Subcommittee for holding this hearing to ensure a more robust national response to the COVID-19 pandemic by expanding access to vaccines, tests, and critical medical supplies.

Premier's Reflections & Learnings from COVID-19 Response Efforts

Premier is a leading healthcare improvement company, uniting an alliance of more than 4,100 U.S. hospitals and health systems and approximately 200,000 non-acute providers to transform healthcare. With integrated data and analytics, collaboratives, supply chain solutions, consulting and other services, Premier enables better care and outcomes at a lower cost.

From the beginning of the COVID-19 pandemic, Premier has been at the forefront of response efforts working around the clock to identify and implement innovative solutions and best practices that ensure hospitals, health systems, and alternate site providers across the country had access to the necessary PPE, medical supplies and pharmaceuticals to treat COVID-19 patients.

Premier has spent significant time reflecting on the experience of the healthcare industry during COVID-19 response efforts to determine elements that worked well as well as areas for improvement for the future. Premier's reflections have found that:

Elements That Have Worked Well:

- Nimbleness and ingenuity of the private sector to anticipate and identify needs as well as respond quickly to fill gaps
- Formation of the Private Sector Supply Chain Coalition to provide a coordinated and collaborative response
- Sharing of supply chain data that accounted for both supply and demand from neutral, vendor agnostic, and value orientated entities
- Regulatory flexibilities and waivers from FDA, CMS, HRSA, and CDC that were delivered rapidly
- Timely and regular access to government leaders and openness to input

Elements That Led to the Current Situation:

- In spite of efforts to counter the trend by some, a focus for the past 20+ years to move manufacturing offshore as a means to reduce costs to offset decreasing reimbursement
- Emerging economies more willing to take greater environmental regulatory risks
- Large populations of low-cost labor
- Incentives provided by other nations to move manufacturing to their markets
- Lack of centralized upstream visibility into supply chain to determine source of raw materials and finished goods. This resulted in a lack of understanding of vulnerabilities, foreign reliance on manufacturing, and impact as export bans and manufacturing shutdowns were announced.

- Unprecedented demand both globally and nationally that led to an imbalance in the supply vs demand (17X increase in surge demand for N95 masks)
- Export bans and manufacturing shutdowns globally
- Insufficient supplies in the Strategic National Stockpile (SNS) and cumbersome process for accessing supplies in the stockpile
- More reactive approach vs a proactive approach by the government at the outset. Product was not allocated to the "hot spots" because there was not clear identification of them until late.
- Fragmented approach to securing supply (private sector vs federal vs states) led to increase in prices as multiple entities competed for the same inventory and out-bid one another
- Lack of clear visibility of distributor fulfillment led to uncertainty on where products were delivered. This continued uncertainty left providers with dwindling confidence in the normal supply chain and proliferated more maverick and forward buying, as well as hoarding. This also led to a rampant gray market and many entities purchasing counterfeit products.
- Insufficient national strategy and plan for addressing global pandemics, including confusion regarding which federal agency was responsible
- Existence of patent restrictions that impeded access to ancillary products needed for care such as viral swabs
- Lack of resources to contain the spread of COVID-19 in nursing homes and proactively identify emerging cases.

Strengthening the Healthcare Supply Chain to Address Future Pandemics

To strengthen the supply chain to address future global pandemics, Premier has robust recommendations on how the existing private sector supply chain can be further enabled and augmented. Premier's guiding principles include:

- Augment the existing private sector supply chain to better respond to global pandemics through diversification and transparency. The private sector supply chain is highly functioning and should be further enabled, not disrupted.
- Develop a cohesive and holistic national strategy for addressing global pandemics and stabilizing the US supply chain to respond to surge demand for critical medical supplies and drugs
- Identify critical medical supplies and drugs needed to treat a global pandemic and associated comorbidities. This identification should occur via a public-private advisory council that includes representatives from manufacturers, GPOs, distributors, physicians, pharmacists, laboratorians, and others. This list must be dynamic and regularly updated as technology advances, best practices are identified, and the practice of medicine evolves.
- Create upstream visibility into the supply chain to understand sources of raw materials and manufacturing facilities. This information is critical to assess vulnerabilities and

prioritize what critical medical supplies and drugs should be focused on initially to assure adequate diversification of the supply chain.

- Design stockpiles to create coordination rather than competition between state, local and national stockpiles.
- Leverage supply and demand data from GPOs, who serve as neutral, vendor-agnostic, and value-orientated entities to drive transparency in the supply chain and forecast demand needs.
- Develop a real-time national surveillance system that includes supply chain data so that there is a real-time means to identify a disease threat as early as possible as well as its implications on healthcare resources.
- Advance payment and delivery system reforms that hold providers accountable for the health of a population, budgets and transparent outcomes. This will incent improving the health of a population, which will both improve patients' comorbidities and attention to care management to sick patients. Acting within a budget helps reduce long-term financial pressure from rising healthcare costs.
- Leverage technology to implement comprehensive infection prevention and antimicrobial stewardship programs in nursing homes to provide meaningful assistance with infection control.

Incentivizing Domestic Manufacturing

To increase domestic manufacturing of critical medical supplies and drugs, there are five major barriers that policy proposals must address. These barriers include: 1) capacity; 2) environmental regulations; 3) labor costs; 4) availability of raw materials, and 5) historical policy decisions that advantaged offshoring. To incentivize domestic manufacturing, Premier recommends Congress consider the following policy proposals:

- Section 3101 of the CARES Act requires a report by the National Academies of Medicine (NAM) on the foreign reliance on manufacturing for critical healthcare supplies, the risk to national security, and recommendations for improving the resiliency of the supply chain. However, these recommendations are not expected to be available in the near future and, therefore, Congress should accelerate the development of this report to strengthen domestic manufacturing in the long-term.
- Offer 0% interest loans to manufacturers of critical medical supplies and drugs to incentivize increasing domestic manufacturing capacity. (for example – investing in automation to offset labor costs)
- Offer tax incentives to manufacturers of critical medical supplies and drugs to incentivize increasing domestic manufacturing capacity, similar to incentives provided during the 1980's and 1990's to incentivize manufacturing in Puerto Rico.
- Ensure there is at least:
    - One domestic supplier of the final form, ancillary products and raw materials for critical medical supplies and drugs.

  - Three global suppliers of the final form, ancillary products and raw materials for critical medical supplies and drugs. Global suppliers should be from geographically diverse regions.
- Incentivize the domestic farming/cultivation of raw materials needed for critical medical supplies and drugs
  - For example: cotton for PPE and swabs, pigs for Heparin, poppy for sedatives, etc.
- Incentivize healthcare providers to purchase domestic manufactured critical medical supplies and drugs through programs such as tax incentives, CMS bonus payments, etc. to create committed purchasing volume for domestic suppliers and offset higher acquisition costs.

Augmenting the Strategic National Stockpile

To develop a truly cohesive and holistic national strategy for addressing future global pandemics and stabilizing the U.S. supply chain to respond to surge demand for essential medical supplies and drugs, Premier recommends the following actions to augment the SNS:

- The SNS should not only focus on the quantity on hand for critical supplies, but also focus on the time to inventory and ensuring the U.S. has contractual relationships established, including contingency and redundancy plans, to ramp up production expeditiously and efficiently upon identification of need.
- The SNS is the supply chain of last resort for health systems, alternate site providers, and first responders. Therefore, the SNS must be built by providers for providers. The SNS must also leverage analytics and insights to assist providers in the delivery of care during global pandemics that is in the best interest of patients and ensure access to the right supplies at the right time.
- The SNS should maintain a minimum of a 90-day supply of critical medical supplies and drugs based upon surge demand from hot spots such as New York, Washington, Detroit, etc.
- The current process for accessing the SNS is cumbersome and state specific. Working alongside private sector partners, the Administration should create a streamlined and efficient process for accessing drugs from the SNS.
- The SNS should work proactively with GPOs to forecast demand and increase capacity/supply to avoid shortages.
- The SNS should work with GPOs to rotate soon-to-expire stock out of the SNS and into health systems at a discounted rate. This rotation is supposed to occur, but GPOs can make this happen and will ensure the SNS is continuously stocked with in-date products and allow the SNS to recoup some of their expenses associated with purchase of these products.
- The SNS should be transparent regarding distribution of supplies and drugs from the SNS. The SNS should provide, at minimum, a detailed monthly report of what supplies were distributed to where and in what quantities.
  - During a public health emergency, reporting should occur weekly

- The SNS, as well as state and local stockpiles, should be encouraged to purchase off GPO contracts to help aggregate purchasing volume and keep prices competitive.
- The SNS should work to ensure that critical medical supplies and drugs are located as close to the delivery of care as possible. This includes exploring opportunities to leverage health system warehouses in major metropolitan areas or in rural areas.
- Create a customized stockpile for nursing homes with appropriate supplies, drugs and other needs.
- Include health systems or regional buying groups as potential stockpile operators. These organizations would be responsible for managing the stockpile for the providers in a region. This would allow an efficient means to rotate inventory and assure accountability for the stockpile.
- To ensure the SNS can deliver during future global pandemics, it is critical to periodically pressure test the system. Annually, without prior notice, the SNS should require all contracted manufacturers to provide the SNS with a specified quantity of product. An annual test allows the SNS to ensure all contracted manufacturers can expeditiously and efficiently ramp up production to meet surge demand, as well as ensure production lines remain operational and are maintained.

Solutions to Environmental Issues Impacting Patient Care

Premier is committed to working with Congress, the FDA, EPA, and stakeholders to find a sustainable approach and path forward that addresses the concerns with sterilization techniques using ethylene oxide while carefully considering the unintended negative consequences that sterilization facility closures would have on patient care. Premier recommends a thoughtful approach to this delicate balance, so we do not hit a tipping point resulting in a greater crisis in medical supply shortages. Premier believes this requires the following steps:

- EPA should reassess requirements specific to the manufacturing of critical medical supplies and drugs and provide clear guidance on the requirements needed.
- The federal government should provide tax credits or incentives for manufacturers to upgrade facilities to meet EPA requirements to begin domestic manufacturing of critical medical supplies and drugs.
- EPA should provide clear guidance on the use of ethylene oxide (EtO) for sterilization of medical supplies. In 2019, several states took action against EtO facilities and closed them. During COVID, Illinois and Georgia permitted EtO facilities to reopen. This was critical to avoid additional shortages of PPE and other medical supplies due to a lack of sterilization capacity. Moving forward, it is critical that EPA define what is required for sterilization with EtO and provide an opportunity for EtO sterilizers to comply with the new requirements.

Maintaining Supply Chain Integrity

During the pandemic, unfortunately a lack of clear visibility of distributor fulfillment lead to uncertainty on where products where delivered. This continued uncertainty left providers with dwindling confidence in the normal supply chain and proliferated more maverick and forward buying, as well as hoarding. This also led to a rampant gray market and many entities purchasing counterfeit products thereby challenging the integrity of the medical supply chain.

To combat the gray market and ensure supply chain integrity, Premier offers the following recommendations:

- Establish a national, centralized clearinghouse to vet all gray market offers regarding vaccine availability. A clearinghouse approach would remove the risk and guess work from efforts by healthcare providers, states and other entities to secure a reliable supply of vaccine. The clearinghouse should:
    1. Hold all payments in escrow until testing is validated;
    2. Test lot samples through a certification process;
    3. Permit the sale of products that are validated; and
    4. Confiscate and take appropriate action against the gray market actor if the product is not validated.
- Require entities associated with the distribution of vaccine and ancillary supplies to implement checks and balances systems, similar to suspicious order monitoring requirements for controlled substances, to identify potential diversion of vaccine to the gray market.
- Promote the reporting of gray market offers to the FDA Office of Criminal Investigations and share reported incidents with the Federal Trade Commission (FTC).
- Implement civil monetary penalties (CMPs) for entities selling vaccine to the gray market.
- Establish best practices for security to minimize diversion from sites.

Expediting COVID-19 Vaccinations of the American People

Working with our provider members to understand the evolving on-the-ground realities, Premier has identified five systemic issues limiting the vaccine rollout that need immediate remediation. Premier urges Congress and the Administration to immediately take the following actions to overcome these obstacles and streamline and expedite the vaccination process throughout the country. We are pleased that the Biden Administration has already adopted some of these recommendations.

#1 Vaccine Hesitancy

On the ground reports suggest that a consistent 30[53]-50[54] percent—and as high as 80 percent[55]—of healthcare workers eligible to receive the vaccine have not been vaccinated. This unanticipated high hesitancy rate has disrupted the CDC's prioritization pathway as providers grapple with finding willing persons to accept the vaccine in the short timeframe that it remains viable.

For healthcare providers, data transparency and an ability to review the data themselves and arrive at their own scientific and evidence-based conclusions is paramount to provider acceptance of new technologies. For the general public, broader education and communication efforts are necessary to explain the necessity of the vaccine and answer individualized questions. What we need is broad and consistent education involving:

- The FDA and vaccine manufacturers making all evidence supporting the safety and efficacy of COVID-19 vaccines publicly available as would normally occur for a new drug;
- A concerted, evidenced-based national public awareness campaign on COVID-19 vaccines that aggressively debunks myths while addressing vaccine safety, efficacy, their role in society, and their importance in our return to normal;
- Encouraging employers to leverage this campaign for their employees and engage in internal peer- to-peer educational opportunities with early adopters;
- Data transparency around vaccine safety and efficacy during phase IV clinical trials, ongoing surveillance for adverse events, and real-world evidence;
- Clear guidance and education on why the US approach to vaccinations may differ from those of other countries;
- Allowing the use of the Medication Therapy Management network for vaccine-related education; and
- Permitting unbranded direct-to-consumer advertising on vaccine availability, safety, and efficacy.

In addition to broad and consistent education to overcome vaccine hesitancy, incentives throughout the entire healthcare ecosystem should be leveraged to encourage vaccination via a multi-faceted approach where multiple parties are incentivized to achieve the common goal of vaccinating the American public as expeditiously as possible. These incentives should include:

- Temporarily waiving the Stark and anti-kickback requirements to allow providers to offer patients incentives to receive the COVID-19 vaccine;
- Urging Medicare Advantage (MA) plans to leverage the Rewards and Incentive Programs to encourage MA enrollees to receive the COVID-19 vaccine; and

[53] https://nypost.com/2021/01/05/around-30-of-ny-medical-workers-refusing-covid-19-vaccine-official/.

[54] https://www.desertsun.com/story/news/health/2021/01/05/half-riverside-county-hospital-workers-refusing-covid-19-vaccine/4118966001/.

[55] https://www.modernhealthcare.com/providers/vaccine-rollout-hits-snag-health-workers-balk-shots?utm_source=modern-healthcare-covid-19-coverage&utm_medium=email&utm_campaign=20210110&utm_content=article4-headline.

- Providing bonus payments to providers and payers and temporary tax incentives for employers for vaccinating a specified percentage of their patient and employee population by the end of fiscal year 2021.

#2 Clinical Staffing Limitations

According to a November survey of Premier members, 53 percent said lack of clinical staff was the top challenge to their COVID-19 response efforts – and that was before the current caseload surge and the added staff needed to administer vaccines that has only exacerbated staffing shortages.

States and the Biden Administration should take the following steps to identify new cohorts of vaccinators to prevent bottlenecks at vaccination sites:

- Recruiting retired pharmacists and pharmacy technicians, as well as student pharmacists who have successfully completed coursework related to the administration of vaccines;
- Leveraging the National Guard to assist with logistical vaccination support, including to support hospitals, retail settings, and community physicians to achieve mass vaccination;
- Temporarily waiving state reciprocity requirements for vaccinators if they are licensed vaccinators in good standing in another state; and
- Appealing to employers to support licensed healthcare workers who are in non-healthcare roles to return to the frontlines.

#3 Distribution Challenges

The current Operation Warp Speed decentralized, opaque distribution process is creating uncertainty for providers around shipments, leading to throughput limits and/or wastage. At the same time, there are proliferating concerns about an emerging counterfeit market for vaccines and the integrity of the distribution channel.

The key to overcoming distribution challenges is building a true end-to-end supply chain that is transparent and resilient. To do this, we need:

- A centralized national real-time tracking and tracing system to provide visibility into the complete vaccine supply chain to replace the current process of states independently reporting this information, a process that is archaic, delayed, and prone to error;
- A data-driven dynamic allocation process to match vaccine allocation with the number of eligible patients in the state based upon the prioritization pathway; and
- Concrete steps to prevent the gray market and ensure supply chain integrity by:
  - Establishing a national, centralized clearinghouse to vet all gray market offers regarding vaccine availability;
  - Requiring entities associated with the distribution of vaccine and ancillary supplies to implement checks and balances systems;
  - Promoting the reporting of gray market offers to the FDA Office of Criminal Investigations;

- o Implementing civil monetary penalties for entities selling vaccine to the gray market; and
- o Establishing best practices for vaccine security to minimize diversion from vaccination sites.

#4 Supply Shortages

Shortages of needles and exam gloves are obstacles limiting the speed of vaccination. Premier members report an inability to order the additional needles needed to administer the maximum number of doses per vial, as well as a 40 percent increase in exam glove demand, which has caused spot shortages.

The key to overcoming supply shortages is to leverage a data-driven approach to drive transparency in the supply chain and forecast demand needs, which can be accomplished by:

- Adding to the ancillary kits accompanying vaccines the additional needles and syringes needed, as well as nitrile exam gloves;
- The Strategic National Stockpile (SNS) releasing any existing supply of needles to Operation Warp Speed to support vaccination efforts and leveraging the Defense Production Act to expeditiously refill the SNS inventory;
- Leveraging public-private partnerships to monitor the rollout, collaboratively discuss challenges, and work proactively to resolve any supply chain challenges that may arise; and
- Ensuring the FDA device shortage list is more specific around the exact product and manufacturer that is impacted.

#5 Communication Gaps

Operation Warp Speed is a large-scale effort but with insufficient coordination. As a result, vaccination sites report widespread confusion, with providers unsure of which state or federal agency is making decisions or where to turn to solve problems.

The key to overcoming communication gaps is establishing a single source of truth with:

- A clear and consistent command and control structure that explains the roles and responsibilities of the various entities involved in the rollout, what decision-making authority they have, and how to engage with them;
- A reconfigured CDC vaccine reporting website to provide data on the first and second dose administered;
- An appointment-based vaccination system with an active waitlist that can be leveraged if there are no shows;
- An administration-led fact-finding process to understand why there are jurisdictional differences in vaccination administration rates and standardized reporting of key administration metrics to allow for data mining to identify best practices to improve vaccination rates in the future; and
- Standardized definitions (e.g., "essential worker") that are applicable across jurisdictions.

Creating Upstream and Downstream Visibility

COVID-19 has exposed one of healthcare's fundamental weaknesses: the fragmented and siloed nature of care delivery and the lack of centralized coordination when it comes to managing and preventing disease spread. The public health system continues to rely on flawed data and obsolete technology that consistently fails to accurately identify and track current cases, monitor disease progression, or predict future surges. Not only do these blind spots create opportunities for the disease to spread, they also undermine the ability to safely plan for economic recovery and re-opening of the country.

The COVID-19 emergency underscores the need for:

- Investing in a robust, real time HIT infrastructure that will provide an on-call, nimble data collection infrastructure that the nation can call upon in any future major crises. Rather than standing up an inadequate and duplicative system as we experienced during the pandemic, the nation needs a system that can track critical product availability - from the raw materials, to manufacturer, to distribution, to hospital inventory. This system would exist behind the scenes and be ready to be "turned on" in a moment's notice. This information would inform dynamic and appropriate product allocation and distribution strategies, minimize hoarding, and enable powerful and accurate prediction, enabling the nation to manage supplies during the crisis.
- Modernizing the nation's public health syndromic surveillance system so that infected patients can be identified earlier through symptom information. Reliance on testing, particularly early on in an emergency, can delay insights for and misinform public health officials.

Expanding Infection Prevention Clinical Surveillance

COVID-19 has brought to the forefront the specific challenges nursing homes face in containing the spread of infectious disease. The virus has accelerated at nursing homes because residents are generally vulnerable to its complications and more susceptible in the contained space of the facilities. While data about infections in nursing homes is limited, the CDC notes that, even prior to the pandemic, a staggering 1 to 3 million serious infections occur every year in these facilities and as many as 380,000 people die of the infections in nursing homes every year.

Infection prevention oversight and training at nursing homes is a challenge in and of itself with limited staffing and several layers or reporting requirements. This challenge is compounded by limited Electronic Health Record (EHR) functionality at the sites. Without a comprehensive infection prevention surveillance workflow, the surveillance, tracking, documenting and reporting of epidemiologically significant organisms and infection is difficult for everyday risks, such as multi-drug resistant organisms, but also when an outbreak like COVID-19 occurs.

Clinical analytics technologies are currently widely leveraged in hospitals and acute setting to detect patient care issues through surveillance, interventions and reporting capabilities that are needed to support antimicrobial stewardship programs. These systems utilize data from

EHRs and have significantly helped clinicians and pharmacists in acute settings identify overuse of antibiotics and drug-bug mismatches, reduce time-to-appropriate therapy and enhance therapy for difficult-to-treat pathogens. Those health systems already utilizing clinical surveillance technology were well positioned to respond to COVID-19 before the pandemic hit.

Unfortunately, clinical analytics technologies are currently not widely used in nursing homes. Nursing homes should have the same access to tools that will help them combat infection spread during any future outbreaks of COVID-19 and during their day-to-day operations, but unfortunately funding remains a significant barrier. Nursing homes are already challenged with meeting their more visible needs, such as testing and securing adequate PPE levels at their sites, but a comprehensive approach is additionally needed to ensure data collection is efficient, non-duplicative and being analyzed in ways that are helpful for facilities.

Conclusion

In closing, the Premier healthcare alliance appreciates the opportunity to submit a statement for the record on the House Energy and Commerce Health Subcommittee hearing on ramping up COVID-19 vaccines, testing, and medical supply chain. Premier is available as a resource and looks forward to working with Congress as it considers policy options to continue to address this very important issue.

Attachment—Additional Questions for the Record, Subcommittee on Health, Hearing on "Road to Recovery: Ramping up COVID-19 Vaccines, Testing, and Medical Supply Chain," February 3, 2021

Luciana Borio, M.D., Vice President, In-Q-Tel,
Former Acting Chief Scientist, FDA,
Former Director for Medical and Biodefense Preparedness,
National Security Council

The Honorable Frank Pallone, Jr. (D-NJ)

1. With the rise of new COVID-19 variants, it will also be crucial to improve our understanding of the impact these variants have on infections, testing, and vaccines. This will require updating our surveillance of the virus, including through genetic sequencing. You noted in your testimony that we are currently only sequencing about 3,000 specimens out of 1.4 million positive tests. What percentage of specimens should we be sequencing, and can you describe what a coordinated national system for sequencing would look like?

A pathogen surveillance system that will keep Americans safe will need to focus on improving the (1) data collection and data systems, (2) workforce and resources to sustain the system, (3) analytical tools (both genomic and phenotypic), and (4) decision-support capabilities.

Some experts have estimated that sequencing 5 percent of representative samples of identified COVID-19 cases would enable the detection of a new variant when the variant represents about percent to 1.0 percent of the country's cases. The CDC has taken steps recently to augment the number of specimens sequenced. CDC's SPHERES program, a consortium of sequencing labs around the country, aims to sequence 20,000 samples per month. The U.K. is aiming to sequencing 10 percent of SARS-CoV-2 positive samples.

There are many U.S. laboratories capable of performing sequencing work, in universities, medical centers, private sector clinical labs, etc., as well as government labs, such as the CDC. One of the most logistically challenging aspect of SARS-CoV-2 sequencing is gathering sufficient numbers of clinical samples from individuals testing positive to make sequencing cost-effective. (Sequencing machines can process thousands of samples at once). New Mexico, for example, has agreed to sequence samples from several other western states.

Another issue is timeliness of results. From the time patients are tested to the collection of clinical samples and delivery to sequencing facilities, to sequencing, to reporting results to local health departments and to the CDC takes days. Ideally, results would be reported within a time frame that is "epidemiologically actionable" – i.e., within 24-48 hours of patient testing. The material and personnel costs of sample collection and sequencing must also be considered, as well as supply chain sustainability and the consequences of re-directing sequencing activity from ongoing studies and clinical work.

The Honorable Lisa Blunt Rochester (D-DE)

1. Because of the disparate access to testing in underserved communities, but also due to a lack of consistent decision-making and guidance out of the federal government, there are a lot of unknowns about the specific impact COVID is having in such communities. I have also heard very little about how high-quality antibody testing can be better deployed in any of these national or state testing plans discussed to date. I have heard very little about what the actual plan is for figuring out how long these vaccines are going to work, or whether there is any variability based on age, or race or ethnicity or co-morbid conditions that impact communities of color. I understand the initial tests FDA let on the market were of varying quality, but now that there are highly specific options out there, how can they be deployed by the new Administration moving forward especially in assessing variability in vaccine response across the population?

For diagnostic and screening tests, the CDC should develop, with input from the FDA, testing guidance so clinicians, public health practitioners and the public are informed of optimal testing strategies for particular scenarios (i.e., screening asymptomatic individual after exposure, pre- and post-travel testing, surveillance testing at the workplace, etc.). There is also a need to provide clearer and more useful explanations about COVID-19 test results to members of the public.

There is little role for antibody-based testing now other than for epidemiological purposes. A positive antibody test does not mean someone is protected from COVID-19 infection. Even individuals who recovered from COVID-19 need to be vaccinated to be optimally protected from re-infection.

Rapid read-out, point-of-use diagnostic tests are being used to screen asymptomatic people in workplaces, schools, etc. One key challenge for public health has been capturing diagnostic test results and analyzing all the aggregate data to guide the public health response. Missing, delayed and incomplete data has hampered the public health response. While mandated by the CARES Act, its enforcement has been limited. This problem will only grow as more tests become available directly to the consumer. Tests that are marketed directly to consumers should include mechanisms to automatically report the results to public health systems. Accurate data reporting is essential for monitoring the trends of disease spread, identifying hot transmission spots, and guiding resource allocation. There remains a need for innovation around ensuring data capture that enhances local, state, and national response.

For vaccine breakthrough cases, the CDC should launch a national surveillance effort to sequence the virus of anyone who develops COVID-19 even after being fully vaccinated. This is important to monitor for vaccine failure that may occur because of waning immunity or because of less protection afforded by the authorized vaccines against the emerging variants of concern.

2. What steps need to be taken by FDA and CDC go about establishing a threshold neutralizing antibody level for protection against COVID-19?

Establishing such a threshold will require clinical research data demonstrating whether there is a threshold at which individuals are likely to be protected from SARS-CoV-2.

The Honorable Brett Guthrie (R-KY)

1. There is growing concern that some of the new strains are more resistant to existing antibody therapies.

a. Do we have the right set of therapies ready to use or will we need additional ones in our stockpile?

The United States lacks a strong therapeutic armamentarium against COVID-19. Although we were very hopeful, the antibody-based therapies have not been successful in treating sicker, hospitalized patients. Thankfully, clinical trials are demonstrating that several monoclonal antibodies are useful in preventing disease progression in certain high-risk individuals.

Nevertheless, most antibody-based therapies are vulnerable to emerging variants that carry mutations that evade or reduce neutralization by these types of therapies. It is possible to develop new antibody therapies that would be effective against variants, but ways of testing such therapies more quickly are needed.

The NIH should establish a national capability for the rapid conduct of streamlined, pragmatic, randomized clinical trials, like what the U.K. has established, to evaluate promising treatments in a suite of common or platform trials that share a common control group. We all hope that the most promising therapies will work but we can't be sure until we study them in properly designed clinical trials. Learning what works and what doesn't is an urgent matter. Broad utilization of unproven therapies, even under FDA's Emergency Use Authorization framework, may end up hurting patients and delays our ability to learn what treatments are most effective.

I'm encouraged that the Biden administration is providing $3.2B to support development of small molecule drugs to address coronaviruses in general. Investments should also include antiviral drugs that may have activity against multiple pathogens. While these are sometimes harder to identify, the time is now to develop these types of drugs in earnest since we do not know what the next pandemic pathogen could be.

b. Do you know if additional antibody therapies are currently under development to respond to these emerging strains and if so, what the status of those therapies are?

Some companies are developing new versions of their monoclonal antibodies to help address the emerging variants. However, the role of highly specific monoclonal antibodies is limited in the treatment of COVID-19 and stand to benefit only a small subset of people (i.e., those with risk factors and who have not developed their own antibodies, and only if the drug is administered soon after infection). However, at least one company, Vir, has a monoclonal antibody, Vir-7831, that seems to retain activity against the variants now circulating as it targets a more conserved part of the SARS-CoV-2. The company is working on formulating the product for intramuscular delivery, which obviates the need for infusion centers that have proven to be a rate-limiting step in the timely delivery of these types of drugs to those who stand to benefit.

c. Can you explain why it is important to have a strong portfolio of therapeutics available, even as more people are able to get vaccinated and what can we be doing to better support the development of new therapies?

No vaccine is 100% effective or work equally well in all patient populations. Patients need access to safe and effective treatments if they become infected. The United States has a formidable and vibrant biomedical research enterprise, but it lacks a national capability to conduct pragmatic, yet rigorous clinical trials required for evaluating the merits of promising treatments quickly. As a result, only a small fraction of patients diagnosed with COVID-19 enroll in a clinical study. The more patients that can be enrolled in such studies, the quicker we can identify winning therapies. I'm encouraged that the Biden administration is providing $3.2B to support development of small molecule drugs to address coronaviruses in general. Investments should also include antiviral drugs that may have activity against multiple pathogens.

2. Last year, Congress provided millions of dollars to be spent on domestic manufacturing capabilities. Focusing on vaccines and therapeutics, how do you suggest we encourage private sector entities to build additional manufacturing capacity or adopt technologies that allow for production to be quickly ramped up in order to respond to future public health emergencies?

Private sector participation is essential to creating a manufacturing ecosystem that's better prepared for tomorrow's public health emergencies. Leading talent and cutting-edge manufacturing technologies, platforms, and processes will be just as important as physical infrastructure.

Historically, limited market incentives have precluded biopharmaceutical manufacturers from investing in the innovation and capacity required for more effective rapid response mechanisms. Today's system is oriented towards discovering new drugs as quickly as possible and bringing them to market. There is little incentive for contract development and manufacturing organizations (CDMOs) or pharmaceutical companies to spend time or resources developing innovative manufacturing processes ahead of a specific product or to take a risk on a novel platform or technology. This dynamic is exacerbated by the lack of regulatory mechanisms to qualify manufacturing technologies outside of product approval processes.

Importantly, expanding existing manufacturing capacity is not sufficient. The current system is reliant on extremely skilled talent and large-scale bioreactors and can only be scaled to a certain point. New technologies are needed that can overcome existing inefficiencies via completely new ways to make vaccines and therapeutics that make it easier to make these complicated products at cost, at speed, and at scale.

U.S. government partnership can help catalyze a modern biomanufacturing ecosystem by providing:

- Near-term investment to offset the cost of new infrastructure, upgrade existing capacity, and advance breakthrough manufacturing technologies.
- Long-term investment in basic and applied research and development for advanced manufacturing technologies.
- Long-term contracts providing commitments to purchase critical vaccines and therapeutics and to the requisite infrastructure for production.
- Tax credits, subsidies, financing, and other support measures for building, modernizing, or revitalizing infrastructure, investing in new technologies, and training the future workforce.
- A regulatory and policy environment that supports greater manufacturing adaptability, including safe and rapid site changes and the adoption of new manufacturing processes and platforms.
- The convening of stakeholders from across government, industry, and academia to collaborate on challenging policy and science problems.

3. While this Committee has long had an interest in exploring ways to increase domestic manufacturing for certain medical products, the COVID-19 pandemic has highlighted even further the desire for a more robust domestic manufacturing infrastructure.

a. How can we best invest in building and maintaining an advanced manufacturing infrastructure to be better prepared for future pandemics?

The COVID-19 pandemic has highlighted longstanding vulnerabilities and inefficiencies in our current manufacturing ecosystem. Insufficient biopharmaceutical manufacturing, particularly for complex biologics (large molecule vaccines and therapeutics), holds readiness at risk and prevents the discoveries of today from reaching patients as quickly and cost effectively as possible.

True preparedness cannot be accomplished through a one-off program or by building in a single stand-alone government facility reserved for emergencies. This would only enhance current supply chain vulnerabilities by consolidating emergency capacity in a single node that could be shut down by a climate event, such as the winter storm recently seen in Texas, or adversary attack. Reserve capacity of this type would also suffer from long lead times to activate the facility in times of need, outdated technologies, and talent that is not trained in leading systems and methods.

As the U.S. looks to build out its domestic production capabilities in the aftermath of COVID-19, it must develop a next generation manufacturing ecosystem that can keep pace with advances in biological sciences and adapt to potential future threats. Rapid, multi-modality manufacturing capacity is vital to creating pathogen-agnostic preparedness for the next pandemic or biological event. At least one company, Resilience Inc., has been established recently and proposes to do just that. We cannot predict what the next threat may be so we must have the systems and tools to quickly counter the widest range of possible disease threats.

The Federal government could set a broad mandate for bolstering U.S. biopharmaceutical manufacturing through sustained investment in manufacturing science, public-private partnerships that create a network of agile capacity, and future-oriented systems that allow us to create lasting preparedness and not a band-aid for today's capacity. A robust network of flexible capacity able to pivot production provides continuous, real-time biopharmaceutical manufacturing capacity with the latest technologies and leading talent that can be available in times of crisis. By also serving industry, the model saves tax-payer dollars and fuels local and national economies through high-paying manufacturing jobs.

b. Do you know if there are there real or perceived regulatory barriers at FDA that prevent investment in advanced manufacturing or maintaining excess capacity that could be activated quickly and flexibly during times of drug shortages or national emergencies?

The remarkable speed with which scientific leaders have readied a COVID-19 vaccine illustrates what is possible with unprecedented public-private partnership and regulatory engagement and flexibility. However, there are regulatory challenges preventing similar speed, flexibility, and innovation in manufacturing.

The current regulatory regime focuses on the approval of individual products. While this has been successful in bringing safe and effective products to market, it does not incentivize investments in new manufacturing technologies that bring enhanced safety, transparency, and quality controls. Product developers take on extensive risk when advancing novel products towards and through clinical trials. Because the FDA does not review manufacturing technologies without a specific product, the only way a new technology would demonstrate compliance to the broader industry is by an individual product developer taking on additional risk.

For products that are already approved, changing the manufacturing location or technique requires FDA review each time. While appropriate to ensure product integrity, there is no system in place to "pre-qualify" multiple facilities in the face of potential disruptions, nor facility agnostic technology. There is also no expedited pathway for manufacturing supplements that use technologies already familiar to the FDA. Combined, the existing framework prevents novel manufacturing technologies moving from research projects to commercial applications as quickly as possible and provides a disincentive for investments in new technologies that can better support preparedness.

Last month, the National Academies of Medicine published an extensive report entitled "Innovations in Pharmaceutical Manufacturing on the Horizon: Technical Challenges, Regulatory Issues, and Recommendations." This report made several recommendations that would help bring manufacturing innovations to fruition faster and change the incentive structure, whether effectuated by Congress or by the FDA under their current regulatory flexibilities. Of particular importance are the following recommendations:

- Advance innovative mechanisms for evaluating technology outside product approvals.
- Expand the scope and capacity of the Emerging Technology Program and the Emerging Technology Team.
- Increase external engagement to facilitate innovation and increase awareness of readiness to evaluate innovative technology.

4. Are there lessons learned from our response to the pandemic that could be extended beyond the public health emergency to support new drug manufacturing innovation, make review processes more efficient, and increase collaboration and communication between FDA and drug manufacturers?

Please see response to question 3.

5. How should Congress balance investments in short-term COVID product production with a strategic longer-term approach to pandemic preparedness?

These short-term investments have been crucial to saving lives and helping restore our economy. There have been many lessons accrued over the course of the COVID-19 pandemic that should be incorporated into a longer-term strategy. The private sector must remain engaged in bio-preparedness even after the immediate emergency subsides, not only because of its collective capacity and bandwidth, but also because it is where innovation resides. Careful attention should be given to supply chain resilience. A resilient supply chain requires more than onshoring manufacturing capacity. It requires a deep understanding of the supply networks and the application of cutting-edge and flexible technologies, including synthetic biology, to manufacture goods on short notice. For example, Antheia, a synthetic biology company based in California, is developing technology that can enable more resilient and agile advanced manufacturing processes for domestic production of key APIs in life-saving medicines.

6. According to Harvard Professor Michael Mina, the appropriate use of rapid antigen tests can curb the spread of COVID, because they are inexpensive, easily scalable, take just minutes to process, and can target populations with higher rates of infection who are unable to access a hospital or lab. They detect people who are currently infectious, so identifying and isolating these individuals could quickly break the chain of transmission. Despite all of this, there is a large misunderstanding of rapid tests.

a. Can you discuss how rapid tests could be used as a public health screening tool?

Rapid tests could play an important role in curbing the pandemic if they are deployed as a screening tool in many different environments. To work, they need to be conducted frequently. For example, individuals must be able to access an antigen test every three or four days to identify they are contagious soon after they are exposed and before they spread to others. While there is some evidence that weekly screenings could be effective, the increase in frequency is optimal to break the chain of transmission. As such, affordability is also key. At home testing of just one test currently costs $25-100, which is out of reach for mot.

One thing that is often overlooked in the discussion around rapid tests is the importance of data reporting. Missing, delayed and incomplete data has hampered the public health response. While mandated by the CARES Act, its enforcement has been limited. This is unfortunate since accurate reporting of mass-testing could allow for a more proactive response. Accurate data reporting is essential for monitoring the trends of disease spread, identifying hot transmission spots, and guiding resource allocation. There remains a need for innovation around ensuring data capture that enhances local, state, and national response.

An option that hasn't been discussed readily is increasing access to at-home testing via the provision of kits that contain multiple antigen tests but doing so in a way that is affordable enough for all Americans. One promising company ContagionNet, by DataRobot, is proposing to provide households with antigen tests in a kit format where individuals can be tested every couple of days to increase the accuracy of the assay and ensure the identification of the contagious period before they have an opportunity to spread the infection to others. Companies should submit data to the U.S. FDA to make sure their screening tests perform as intended.

b. How can we better utilize rapid tests in school and work settings and not just focus on PCR tests?

Antigen tests and PCR tests are different tools. While PCR can be highly accurate and detect and amplify small amounts of SARS-CoV-2 RNA, it is not positioned well to help reduce transmission rates. It is typically expensive, requires trained personnel and laboratory equipment to administer, and the time to turnaround results can be several days. Therefore, PCR tests are much better positioned to confirm someone is sick as opposed to stopping or slowing the spread. Today, antigen screening is better poised as a way to stop transmission. In the future, we should expect tests that retain the accuracy of PCR tests and the convenience, speed, and ease of use as antigen tests.

Antigen tests can be used to screen people upon entry into a space or event or provided to children to take at home on a regular basis. This is being done right now in the Philadelphia region with Assisting Childhood Education through Increase Testing or Project (ACE-IT), which aims to reduce the risk of the spread of COVID-19 within schools. ACE-IT is a collaboration with the Children's Hospital of Philadelphia, PA-Department of Public Health, United States Digital Services, DataRobot, and Southwest Texas Regional Advisory Council. The program serves staff and students in school districts across the five-county southeastern Pennsylvania region. As of March 12, over 300 schools in the Philadelphia area have been reopened for in person-learning and over 300,000 tests have been conducted under the program. A similar program is being launched in Seattle, and a playbook has been developed for how this can be done for every county and metro in the country.

The United Kingdom is about to roll out mass testing to reopen all schools. The students will then get kits so they can test themselves at home. The U.K. government has distributed nearly 57 million rapid test kits to schools across the country.

Similar programs, screening upon entry or ensuring the ability to check for contagiousness at home, can be done as part of re-opening congregate work settings. Companies should submit data to the U.S. FDA to make sure their screening tests perform as intended.

The competitor to antigen-based testing is broad access to lab PCR testing using pooled samples. Although time to result is significantly longer, accuracy is improved. All strategies should be considered.

7. Serology tests continue to be underutilized, even though they are an important tool in understanding the true spread of the virus. They could be also useful at the patient level - for example, if a patient presents with a heart condition, lung condition, diabetes, their doctor may want to know if they had COVID and developed their condition because of the infection.

a. In your opinion, should appropriate use of serology testing be further leveraged in a testing strategy?

Serology testing is a useful public health tool but of limited utility for testing of individuals. The most valuable tests are the ones that lead to a specific course of action. The results of a serology test, whether positive or negative, do not tend to inform courses of action, such as a decision to isolate, quarantine, or be vaccinated.

b. Would it make sense to include a COVID serology test in wellness panels, for example?

As I described above, the results of a serology test do not impact individual decision-making and has little use for wellness panels.

8. Some serology tests can measure the approximate level of antibodies in a person's body. These tests can potentially be used to track the immune response to a COVID vaccine – helping to identify when a booster shot may be needed among other benefits.

a. How should these tests be leveraged as part of the vaccine roll-out and follow-up?

There is no role for antibody tests to be used in the vaccine roll-out or follow-up. There is insufficient data to rely on antibody levels to inform vaccine boosting strategies.

There is accruing evidence that individuals who have had COVID-19 may only need one dose of the mRNA-based vaccines. Even if the U.S. where to adopt such a strategy, it would likely rely on a history of a positive COVID-19 test. It would be impractical to do an antibody test on everyone before vaccinating.

b. Do you see a benefit to tracking the durability of the immune response, particularly considering some of the mutated strains like those from South Africa, Brazil, or United Kingdom?

Yes, we must track the durability of protection, carefully monitor for vaccine failures, and asses the prevalence of vaccine-failures that are due to infection with variant strains.

The Honorable Michael C. Burgess, M.D. (R-TX)

1. The current vaccine distribution chain only involves one distributor. Have there been capacity issues with distribution that could be solved by involving more private distribution companies? Are there certain areas, for example rural, that are more difficult to reach under the existing distribution channels?

I am not aware that the distribution chain only involves one distributor. I strongly believe in leveraging all capabilities that exist in the private sector to allow for a more timely and robust public health response, and allow for vaccine to reach all areas of the United States.

The Honorable Neal P. Dunn, M.D. (R-FL)

1. What steps should the Biden administration take to guarantee that leading American vaccine and vaccine raw material manufacturers will be approached by the Administration's COVID-19 Response Team to ensure that our Nation's vaccine manufacturing capacity and supply chain can meet expected demands and that Americans have timely access to a vaccine?

a. What recommendations do you have for the Biden administration to sustain those relationships and engagement strategies post the COVID-19 pandemic to make certain we have rapid vaccine manufacturing capabilities for potential future pandemics and other global health challenges?

The Biden administration is reportedly looking at end-to-end solutions for rapid vaccine manufacturing for both the current pandemic and what infrastructure needs to be supported now so that we do not find ourselves in the same situation in the future. The solutions are complex. We need to increase capacity for raw materials, consumables and equipment in addition to capacity for drug substance and drug product. The key will be sustainment of these efforts when the pandemic wanes. Please also refer to my answers to questions 2-5, above, posed by the Honorable Brett Guthrie.

2. What steps should the Administration's COVID-19 Response Team take to ensure that drug identification platforms that can help to protect the public from the next pandemic will be funded over the next few years?

a. As we continue in the fight against COVID-19 and witness the rise of new virus variants, would you support the development of an oral broad-spectrum host direct antiviral (HAD) for immediate deployment in response to viruses, their variants and other potential pathogens?

Theoretically, yes. In practice, these types of therapies have eluded us. For example, randomized controlled clinical trials have shown that neither ivermectin nor colchicine are effective in the treatment of COVID-19. Most drugs that appear to be active in cell lines or even in animal models do not work when subjected to proper clinical trials. It is critical to expand our national capability for the study of such promising therapies.

The Biden administration is providing $3.2B to support development of small molecule drugs to address coronaviruses in general. Those can be considered pan-coronavirus antiviral drugs. Investments should also include antiviral drugs that may have effectiveness against multiple pathogens. While these are sometimes harder to identify, the time is now to develop these types of drugs in earnest since we don't know what the next pandemic pathogen could be.

3. Given that Federal, state, and local officials are grappling with the effects of vaccine shortages, lack of transparency about stockpiles, and instability in the supply chain, what steps should the Administration's COVID-19 Response Team take to introduce additional COVID-19 vaccine candidates into market that are easier to distribute, remain stable at more favorable temperatures and only require a single dose?

From public reports, the administration is taking all of the necessary steps to secure COVID vaccines to all Americans who want them. On February 27, 2021, the U.S. FDA issued an emergency use authorization (EUA) for the Johnson & Johnson vaccine. This is the third EUA for a COVID-19 vaccine and the first for a vaccine that can be stored and distributed at refrigerator temperatures between 2°C and 8°C (36°F and 46°F) and requires a single dose. From public reports, mRNA-based vaccine companies are working on strategies that could improve the thermostability of their vaccines. Given the breadth of technologies in the U.S. Government supported COVID vaccine portfolio, and the emergency of variants, there could be a greater focus on the development of universal coronavirus vaccines that could address all of the different species and variants of coronaviruses.

Attachment—Additional Questions for the Record, Energy and Commerce, Subcommittee on Health, Hearing on "Road to Recovery: Ramping up COVID-19 Vaccines, Testing, and Medical Supply Chain," February 3, 2021

Julie Morita, M.D.,
Executive Vice President,
Robert Wood Johnson Foundation

The Honorable Frank Pallone, Jr. (D-NJ)

The pandemic has laid bare vast disparities amongst our most vulnerable populations, as well as highlighted severely under resourced state and local public health departments. You commented in your testimony that both our public health system was underfunded prior to the pandemic and that we cannot accept these deficiencies as status quo while moving on to address the next crisis. Will you please describe how a lack of core baseline public health funding impacts the ability of local public health departments to plan and carry out their mission?

We often think of health in terms of healthcare, and with good reason: high quality, affordable healthcare is an essential component in how well and how long we live. It should not be reserved only for those wealthy enough to afford or fortunate enough to access it, yet nearly 30 million people in the United States were uninsured prior to the pandemic and millions of job losses over the past year have exacerbated these trends. Achieving universal healthcare coverage in the United States is long overdue.

Nevertheless, access to and quality of clinical care only accounts for approximately 20 percent of a person's overall health picture, with the other 80 percent dependent upon social and economic factors, health behaviors, and the physical environment. That is where public health comes in.

As the American Public Health Association explains, whereas doctors treat those who are hurt or sick, those who work in public health "try to prevent people from getting sick or injured in the first place." So much of what affects our health happens outside the doctor's office, such as whether our air and water are clean, if we have enough healthy food to eat and opportunities for physical activity, and if the homes where we live and buildings where we work are safe and secure. Public health has a hand in all of those elements, and others, of daily life.

As we have seen over the past year, public health also plays a critical role responding to emerging threats and diseases. That includes monitoring and collecting data on where outbreaks are occurring and who is being affected; crafting and explaining guidance for how people can keep themselves, their families, and their communities safe; and ensuring vaccination efforts to prevent infection are efficiently and equitably managed.

Nevertheless, investments in public health in the United States are woefully lacking. Healthcare spending in the United States reached $3.6 trillion in 2018, yet public health funding accounted for less than three percent of that total. Even more troublingly, public health funding at all levels has declined dramatically over the past several years, including a 50 percent decline in the CDC's public health and preparedness response budget over the past 10 years and a 33 percent decline in state and local public health funding since 2003.

During the COVID-19 crisis, we have seen the consequences of this underinvestment. To take one salient example, it is essential that we collect Covid-19 vaccine data by race and ethnicity to ensure that shots are being administered to those populations and communities that have been hit the hardest by the pandemic. Yet race and ethnicity is known for only about half of all those who have received at least one dose, a direct result of underfunded and antiquated public health reporting systems. Gaps can only be addressed sufficiently if they are identified sufficiently.

The American Rescue Plan Act includes $160 billion in additional public health spending that will bolster vaccine administration, improve testing and contact tracing efforts, and help modernize public health data systems. It also provides $7.6 billion to expand the state, local and territorial public health workforce. These significant investments will help frontline public health workers address the immediate challenges presented by the pandemic as well as manage long-term needs and future outbreaks.

However, it is essential that we not treat these investments in public health as a one-off. The trend in the United States is to invest in public health during and immediately after a crisis, and then revert to an underfunded status quo once an immediate threat has passed. For us to ensure that we can effectively manage future outbreaks, as well as the daily public health needs of more than 300 million people, that trend must end with this pandemic.

Community vaccination sites are a critical part of the American Rescue Plan that has been proposed by the Biden Administration. Specifically, a $20 billion investment has been included to help set up these sites, some of which will be able to vaccinate thousands of individuals per day when we have adequate supply. What are the important logistical steps that will need to go into preparing these sites and using them to get more vaccines into arms?

After a slow start, the Covid-19 vaccination effort has picked up considerably. To date, we have successfully administered more than 109 million shots, with more than 20 percent of our nation partially vaccinated and more than 10 percent fully vaccinated. Over the past week, we have averaged well over two million shots administered per day. The increased pace of vaccination, combined with rates of new cases that are at considerably lower levels compared to just a few months ago, give me hope that we may finally be turning a corner against this devastating virus.

Yet the benefits of vaccination are not being shared equally. As we have seen since the start of this pandemic, Black and brown communities have suffered the highest case, hospitalization, and death rates. Given those trends, as well as the fact people of color make up a significant proportion of frontline workers who have among the highest risks of exposure are, it is both a practical and moral imperative that people of color be at the front of the vaccine line. Yet per CDC data, of those who have received at least one vaccine dose, 65 percent of recipients are White, compared with 9 percent Hispanic, 7 percent Black, 5 percent Asian, and 2 percent American Indian or Alaska Native.

Those trends are deeply troubling. As I remarked in my testimony before the subcommittee last month, "vaccines are only as effective as people's ability to obtain them and willingness to access them." I explained how, during my time at the Chicago Department of Public Health during the H1n1 crisis in 2009, we made it a priority to bring vaccines directly to neighborhoods that had the biggest needs and the least access to ensure that priority populations were not being left behind.

I am hopeful that the funding in the American Rescue Plan Act devoted to setting up community vaccination sites will go a long way toward ensuring that the next phase of the vaccination rollout is both swift *and* equitable. These funds will scale up federally run centers and complement ongoing state, local, tribal and territorial efforts. More than 750 additional community health centers are going to receive vaccine doses, for a total of 950 sites, while pharmacy sites and pop-up clinics are doubling. In the not too distant future, we can also expect both a national vaccine website and a 1-800 number for people to call, which will hopefully make it easier for people to secure appointments and can reach destinations easily.

Most people across all races and ethnicities want to be vaccinated, but they are having trouble navigating a very complicated system. Principles to follow for this next phase should include:

- Locating sites in easily accessible and trusted places.
- Offering appointments before and after hours, and on weekends, for those who cannot take time off of work to get vaccinated
- Ensuring systems for making appointments are accessible to low literacy, non-English speaking individuals
- Providing phone and walk-in registration for those who do not have Internet access.

- Collaborating with trusted community voices and existing grassroots efforts to address people's questions and concerns and help people navigate the registration process.

During a public health emergency, one of the most important roles of the federal government is to provide clear, consistent, and fact-based communication. The CDC has played a key role in federal messaging during this pandemic by publishing guidelines that all Americans can utilize to improve safety for themselves and others. Why is it so important that our federal agencies are communicating a clear and consistent message throughout the COVID-19 pandemic?

Whenever a new threat like Covid-19 emerges, what we do not know in the beginning far outweighs what we do know. That changes over time, as more information becomes known. As such, recommendations for how people can keep themselves, their families, and their communities safe evolve as well.

We have seen that play out during Covid-19. Perhaps the most salient example is masks. At the start of the pandemic, the CDC did not recommend universal mask wearing. This was partly due to lack of supply, in particular with respect to N95 masks, and the immediate need to ensure that frontline healthcare workers with the highest degree of exposure had enough supply to keep them safe. It was also partly due to lack of evidence, as we did not know early on whether universal mask-wearing would be a successful deterrent to this new threat. Over time, of course, research has shown that universal mask wearing is an exceptionally effective response, which led CDC to change its recommendations to encourage all people in the United States to wear masks in public.

Unfortunately, for much of the pandemic, the CDC and other public health agencies were sidelined. When the CDCs guidance on masks changed, agency leaders were not permitted to explain to the American people why the guidance changed. As a result, mask wearing became a political litmus test rather than a public health imperative. In some places, state and local leaders followed public health guidance and adopted mask mandates. In others, however, state and local leaders followed political winds by either not mandating masks at all or lifting mandates far too quickly. We still have not fully recovered from the politicization of the pandemic, and thousands of lives have been consequently and needlessly lost.

A situation like this shows why it is so critical for public health to take the lead on a response to a new threat and why policymakers at all levels must follow the public health roadmap for both better health outcomes and economic recovery. The CDC is arguably the most renowned public health institution in the world; I am deeply proud to have worked there. I am heartened that CDC has become significantly more visible during the response in recent months, but we are still paying the price for how long it took us to reach this point.

How do you think CDC's approach to communication throughout the last year has impacted the public's willingness to be tested for COVID-19 and participate in local contact tracing efforts?

Contact tracing is a critical component of public health. At its core, the goal is to ensure that one case of a disease or virus does not lead to a widespread outbreak. Public health agencies do so by tracking persons who test positive, reaching out to that person's close contacts, and encouraging those contacts to be tested and quarantine/isolate following a confirmed exposure. In most public health emergencies, CDC establishes and promotes guidance related to testing and contact tracing, guidance that is followed by state, local, tribal and territorial health agencies and healthcare providers.

Unfortunately, contact-tracing efforts in the United States in response to Covid-19 have been rendered less effective by a variety of factors, including:

- Rapid increases in caseloads that made following each individual case difficult, if not impossible, in most parts of the country.
- A lack of funding for state and local public health departments to implement facets of contact tracing plans, such as hiring investigators and interviewers.
- Hesitancy on the part of contacts to speak with contact tracers, particularly those in communities of color and immigrants who have suffered past or current mistreatment from medical and/or public health systems.
- Millions of workers lacking paid sick and family medical leave, meaning that a 14-day quarantine period could cost a person his or her job and the ability to put food on the table or pay rent.
- A dearth of reliable and accessible testing, particularly early in the pandemic and significant delays in receiving results.

These barriers to successful testing and contact tracing programs were exacerbated by CDC not being permitted to assume its typically prominent public platform for much of the past year to explain its guidance on contact tracing and other matters. As a result, confusion on contact tracing often reigned among public health agencies, healthcare providers and the public, leading to inconsistent approaches being implemented in various parts of the country.

Despite the difficulties with respect to testing and contact tracing efforts, it remains essential for us to track the virus—even as new cases decline, particularly in light of new variants that may be more transmissible and lethal. I am hopeful that the public health funding in the American Rescue Plan Act, a stronger commitment to genomic sequencing, and a continued decline in the numbers of new cases will all make it easier for CDC and other public health agencies to more effectively and efficiently track the spread of the virus in the coming months.

In what ways do you think CDC is succeeding in their approach to communicating about the COVID-19 vaccine and in what ways do you think they can improve?

I have full confidence in Dr. Rochelle Walensky and the thousands of devoted public servants at the CDC to help lead us out of this crisis. I am pleased that CDC has been permitted to communicate more consistently with the public in recent months. Dr. Walensky's regular opportunities to brief the media and the public have been critically important, and those opportunities will continue to be essential over time.

The fact that we have three highly safe and effective vaccines against Covid-19 just over a year after this new virus was identified is an astounding scientific achievement. President Biden has directed that states make all adults in the United States eligible for vaccines by May 1. Majorities of people across all races and ethnicities want to be vaccinated. As supply increases and accessibility improves, tens of millions of additional people in the United States will likely be vaccinated in the coming months.

CDC must use that time to continue regularly reporting vaccine administration data and help encourage and enable states to report that data by race, ethnicity, occupation, and neighborhood. The CDC should also continue its efforts to support and partner with existing community-based and grassroots efforts to understand people's concerns and help move those on the fence from vaccine hesitancy to vaccine confidence.

The Robert Wood Johnson Foundation is pleased to do its part to assist with these kinds of efforts to help build trust and confidence in the safety and effectiveness of the COVID-19 vaccines and increase COVID-19 vaccinations in communities most affected by the pandemic. Our Foundation has provided grant support for several such projects, including:

- Center for Strategic and International Studies Panel on Vaccine Confidence and Misinformation
- Ensuring Equity: State Strategies for Monitoring COVID-19 Vaccination Rates by Race and Other Priority Populations
- Ensuring Access to the COVID-19 Vaccine for Adult Medicaid Enrollees: A Roadmap for States
- Anticipating COVID-19 Vaccination Challenges through Flu Vaccination Patterns

Recently, CDC issued interim guidance for what fully vaccinated individuals can do, which will allow those individuals to see and hold loved ones, engage safely with others in small groups, and begin a return to the joys of daily life we have all missed over the past year. I am hopeful that CDC will be able to update that guidance regularly in the coming months. CDC's initial guidance was delayed, and while I understand and appreciate the fact that the science on which this guidance is based is constantly evolving, tens of millions of additional people will be turning to this guidance in the not-too-distant future as supply and accessibility increase. My hope is that updates to this guidance, such as travel protocols and recommendations for those fully vaccinated, will soon be forthcoming.

The Honorable Michael C. Burgess, M.D. (R-TX)

The CDC's Advisory Committee on Immunization Practices (ACIP) made its vaccine prioritization recommendations to assist jurisdictions in decision making on how to allocate the limited doses of available vaccines. The ACIP recommendations identify non-health care frontline essential workers should be vaccinated during jurisdiction's phase 1b. Should individuals who work in vaccine, therapeutic, or related medical countermeasure industry, who are essential to the production of vaccines be prioritized during phase 1b?

The Advisory Committee on Immunization Practices (ACIP) is an independent advisory group that makes recommendations to the CDC—and in turn, to states—on who should receive vaccinations. ACIP is composed of scientists, infectious disease experts, and medical organizations. As a former member of ACIP, I can state with full confidence and firsthand experience that the committee's operations are built on transparency and research, with no political agenda.

As such, while the ACIP recommendations do not carry the force of law, states typically adhere to them. When the Pfizer and Moderna COVID-19 vaccines were approved for emergency use, ACIP issued recommendations that took into account risk of both exposure and severe disease or death. They started with frontline healthcare workers and people who live in long-term nursing care, followed by those over age 75 and essential workers. The phased approach was also designed to promote an equitable rollout.

Unfortunately, ACIP's guidance was largely abandoned in short order. Before supply increased or accessibility improved, many states quickly opened up vaccine eligibility to anyone over age 65 after healthcare workers and long-term care residents and workers. In doing so, there has been less focus on vaccinating essential workers, despite their high risk of exposure and the fact that a significant proportion of those workers are people of color. States should work to ensure that frontline and essential workers are at the front of the line.

The current vaccine distribution chain only involves one distributor. Have there been capacity issues with distribution that could be solved by involving more private distribution companies? Are there certain areas, for example rural, that are more difficult to reach under the existing distribution channels?

Issues of inequity have long plagued people living in rural America — from a lack of broadband access to food insecurity to underfunded schools. These economic and geographic barriers to opportunity have been exacerbated during the pandemic, with rural communities experiencing disproportionate rates of cases due to a generally older population and higher rates of underlying medical conditions.

These inequities have extended to the vaccine rollout. In rural counties in the center of the country, a shortage of pharmacies is hampering the distribution of COVID-19 vaccines, potentially extending the pandemic in these communities. The American Rescue Plan's additional funding to increase the number of community health centers and double the number of pharmacy and pop-up clinics, which will include mobile units, will benefit rural communities as well. A recent poll finds that upwards of 40 percent of people living in rural areas would choose not to be vaccinated, which is concerning. Increasing access to the vaccine in rural parts of the country should go hand-in-hand with efforts to increase confidence in the vaccine as well.

The Honorable Gus Bilirakis (R-FL)

Obesity has proved to be a major risk factor in the COVID-19 pandemic and past pandemics, such as the H1N1 pandemic in 2019. Over 40% of Americans have obesity, and that number is projected to continue to grow. In addition to hampering our public health preparedness, obesity leads to chronic diseases that account for nearly $500 billion in direct medical costs and over $1 trillion in lost productivity. Doesn't that indicate we need to put all resources to bear, from intensive behavioral counseling, to anti-obesity medications, to bariatric surgery, to help those with obesity and improve our ability to respond to future public health threats?

Obesity is linked to increased risk for serious health conditions, including heart disease, diabetes, and certain types of cancer. In the U.S., childhood obesity—which impacts roughly one in seven youth ages 10-17—is estimated to cost $14 billion annually in direct health expenses. As a result, since 2007, the Robert Wood Johnson Foundation has pledged a total investment of more than $1 billion to address childhood obesity and help ensure that all children in the United States grow up at a healthy weight.

Obesity is a significant underlying condition with respect to Covid-19. Obesity increases the risk for severe illness from COVID-19 among people of any age, including kids. Moreover, people with obesity tend to become sicker, are more likely to be hospitalized, and are even more likely to die if they get sick with COVID-19.

One of the underlying causes of obesity is a lack of access to healthy foods. Prior to Covid-19, millions of families were living in poverty, with hunger, in unsafe homes and without health care. School closures, jobs losses, and wage reductions during the pandemic have exacerbated these trends. Feeding America estimates that 45 million people, including 15 million children, experienced food insecurity in 2020, with 42 million (and 13 million children) projected to experience food insecurity in 2021. Again, significant racial disparities exist; approximately 21 percent of Blacks individuals may experience food insecurity in 2021, compared to 11 of white individuals.

Congress and USDA have taken important legislative and regulatory steps to address food insecurity over the past year, including a 15 percent increase in SNAP benefits and free school meals for all students. However, those provisions are currently slated to expire on September 30, 2021. Per our recent policy brief, RWJF believes that Congress should permanently increase SNAP benefits. Moreover, we should work to ensure that students—particularly where schools remain closed—do not lose access to nutritious school meals that improve their health.

Attachment—Additional Questions for the Record, Subcommittee on Health, Hearing on "Road to Recovery: Ramping Up COVID-19 Vaccines, Testing, and Medical Supply Chain," February 3, 2021

The Honorable Michael O. Leavitt,
Founder and Chair, Leavitt Partners,
Former Secretary of Health and Human Services,
Former Governor of Utah

The Honorable Frank Pallone, Jr. (D-NJ)

Gov. Leavitt, I appreciated in your testimony your suggestion that government at all levels needs to prepare for the next pandemic. As someone who has had to worry about balancing a state budget, can you describe the challenges that states have in funding core public health activities that can help ensure they are prepared?

Governor Leavitt Response

States have faced a number of challenges in sustaining for funding for core public health and pandemic preparedness activities. Yet, with leadership, planning, and partnership at the state and local level, our state leaders are quite capable and able when given the right tools.

Most notably, pandemic preparedness often does not feel like an urgent priority when everything is going well. As you may have heard me say, everything we do before a pandemic will seem alarmist. Everything we do after will seem inadequate.

However, in my verbal testimony, I believe I also mentioned that the growth of the Medicaid program as a large portion of the average state budget also puts pressure on states who want to make investments in public health and pandemic preparedness. One way this Committee could help address that issue is to identify a handful of once well-intended but perhaps now-outdated requirements that CMS still requires states to adhere to in Medicaid. Even small changes to remove outdated federal requirements can help free up limited state dollars and make a notable difference at the state level.

Let's be clear: public health is often a forgotten function of government, working quietly behind the scenes and not drawing attention to the part it plays when things are going well. But the COVID-19 pandemic has thrust public health into the spotlight, and it is now getting the attention it warrants. The public health function of our state and local governments is being tested in many ways through the current public health emergency, and it is in desperate need of modernization.

As I said during the Committee hearing, in my judgement, now is the time not just to note important lessons, but to harvest them. I hope that funding provided by Congress to states is used *wisely* to help states and local agencies make long-term improvements. It is not enough to simply issue a funding notice or hold some listening sessions or publish a report. The hard work of state and local improvements need to be well-designed and carefully thought-out, embedded in relationships, and connected to a strategic vision and operational plan. For example, if state and local public health agencies had steady funding to maintain their capacity to trace contacts for emerging infectious diseases, well-trained personnel, IT infrastructure, and surge capacity, it would not be as great of a strain to respond to a pandemic or any other health emergency.

Finally, one significant opportunity state leaders have at the moment is to help take advantage of the "teachable moment" in their states to show how investment in long-term public health capacity has positive economic impacts on the private sector. Over the past year, the livelihoods of many employers and workers are threatened by the economic impacts of COVID-19. Never before have we seen such a stark economic argument for public health infrastructure that can help mitigate and reduce risks. Seeing this visceral connection between public health and private sector wellbeing should spur employers and leaders in the business community to step up in new ways to partner with and support state and local public health agencies, not only during the COVID-19 pandemic, but on a going-forward basis.

The Honorable Nanette Diaz Barragán (D-CA)

The Port of Los Angeles, which is in my district, is currently experiencing one of the most serious outbreaks of COVID-19 in the nation. Numerous Southern California longshore workers have been unable to work due to contracting the virus, potential exposure, or remaining in their home out of concern of infection because of a pre-existing medical conditions. The total number of positive cases in the last two months of 2021 is greater than all of 2020 combined. The Port of Los Angeles' COVID-19 test positivity is accelerating at an alarming rate, and 12 longshore workers have lost their lives.

1. Given the severity of this situation and the very real risk of terminal shutdowns at one of America's most critical ports, should national vaccination prioritization be considered for frontline logistics workers such as the longshore workforce, truckers, railroad workers, etc.?
2. If not, why not, and what can we do to ensure these workers are vaccinated as quickly as possible?

Governor Leavitt Response

I am genuinely saddened to hear about the hardship of the longshore workers in your district and the increased number of positive COVID-19 cases early this year. I hope the situation has been much improved in recent weeks.

Certainly, we do need to recognize the challenges and hardships faced by the longshore workforce, truckers, railroad workers, and others. While I know it was so hard for many to wait as the early vaccines went to our first responders, physicians, nurses, and the elderly at the greatest risk from COVID-19, I think the last few months generally have shown that the CDC's recommendations were based in science, and also gave states the ability to prioritize limited supplies for the most at-risk individuals and needs of populations in their own states. The prioritization is very challenging and imperfect, but it is necessary.

Thankfully, the last number of months have been a tremendous success with regard to the increased supply of and access to COVID-19 vaccinations. This is due to the tireless efforts of literally thousands of men and women—from scientists and researchers, to manufacturers and distributors, to unprecedented partnerships and collaboration across the private sector and all levels of government. From retail pharmacies to primary care physicians offices, from federally qualified health centers to large health care systems – there has been an unprecedented effort to convert *vaccines* into *vaccinations* by getting shots in arms. We have so many of our fellow Americans to recognize and thank for their service and assistance during this period.

The Honorable Michael C. Burgess, M.D. (R-TX)

Technology has become an integral part of our public health response to COVID-19. County health departments in Texas have been standing up their own websites to allow for online vaccine registration. This seems like a prime opportunity for private sector entrepreneurial leaders to help develop products to streamline this process.

State flexibility to choose what works best for the state is key, but would it be helpful to disseminate a list of best practices or guidelines to states regarding the development and use of technology for testing and vaccine registration?

Governor Leavitt Response

The development of a set of best practices for states, counties, and cities regarding the use of technology would be a valuable exercise. Incentives to leverage these best practices that are tied to increased funding opportunities associated with modernizing state public health technology infrastructures would also be helpful.

Assuming states would like the flexibility to provide their residents with voluntary, digital proof of their vaccination status, here are some thoughts on best practices for how to do that:

- *Identity Proofing:* Ensure that when an individual is receiving a vaccine their identity is validated and accurate demographic information is included in the initial vaccine administration record that can tie that vaccine administration to the individual. Their legal first and last name, mobile phone number, email address, and date of birth are all identifiers that can assist in helping to identify the individual. If possible, include their vaccine information as part of their electronic health record.
- *Use of open standards:* Each vaccine administration system of record should use open standards (e.g., HL7® FHIR®, W3C, etc.) to transmit data between systems. The health care industry is supporting the SMART Health Cards Framework to transmit data between systems in a secure, privacy-by-design method. Each vaccination system of record should implement the standard to ensure citizens of their state can securely and voluntarily access their vaccination information on an application of their choice for a variety of different use cases.
- *State Immunization Information Systems (IIS):* All states should require that when vaccination information is recorded, that information is automatically sent to the state immunization information system via the use of open standards. Currently, many states don't require all vaccinations to be reported to the state IIS therefore when adults are looking for a digital proof and representation of their vaccination information they can access it similar to how they access the information for their children's vaccination information when they enter the school system.

I have heard that some state vaccination and testing sites have been struggling to identify patients who are truly uninsured compared to those who have other insurance available. Either insurance is not captured at scheduling or onsite, and/or is unknown to the patient or the testing/vaccine administrator. What are states doing to ensure program integrity and maximization of insurance coverage for their COVID testing and vaccines?

Governor Leavitt Response

As you are identifying, with the breadth, complexity, and speed of the vaccination efforts that states have been leading in partnership with their local organizations, there will be challenges identified along the way. As you know, there is wide variation amongst states practices and approaches even before the public health emergency, so I don't know that I can characterize current practices with precision. But as a former Governor, I always think the best way to understand the challenges states face is to talk with governors and other state officials leading the relief effort. I do think it helps to keep the challenges in context by realizing that the vast majority of Americans have health coverage, the vaccinations are not only life-saving, but they are essential to helping us advance along the road to recovery and soon find a greater sense of normality.

The current vaccine distribution chain only involves one distributor. Have there been capacity issues with distribution that could be solved by involving more private distribution companies? Are there certain areas, for example rural, that are more difficult to reach under the existing distribution channels?

Governor Leavitt Response

The challenge in effective distribution of vaccines is high, and especially when usual methods are disrupted by the very pandemic itself. As is obvious, the pandemic impacts the very workforce and availability of equipment and supplies required for the response. It is an insidious, inherent consequence of a pandemic. While I am not directly familiar with all of the channels used, let alone the challenges experienced, it is evident that more than one channel was available even in the early stages of the pandemic. For example, one of the early vaccine manufacturers deployed its own distribution system for its product, and the other relied on a government-procured system. This diversification has its own risks. But the advantages became apparent during our own pandemic preparations in 2005 despite the complexity and risks of such diversification across systems, and even across public and private actors. Such diversification can in fact lead to a stronger response capacity when it optimizes relative strengths in access to financing and diverse human and other essential resources, nimbleness in response, innovations in technology, capacity to convene and call to action, and even the incentives to excel when measured against others.

The Honorable Brett Guthrie (R-KY)

1. Your testimony mentions the need for open communication with manufacturers and stakeholders to ensure COVID vaccines and therapeutics remain available. Can you elaborate as to why it is important for the government to maintain an open dialogue and why it would be helpful to extend those channels of communication to manufacturers of non-COVID products?

a. You recommend this communication be collaborative and use innovative, non-compulsory procurement tools, can you provide an example of what this would look like?

Governor Leavitt Response

As a nation, our culture and our economy have thrived when grounded in an ethic that balances our instinct for compassion to those in need with a passion for economic excellence and innovation. We have a history of responding best to those who inspire and propose, and not so well to those who impose and compel. We have seen the best of this culture and ethic in the nation's response to this pandemic. Health care providers came to service of the nation, at great peril to their own health. Essential workers continued to produce and deliver essential products and services. The nation's manufacturers of vaccines, diagnostics and tests, therapeutics, and devices stepped up to innovate and to deliver life-saving products that responded to the pandemic, while keeping non-COVID products available to patients. Many of the supplies, supply chains, products, and people involved in COVID response are also used with non-COVID response. Government plays its role best when it communicates the need, helps organize the field of play, sets basic rules of conduct, and provides the essential financing and resources needed, not just for the immediate response but also for genuine and enduring preparedness for the future. I have some confidence that the example we provided in the run up to the avian flu threats in 2005-2009 may serve as one example for how this might look, using many of the tools that Congress provided in the aftermath of 911 and the anthrax attacks.

2. How to best incentivize the development of new antimicrobial drugs has long been an interest of Members on this Committee. As you mention, the pipeline of drugs to fight these infections is thin, making the threat of an antimicrobial-resistant superbug even more

dangerous. As you likely know, encouraging this type of research and development, while critical, is challenging given that we are asking companies to invest heavily – both their time and resources – into products we hope to never have to use and for which there is a limited market. What lessons realized from the response to this pandemic should inform our efforts to advance the development of antimicrobial drugs and be best prepared for an antimicrobial-resistant threat?

Governor Leavitt Response

Thank you for that important question. As I have said before, we are immensely fortunate that because of scientific advancements, dedicated leadership, intense collaboration, and private and public sector investments in American innovation before and during the current health emergency, we have multiple very safe and highly-effective vaccines approved to prevent severe COVID-19. This accomplishment is unprecedented and historic, and worth celebrating.

This accomplishment is also worth learning from – and not just learning from, but we should be seeking to replicate the best successes and most effective collaborations from 2020 to prepare for the threat of antimicrobial resistance.

One success from the past year has been the federal government investing in multiple platforms in a portfolio approach. It seems to me that funding should be prioritized in a manner that ensures a diversified approach with a stable time horizon. Clearly one of the lessons for this Committee from COVID-19 is that investment in combatting known threats can save thousands of lives and livelihoods and therefore merits Congress's focus to act now.

Another success has been the unprecedented collaboration of scientists, researchers, clinicians, and regulators across the private and public sector. Another one of the lessons for this Committee is that honest collaboration which prioritizes the common scientific challenges helps avoid knee-jerk institutional reactions and foster trust.

We have to acknowledge that the threat of antimicrobial resistance is not a distant hypothetical; it is a present threat that grows with time. The CDC has reported that more than 2.8 million antimicrobial-resistant infections occur in the U.S. each year, and an estimated 35,000 Americans die as a result[56] Imagine how much worse the problem would be if we had no new drugs to combat antimicrobial resistance. Unfortunately, such an dire outcome is possible because the pipeline of drugs to fight these infections is tepid. So, if an antimicrobial-resistant superbug were to cause the next pandemic, the U.S. would not have the ability to fight it like we did COVID-19. Antimicrobial resistance is already a challenge –so its danger and deadliness as a threat to American lives grows in direct proportion to our inaction.

3. In your discussion about Immunization Information System, you point out that several states that do not require everyone who administers a vaccine to report that information to a state Immunization Information System. What federal policies could incentivize and encourage the reporting of more complete information to state Immunization Information Systems?

Governor Leavitt Response

Any federal policies that provide additional funding to states to modernize their public health technology infrastructure should include a requirement to ensure the following:

[56] https://www.cdc.gov/drugresistance/biggest-threats.html#:~:text=According%20to%20the%20report%2C%20more%20least%2012%2C800%20people%20died.

- *Digital reporting by vaccine administrators:* All states should require that when vaccination information is recorded, that information is automatically sent to the state immunization information system via the use of open standards. Currently, many states don't require all vaccinations to be reported to the state IIS therefore when adults are looking for a digital proof and representation of their vaccination information they can access it similar to how they access the information for their children's vaccination information when they enter the school system.
- *Ongoing funding for state public health:* One of the major issues state public health agencies have today is they only receive significant funding when a pandemic or significant public health event occurs. Ongoing incentive-based funding could be provided to states if they commit to implementing a modern, Application Programming Interface (API)-based architecture that would allow individual consumers to access their testing and vaccination information from an application of their choice.
- *CMS Interoperability rules:* Recently, CMS issues an interoperability rule (9115-F) that discussed the need for payers (including state Medicaid agencies) to build a modern, API-based infrastructure that would help to modernize the ability for payers to transmit data in the 21st Century. HHS could develop additional federal regulatory policies incentivizing states to implement the same modern technology open standards that were discussed in the CMS rule.

4. In many cases, targeted upfront investments in public health modernization at the state and local levels can save the federal government money over time. Can you further explain why increased state and local funding for public health would reduce the strain to respond to a pandemic or any other health emergency?

Governor Leavitt Response

In addition to my reply to the full Committee Chairman on a very similar question, it is worth saying that funding for state and local public health activities does need to be increased, but it must also be sustainable. We all know the familiar story of Congress or a state legislature passing a bill and declaring victory. Such an approach is well intended but overlooks the continued focus over time that is needed to repair and restore public health. Think of a holistic vision of dedicated attention that covers a wealth of services and activities, like training and retaining qualified staff, developing and maintaining 21st century data and surveillance systems, and ensuring the proper expertise and experience of public health professionals is retained. In its best sense, funding can help build public and private sector partnerships, support learning collaboratives, and support pandemic planning and readiness response activities.

5. Federal and state officials have a unique responsibility to prepare for pandemics, but they are not the only leaders who need to be prepared. You recommend that preparedness exercises must be done regularly at the federal, state, and local government levels, as well as by the private sector, communities, and families. Where are these preparedness exercises not standard practice, and how can we make these exercises more widespread, more frequent, and flexible in preparing states and localities for both known and unknown threats?

Governor Leavitt Response

Many state, local, and business leaders periodically conduct readiness assessments and update protocols that focus on continuity of operations in the event of a natural disaster (such as a wildfire, hurricane, or tornado) or a security incident (like an act of terrorism or an active shooter). These exercises are seen as prudent steps that responsible leaders take to anticipate known threats, identify measures that can be put into place to be prepared to respond to known risks, and implement practices to protect the safety and welfare of the individuals for whom they are responsible. In many respects, state and local leaders – as well as business leaders – need to approach pandemic preparedness the same way.

As I have often said, pandemics are a fact of biology and a reality of history. While the world has not witnessed a pandemic as deadly or disruptive as the COVID-19 public health emergency in many years, they have occurred.[57] in certain regions and locations around the world, there have been some pandemics certainly have been very serious outbreaks. In the years since I began my tenure as Secretary of Health and Human Services through today, the world has witnessed a number of very serious, deadly, infectious diseases, ranging from SARS in 2003, to H1N1 in 2009, from Ebola in 2014, to Zika in 2015.[58] While none of those infectious diseases resulted the widespread disruption that COVID-19 has caused, each posed a serious threat.

We must be clear eyed that with worldwide commerce and travel, biological agents from one corner of the globe can be on our doorstep in a matter of hours. Thus, state, local, and business leaders need to anticipate future pandemics and future scenarios where infectious disease spreads and promote a culture of readiness reviews and continuity of operations planning.

States and businesses need to be prepared for different types of challenges, and need to think categorically about preparedness through the lens of continuity and protection of personnel, access to data and files, physical building security, and other such divisions of operations and service. State and local leaders have a tremendous opportunity to collaborate with the private sector to foster a sense of shared ownership and collaboration for preparing for challenges that we all hope never occur.

6. In your testimony, you discuss "long haulers" or individuals who virologically have recovered from infection, but still suffer from persistent symptoms, such as fatigue, muscle pains, and cognitive abnormalities. How can federal and state health programs such as Medicare, Medicaid and the Children's Health Insurance Program help meet the needs of long haulers?

Governor Leavitt Response

I appreciate your question because it is an important one. As you may know, Nancy-Ann DeParle and I co-convene the COVID Patient Recovery Alliance[59] We just recently publicly announced our efforts (April 2021), but have been organized as a group and working since last fall (2020). We certainly commend you and your colleagues for your recent hearing on long-COVID.[60]

[57] https://www.cdc.gov/flu/pandemic-resources/basics/past-pandemics.html.
[58] https://www.cdc.gov/globalhealth/infographics/global-health-security/global-disease-detection-timeline.html.
[59] https://covid19patientrecovery.org/about-us/.
[60] https://tinyurl.com/HouseECletter.

Our multi-sector alliance is a collaboration of leading organizations whose mission is to define, develop, and assist in implementing a national strategy to characterize, diagnose, ensure care for, and sustainably fund the full recovery of individuals with long-COVID. Our Alliance is linking diverse data sources to inform the development of models of care and assess whether current payment structures are adequate for the care and full recovery of these patients.

The Alliance is building out a comprehensive list of ideas and actions that federal policymakers in Congress and the Administration can take to help respond to the needs of individuals with long-COVID. While the Alliance does not yet have a consensus-based, comprehensive blueprint of actions to share externally with you and your colleagues, we would welcome the chance to be in touch with you and share ideas as we move forward. In broad strokes, we see the need for

1. Efforts that promote iterative learning and direction insights from data in the nearer-term (rather than wait years for ideal precision in a way that could miss out on informing the health care system's near-term response to current needs);
2. Collaborative efforts from medical and scientific leaders to better understand long-COVID and develop clinical care pathways for long-COVID;
3. A focus on the delivery system to ensure models of care that ensures patients can get the appropriate care from the right providers and reaches patients regardless of their source of health care coverage – especially prioritizing individuals who already are underserved, face disparities, or face inequities.
4. A careful assessment regarding the degree to which our current payment systems and strategies adequately resource and account for the delivery of appropriate care for patients with long-COVID.

More generally, as you think about this issue, here are a few ideas to start:

- Perhaps one of the simplest but most impactful things that Medicare, Medicaid, Marketplace plans, and the Children's Health Insurance Program can do is to recognize that many of the individuals served by these programs (and the plans with whom they contract) will have long-COVID – a range of ongoing symptoms for some period of time. As clinical understandings of long-COVID increase and clinical care pathways emerge, these programs can help amplify efforts that educate providers, inform patients of how to get the care they need, and reduce any potential stigma from long-COVID. Given the scope of those programs and the likely size of patients experiencing long-COVID, there are likely millions of such patients.[61]
- The Committee's hearing on long-COVID was important way to both educate members and draw attention to this evolving issue. The Committee's continued engagement with the health care community – medical leaders, scientific researchers, data analysts, health plans, and others – to closely monitor the evolution of the science, emergence of clinical care pathways, and efforts of the health care community to address this issue.

[61] Based on estimates from CDC and the Institute for Health Metrics and Evaluation, it is thought that roughly 100 million Americans have been infected by the virus causing COVID-19. Published studies indicate 10-30 percent of people diagnosed with COVID-19 may have ongoing symptoms (long-COVID) after acute infection, many of which can impact return to work and life.

- Policymakers could work with researchers to support surveys of patients enrolled in those programs to better understand their needs.
- Given the disproportionate impact that COVID-19 has had on communities of color and underserved populations, it is likely there are more individuals with long-COVID who already faced disparities and inequities. Policy strategies should be responsive to this dynamic. For example, consider the value of targeted resources to Federally Qualified Health Centers to help scale up care pathways for patients with long-COVID.
- Consider what types of grants and funding can help scale up delivery system efforts when clinical care pathways emerge.
- As data and evidence becomes clear, CMMI may have a role to play in supporting the primary care workforce and advancing payment models that support value-based strategies for the care that patients with long-COVID will need.

The Honorable Gus M. Bilirakis (R-FL)

1. As policy makers consult the data to direct response efforts, where should the goal posts be erected – in other words, where should the bulk of our attention and resources be directed as states reopen? Does a response addressing mortality have different considerations than one that prioritizes transmissibility?

Governor Leavitt Response
The unprecedented collaboration across the health care community and beyond to make available and promote widespread vaccination against COVID-19 helps reduce both the mortality associated with COVID-19 and the transmissibility of COVID-19. Vaccination is critical to safely returning to a sense of normality and the continued widespread vaccination of individuals against COVID-19 should be a priority for policymakers.

2. One of the issues we hear about is the difficulty states and providers are having at the last mile, actually getting shots into arms. Once phase 1 has been completed, do you agree that we should have an all-hands-on deck approach, using all of America's commercial distribution resources, customer connectivity, expertise and end-to-end logistics across a multitude of provider settings, to ensure the American public has expedited and equitable access to a vaccine once we get to broad distribution?

Governor Leavitt Response
The last number of months have been a tremendous success with regard to the increased supply of and access to COVID-19 vaccinations. This is due to the tireless efforts of literally thousands of men and women—from scientists and researchers, to manufacturers and distributors, to unprecedented partnerships and collaboration across the private sector and all levels of government. From retail pharmacies to primary care physicians offices, from federally qualified health centers to large health care systems – there has been an unprecedented effort to convert *vaccines* into *vaccinations* by getting shots in arms. As we have entered a phase in which there is less demand than supply in some areas, it is critical that vaccines be available in multiple settings to eliminate barriers to vaccination and ensure equitable access to vaccines. We are seeing many success stories in this respect, thanks to the unprecedented collaboration

of employers, community leaders, non-profits, educators, state and local leaders, and so many others.

Attachment—Additional Questions for the Record, Subcommittee on Health, Hearing on "Road to Recovery: Ramping up COVID-19 Vaccines, Testing, and Medical Supply Chain," February 3, 2021

Mr. Greg Burel,
President and Principal Consultant, Hamilton Grace,
Former Director,
United States Strategic National Stockpile

The Honorable Frank Pallone, Jr. (D-NJ)

1. Mr. Burel, can you explain the history of preparedness funding? Has funding in this space been consistent over the years?

Funding for preparedness has not been consistent over the years. It is imperative that the SNS receive consistent funding to allow for appropriate investment in countermeasures of all types. SNS must be funded for both its Chemical Biological Radiological and Nuclear (CBRN) defense mission as well as for Emerging Infectious Disease (EID) threats. SNS funding has not kept pace with the requirements for just the CBRN mission. Based on my professional judgement and similar professional judgement budgets previously provided Congress, I believe that SNS needs a one time infusion of up to $1 billion to bring all stocks up to meet requirements and then approximately $800 million in annual appropriations to maintain those stocks. This amount would improve our posture for CBRN response. EID response should be funded in an amount I would defer to HHS for answer.

The following table shows the funds appropriated since 2000 in millions:

FY 2000	52.0
FY 2001	52.0
FY 2002	645.0
FY 2003	298.050
FY 2004	397.640
FY 2005	466.7
FY 2006	524.339
FY 2007	496.348
FY 2008	551.509
FY 2009	570.307
FY 2010	595.661
FY 2011	591.001
FY 2012	533.792
FY 2013	477.577
FY 2014	549.343
FY 2015	534.343
FY 2016	569.250
FY 2017	573.907

FY 2018	610.0
FY 2019	610.0
FY 2020	705.0
FY 2021	705.0

The Honorable Michael C. Burgess, M.D. (R-TX)

1. Mr. Burel, what currently happens if the Defense Production Act is invoked and we end up with too many of a particular medical item – for example, ventilators?

a. What can the federal government do to better equip the Strategic National Stockpile to handle such a scenario?

When the government holds material that is ultimately no longer required, that material may be declared "excess" and disposed of in accordance with statute that governs government property and its ultimate disposal. The General Services Administration (GSA) is charged with property disposal. Property may be declared as excess and offered through GSA sales authority with funds realized from sales being returned to the US Government but not to the "selling" agency. (https://www.gsa.gov/policy-regulations/regulations/federal-management-regulation/federal-property-management-regulation-fpmr-related-files).

It is also permissible under statute for SNS and other government programs to offer excess property to other federal agencies directly when there is a known or potential requirement. For example, if SNS has medical material that may be of use to the Veterans Administration (VA), SNS can contact VA officials and offer to transfer that property to them. In practice, it is uncommon for SNS to find another agency that will accept such a property transfer. In these scenarios the receiving agency does not reimburse SNS for the value of the property.

In normal operations, as it may be unclear immediately if such property may be needed in a future response, SNS will hold that property until the normal end of its useful life. When the property is no longer serviceable, or in the case of expiry dated product when it reaches its expiration date, it is destroyed in accordance with all applicable law and regulation. The disposal of such products also presents a cost to SNS.

To better equip the SNS to dispose of unrequired material, the Congress should provide SNS with authority to sell excess material and realize that income through an authorized Working Capital Fund. Such a fund would allow the SNS to use income realized from sales of unrequired property to purchase other required material.

It is my recommendation that the Congress authorize the SNS to sell excess property and further that the Congress authorize a Working Capital Fund for SNS to realize the income of such sales. Further, I would recommend Congress through the Department of Health and Human Services commission the National Academy of Public Administration (NAPA) to consider and propose the best way to implement such authorities for the SNS. I and other NAPA fellows have considered just such a scenario recently.

2. Access to COVID-19 testing is still an issue. A limiting factor has been access to swabs, viral transport medium, lateral flow membrane, and the raw materials for producing these essential components of testing. As Congress and the administration review and take actions to revitalize the Strategic National Stockpile (SNS) how can the SNS play a role in ensuring the medical supply chain has adequate supplies of raw materials necessary to produce necessary testing supplies and PPE?

It is imperative that more manufacturing capability be available "on-shore" or "near-shore." The current medical supply chain has little flexibility to respond to large surge requirements due to its "just in time" nature. This operational norm is well designed for cost management but does not lend itself to any flexibility.

I propose Congress enact authorities and appropriate funds to allow SNS to invest in manufacturing capabilities including the acquisition of raw materials held by manufacturers to increase manufacturing in surge need. Authorizing language in the Public Health Service Act to direct the SNS to undertake these investments should be coupled with the creation of an investment fund with "no-year" monies.

3. The current vaccine distribution chain only involves one distributor. Have there been capacity issues with distribution that could be solved by involving more private distribution companies? Are there certain areas, for example rural, that are more difficult to reach under the existing distribution channels?

Limiting vaccine distribution to a single company and a limited number of dispensing sites creates barriers for vaccination. For example, in the case of pediatric patients and other vulnerable population members, there is significant trust in the regular healthcare providers with whom these individuals and families seek to provide care. With a single distributor and the accompanying challenges in requesting small packages of doses that may be administered to patients it is difficult if not impossible for these physicians to deliver vaccines. The normal supply chain that provides these professionals with vaccines and other medications for their patients should be used to the fullest extent so that persons seeking vaccines can be inoculated by their primary providers. Utilizing the existing supply chain will alleviate problems and barriers associated with having all vaccine flow through a single distributor.

The Honorable Gus M. Bilirakis (R-FL)

1. Today's lean manufacturing supply chains often operate "just in time" instead of "just in case" to reduce costs and maximize efficiency; however, this is a duel edge that can present challenges in the midst of a pandemic response – as we saw with personal protective equipment. How can supply chains balance resiliency with value moving forward?

The government should provide incentives to manufacturers and distributors to hold more essential products than needed for just in time order fulfillment. A number of manufacturers made investments to provide on-shore manufacturing of material during COVID that have not seen good uptake on available products. FDA needs to move rapidly to grant full approval to these on-shore manufactured products. These manufacturers need incentives to continue their work and achieve pricing competitive with foreign made products.

SNS should be provided funding and authority to enter into joint ventures or other financial arrangements with manufacturers to cover costs of new on-shore lines and to invest in margins for holding above immediately needed products.

The Honorable Billy Long (R-MO)

1. Mr. Burel, your testimony touches on the concept of increasing the flexibility of the supply chain through domestic production and a cushion with distributors to meet future surges. Can you share additional details on what that type of framework looks like?

It is imperative that more manufacturing capability be available "on-shore" or "near-shore." The current medical supply chain has little flexibility to respond to large surge requirements due to its "just in time" nature. This operational norm is well designed for cost management but does not lend itself to any flexibility.

I propose Congress enact authorities and appropriate funds to allow SNS to invest in manufacturing capabilities including the acquisition of raw materials held by manufacturers to increase manufacturing in surge need. Authorizing language in the Public Health Service Act to direct the SNS to undertake these investments should be coupled with the creation of an investment fund with "no-year" monies.

Congress should create priorities for federal government purchase of medical supplies to favor US based manufacturing. These priorities, however, should not disallow purchase of non-US supplies when that presents a particularly favorable position for the government.

The Honorable Larry Bucshon, M.D. (R-IN)

1. Mr. Burel, with regard to ongoing PPE and other critical medical supply constraints, how can the public and private sector better cooperate to enhance last mile distribution?

The major medical supply distributors and the SNS should work together to determine how best to accomplish a long term successful partnership during crisis. SNS has had success working with industry in exercises to help increase awareness of needs during public health emergencies of various types. I would propose a study to be conducted jointly by HHS/SNS, the National Academy of Science and the National Academy of Public Administration be sponsored to consider how best to create a routine partnership between government and industry to act immediately upon a public health emergency declaration.

2. Mr. Burel, I am hearing that the lack of visibility when critical medical supplies are shipped from the Strategic National Stockpile (SNS) to healthcare systems around the country has impeded private sector allocation efforts and has even led to duplicative shipments. How can we ensure greater transparency of shipments going from the SNS out to the States?

This question is complex and the need to protect specific SNS material holding so as not to disclose potential weaknesses to determined actors can somewhat impede full transparency. I would defer this question to HHS for SNS and HHS Security Personnel for response based on current threat information.

3. Mr. Burel, I've heard concerns about states mandating that hospitals maintain 90-day stockpiles of PPE which, while well intended, distorts demand throughout the country and potentially siphons off needed PPE. Can (should) the Federal Government coordinate with the States to standardize these practices in a way that reflects the on the ground realities and true demand (i.e., based on the burn rate) for PPE?

I would suggest rather than distorting demand, such requirements may effectively drive a higher demand to result in more manufacturing These stocks would allow these healthcare facilities to be self sufficient in certain scenarios without having to reach back to the supply chain for material. Combining marginal additional stocks at healthcare facilities, marginal additional stocks at distributors and manufacturers and stocks held at state and federal levels for the truly catastrophic need will better prepare the nation and spread that responsibility and cost logically.

The Federal Government needs to engage in stronger coordination with states and localities for Public Health Preparedness overall. Additional funds are needed at the state and local level to be better prepared. These funds can be provided through the Public Health Emergency Preparedness Cooperative Agreements managed by CDC. SNS should be directed, funded and staffed to return to regular consultation with state and local preparedness professionals. This support from the federal government has become fractured and inefficient after the responsibility was removed from the SNS. The SNS incorporates the public health preparedness expertise as well as supply chain and general medical logistics expertise required to support this consultative work.

Chapter 2

Compensation Programs for Potential COVID-19 Vaccine Injuries*

Kevin J. Hickey and Erin H. Ward

More than 200 million Americans have received one or more doses of a Coronavirus Disease 2019 (COVID-19) vaccine, along with billions of people worldwide. The Food and Drug Administration's (FDA's) emergency use authorizations for the Pfizer-BioNTech, Moderna, and Johnson & Johnson COVID-19 vaccines were based on months-long clinical trials (including safety monitoring) of each vaccine, involving tens of thousands of participants. These trials did not identify any safety concerns that would preclude such authorization. (The Pfizer-BioNTech COVID-19 vaccine subsequently received full approval from FDA.) Post-authorization, the COVID-19 vaccines have been subject to safety monitoring requirements by FDA and the Centers for Disease Control and Prevention (CDC) to detect long-term or rare adverse health events.

The most common side effects of COVID-19 vaccines are mild—such as local pain around the injection side, tiredness, or fever—and usually resolve within a few days. As with most vaccines, however, a very small percentage of inoculated individuals experience serious adverse reactions to a COVID-19 vaccine.

For example, approximately two to five people per million receiving mRNA COVID-19 vaccines experience anaphylaxis, a severe allergic reaction, following vaccination. (For this reason, the CDC recommends that all individuals be monitored for at least 15 minutes following their vaccinations, and that all vaccination sites have epinephrine available for treatment of anaphylaxis.) Other serious adverse events reported following vaccination, such as myocarditis and Guillain-Barré Syndrome, are similarly rare and may be associated with COVID-19 vaccines.

Federal law has two distinct compensation regimes that may compensate individuals harmed by adverse reactions to vaccines. In general, the National Vaccine Injury Compensation Program (VICP) may provide compensation for injuries or deaths associated with most vaccines routinely administered in the United States (such as pediatric and seasonal influenza vaccines). During certain public health emergencies, the Countermeasures Injury Compensation Program (CICP) may provide compensation for injuries and deaths resulting from the administration of "covered countermeasures" under the Public Readiness and Emergency Preparedness Act (PREP Act), which may include vaccines.

Under the Secretary of Health and Human Services' (HHS's) PREP Act Declaration for COVID-19 (and its amendments), COVID-19 vaccines are covered countermeasures within the

* This is an edited, reformatted and augmented version of Congressional Research Service Publication No. LSB10584, updated October 20, 2021.

PREP Act's scope. As a result, CICP—and not VICP—will apply to injuries resulting from COVID-19 vaccinations while the public health emergency persists and the Declaration remains in force. Compensation through CICP is generally somewhat more limited than through VICP. This chapter will review and compare the compensation regimes available for vaccine-related injuries under CICP and VICP, and describe the procedures for injured individuals to obtain compensation under each program. The chapter ends with a *Table* comparing the two regimes.

The Countermeasures Injury Compensation Program

To encourage expeditious development and deployment of medical countermeasures during a public health emergency, the PREP Act authorizes the Secretary of HHS (the Secretary) to limit legal liability for losses resulting from the administration of medical countermeasures such as diagnostics, treatments, and vaccines. In a declaration effective February 4, 2020 (the PREP Act Declaration), the Secretary invoked the PREP Act and declared COVID-19 to be a public health emergency warranting liability protections for covered countermeasures. Pursuant to the PREP Act Declaration and its subsequent amendments, manufacturers, distributors, and health care providers are generally immune from legal liability (i.e., they cannot be sued for money damages in court) for losses related to the administration or use of covered countermeasures against COVID-19.

In addition to providing immunity from liability, the PREP Act established CICP, a compensation program for individuals seriously injured or killed as a direct result of the administration or use of a covered countermeasure. CICP is a regulatory process administered by HHS's Health Resources and Services Administration (HRSA). HRSA regulations govern CICP's procedures and eligibility determinations.

Covered Vaccines and Injuries

Under the PREP Act and the amended Declaration, covered countermeasures for COVID-19 may include drugs, biological products, and medical devices that the FDA approves, licenses, or authorizes for emergency use "to diagnose, mitigate, prevent, treat, or cure" COVID-19, or used "to limit the harm that COVID-19 . . . might otherwise cause." For example, personal protective equipment (PPE) (e.g., respirators), ventilators, therapeutic drugs (e.g., remdesivir), and monoclonal antibody treatments approved or authorized by FDA to treat or prevent COVID-19 are covered countermeasures under the PREP Act. Notably, FDA-authorized or -approved COVID-19 vaccines—such as those produced by Pfizer, Moderna, and Johnson & Johnson—are covered countermeasures under the PREP Act Declaration.

Under the PREP Act, CICP remedies "shall be exclusive of any other civil action or proceeding" for injuries directly caused by administering covered countermeasures, with limited exceptions. Thus, while the current PREP Act Declaration and public health emergency remain in effect, CICP is the exclusive remedy for claims within the PREP Act's scope, including injuries resulting from COVID-19 vaccinations. (As discussed in detail below, VICP may eventually apply to COVID-19-vaccine injuries after the public health emergency terminates, contingent on certain statutory and regulatory changes.)

CICP compensation is limited to eligible individuals, such as persons injured by countermeasures or their survivors. CICP only provides compensation for death or "serious physical injuries," that is, injuries that warrant hospitalization or lead to a significant loss of function or disability. Thus, individuals who experience only minor side effects from a COVID-19 vaccine—such as soreness, headache, or fatigue— would not be eligible for CICP compensation.

Procedure for Obtaining Compensation

To apply for CICP compensation, a claimant must file a request for benefits within one year of the date the countermeasure was administered. (If the Secretary publishes a new Countermeasure Injury Table, a newly eligible claimant may file within one year after the new table is established.) In addition to the request form, claimants may need to submit medical records and other evidence to establish eligibility. If determined to be eligible, claimants may submit additional documentation to demonstrate the compensation amount. Eligibility and compensation determinations are made by CICP, as the delegate of the Secretary. Claimants may seek reconsideration of an adverse eligibility decision by CICP, but the ultimate decisionmaking authority lies with the Secretary. The PREP Act precludes judicial review of the Secretary's eligibility and compensation decisions.

CICP claimants can prove eligibility for compensation in one of two ways. The first only applies to injuries listed on a Countermeasure Injury Table, which the Secretary must establish by regulation when compelling medical and scientific evidence shows that administration or use of a covered countermeasure directly causes particular injuries. (The table established for the H1N1 pandemic influenza vaccine is one example; no such table has yet been promulgated for COVID-19 vaccines or other COVID-19 countermeasures.) For injuries listed on a Countermeasure Injury Table, if the claimant can show that the countermeasure recipient's injury is listed on the table and was sustained within the relevant time interval (and meets any other requirements set forth in the table), CICP will presume the injury was a direct result of the covered countermeasure. For injuries not on a Countermeasure Injury Table (or outside its scope), the claimant must prove the non-table injury was the "direct result" of the countermeasure's administration based on "compelling, reliable, valid, medical and scientific evidence" beyond mere temporal association.

Available Compensation

Compensation under CICP is limited to (1) reasonable medical expenses (e.g., unreimbursed hospitalization costs); (2) loss of employment income (e.g., income lost from inability to work due to disability); and (3) a set death benefit where the death is a direct result of the administration or use of a covered countermeasure. Attorneys' fees and pain-and-suffering damages are not available. CICP awards are also subject to various annual and lifetime limits. For example, annual lost employment income awards are capped at $50,000 per year, and the standard maximum death benefit is the same as that under the Public Safety Officers' Benefits program (currently $370,376).

Given the limited number and scope of past PREP Act declarations, CICP has been used relatively infrequently since the PREP Act's 2005 enactment. The majority of these non-COVID-19 claims were related to the H1N1 influenza vaccine. According to HRSA, for fiscal years 2010 through 2021, CICP received 491 claims unrelated to COVID-19, of which 39 (8%) were determined to be eligible for compensation; 29 claims (6%) have been paid out by CICP, amounting to $6 million in awards.

In light of the COVID-19 pandemic, HRSA has received a larger number of CICP claims than it has received historically. As of September 1, 2021, CICP has received 2,392 claims alleging injury or death relating to COVID-19 countermeasures, of which 1,031 claims (43%) relate to COVID-19 vaccines.

CICP has not yet compensated any claims relating to COVID-19 countermeasures; it has denied three claims because the standard of proof for causation was not met and/or a covered injury was not sustained. The remainder of the COVID-19 countermeasure claims (2,389 or 99.9%) are in review or pending CICP review.

Several COVID-19 emergency appropriations allow the Secretary to transfer funds to the Covered Countermeasure Process Fund. Such funds, in addition to prior year fund balances, can be used for CICP compensation awards.

The National Vaccine Injury Compensation Program

After the Secretary terminates the PREP Act Declaration for the COVID-19 pandemic, any injuries or death from COVID-19 vaccines administered after the declaration ends would be addressed in court under tort law unless the COVID-19 vaccines are added to the National Vaccine Injury Compensation Program (VICP; 42 U.S.C. §§ 300aa-10–300aa-44). VICP provides compensation for injuries and deaths caused by certain vaccines that are subject to an excise tax and listed on the Vaccine Injury Table.

VICP was created by the National Childhood Vaccine Injury Act of 1986 (NCVIA) amid concerns that lawsuits against vaccine manufacturers and health care providers alleging vaccine injuries could lead to vaccine shortages and lower immunization rates. Under a typical state tort law framework, the injured person must generally prove that a vaccine caused the injury and that either the vaccine manufacturer is at fault (e.g., negligent, failed to warn adequately) or, under products liability doctrines, that the vaccine was defective. If the person cannot prove one of these elements—for example, if the manufacturer adequately warned of side effects or it is unclear whether the vaccine caused the injury—the claimant receives no compensation. If the vaccine manufacturer is found liable, however, it may be responsible for compensatory damages and potentially punitive damages as determined by a jury. Regardless of the outcome, both sides generally would be responsible for litigation costs.

The NCVIA created a no-fault alternative compensation program for deaths and injuries caused by certain vaccines that are recommended by the CDC for routine administration in children or pregnant women.

The program shields manufacturers of certain vaccines from most liability for vaccine-related injuries and deaths, while providing compensation to those injured by vaccines from a trust fund funded by excise taxes paid by the vaccine manufacturers. By limiting liability exposure for vaccine manufacturers, expanding the availability of compensation for injured parties, and lowering the burden of proof, the program reduces uncertainty for both injured persons and vaccine manufacturers. From implementation of the program in 1988 through October 1, 2021, more than 24,441 petitions for compensation have been filed, of which 20,300 have been adjudicated, and 8,353 determined to merit compensation. The program has paid out approximately $4.7 billion in compensation since its inception.

Covered Vaccines and Injuries

To receive compensation, an injured party must show he or she received a "covered vaccine." Not every FDA-approved vaccine is covered by the VICP. The NCVIA included an initial Vaccine Injury Table listing vaccines covered by the program. The statute provides that vaccines can be added to the program by the Secretary amending the Vaccine Injury Table to add vaccines recommended by the CDC for routine administration to children or pregnant women within two years of such a recommendation. To receive compensation through the VICP, the injured person must have received a vaccine that is (1) recommended by the CDC for routine administration to children or pregnant women, (2) listed by the Secretary on the Vaccine Injury Table, and (3) subject to an excise tax that funds the Vaccine Injury Compensation Trust Fund from which compensation is paid. The types of vaccines subject to the excise tax are specified in statute and therefore can only be amended by an act of Congress.

In addition to having received a covered vaccine, the injured party must show either that (1) he or she experienced an injury listed for the vaccine in the Vaccine Injury Table and the first symptom of the onset or significant aggravation of the injury occurred within the time frame specified in the table, or (2) the vaccine caused the injury. The Vaccine Injury Table accordingly allows injured persons to avoid having to prove a vaccine caused their injuries by allowing them instead to show they received an injury that has been associated with the vaccine soon after receiving the vaccine. Nonetheless, injured persons still have the option of directly proving that a vaccine caused their injuries if they experience a less-common injury or the onset or aggravation of the injury is delayed.

Procedure for Obtaining Compensation

To receive compensation through VICP for a vaccine-related injury or death, the injured person (or the estate in the case of a death) files a petition with the U.S. Court of Federal Claims (Claims Court). The petition must generally contain an affidavit and supporting documentation, including relevant medical records, showing the person

- received a vaccine listed in the Vaccine Injury Table;
- sustained an illness, disability, injury, or condition set forth in the Vaccine Injury Table for the particular vaccine, and
    - the first symptom or manifestation occurred within the required time period; or
    - the vaccine caused the injury;

- suffered residual effects or complications that lasted for more than six months or required inpatient hospitalization and surgery, or died; and
- has not collected another award or settlement for the injury or death.

Petitions for vaccine-related injuries must generally be filed within three years of the first symptom or significant aggravation of the injury. Petitions for vaccine-related deaths must be filed within two years of the death and within four years of the first symptom or significant aggravation of the injury from which the death resulted. If the Vaccine Injury Table is amended such that a person qualifies for compensation who previously did not, that person has two years from when the table is revised to seek compensation for injuries or deaths that occurred up to eight years before the table was revised.

When a person files a petition with the Claims Court, the clerk of the court forwards the petition to the chief special master to assign the petition to one of eight special masters. The special master conducts a proceeding to evaluate whether the petition merits compensation under the VICP and, if so, how much.

The proceedings resemble trials in allowing the presentation of evidence and submission of testimony, but they operate under more flexible, informal procedures to allow for expeditious resolution. Once a petition is filed, the special master has 240 days to issue a decision that includes factual findings and legal conclusions, though the parties may suspend the proceedings by motion for up to 150 days if necessary.

Following the decision, the petitioner has 30 days to appeal a special master's decision to the Claims Court for review. The court then has 120 days to uphold the decision, issue its own decision, or remand to the special master for further proceedings. Once the court issues its judgment, either because the petitioner does not appeal the special master's decision within 30 days or the court issues a decision after review, the petitioner has 60 days to appeal the judgment to the U.S. Court of Appeals for the Federal Circuit (Federal Circuit). If the petitioner chooses not to appeal the decision, the judgment becomes final.

After a final judgment, the petitioner has 90 days to inform the Claims Court whether the petitioner accepts the judgment or will file a civil action for damages in court. A petitioner may also withdraw its petition and file a civil action if the special master fails to act within 240 days or the Claims Court fails to enter the judgment within 420 days, both time frames excluding any suspended time. (Petitioners may opt not to withdraw their petitions if they do not want to risk proceeding in civil court.) Petitioners who neither rejected a judgment nor withdrew their petition due to the court's failure to act in time are barred from filing civil claims.

In addition to limiting the availability of civil actions to parties who have gone through the petition process, the VICP imposes certain limitations on vaccine manufacturers' liability. For example, vaccine manufacturers are not liable for injuries or deaths due to unavoidable side effects from properly prepared vaccines accompanied by proper directions and warnings. Any action that proceeds against a vaccine manufacturer is tried in three stages: (1) liability, (2) general damages, and (3) punitive damages.

Trifurcating the trial in this manner limits the evidence presented to the jury in the first and second stages to the evidence relevant to each stage of the trial.

Available Compensation

The VICP allows individuals to receive compensation for

- actual and reasonably projectable unreimbursable expenses directly related to the vaccine-related injury, including the cost of diagnosis, medical care, rehabilitation, counseling, and vocational training, among others;
- actual and anticipated loss of earnings;
- actual and projected pain and suffering and emotional distress, capped at $250,000;
- vaccine-related death, in the amount of $250,000; and
- reasonable attorneys' fees and other costs associated with proceeding on the petition.

The NCVIA authorized appropriations to compensate individuals injured by vaccines administered before October 1, 1988. Compensation for injuries for vaccines administered after October 1, 1988, is paid out of the Vaccine Injury Compensation Trust Fund (Trust Fund). Vaccine manufacturers pay into the Trust Fund through excise taxes imposed on covered vaccines. The Trust Fund may only be used to pay for vaccine- related injuries from vaccines subject to the excise tax at the time of payment, and for certain government administrative expenses incurred when administering the program. As a result, only vaccines subject to the excise tax are included in the VICP.

Considerations for Congress

The future of the COVID-19 pandemic, the impact of SARS-CoV-2 variants, and the vaccines authorized to prevent COVID-19 remain uncertain. COVID-19 vaccines are currently only authorized and CDC-recommended for individuals 12 years and older or 18 years and older, depending on the vaccine. In addition, the CDC recommends that people who are pregnant receive a COVID-19 vaccine, and recently recommended booster shots of Pfizer's COVID-19 vaccine for some groups. It remains to be seen, however, whether additional inoculations will be needed for the general population on a regular basis as the virus evolves.

Accordingly, it is unknown whether COVID-19 vaccines will be recommended for routine administration after the public health emergency ends, and specifically whether the CDC will recommend any such vaccine for routine administration to children or pregnant women. If so, Congress may consider whether to add COVID-19 vaccines to the excise tax list, which would include them in the VICP. Alternatively, Congress might consider a broader amendment to the excise tax statute to allow any vaccine recommended for routine administration to children or pregnant women to be automatically subject to the excise tax and therefore eligible for the VICP. Or, if Congress decides that COVID-19 injuries should be compensated through VICP even while the public health emergency persists, Congress could amend the PREP Act and NCVIA accordingly.

Congress could also implement an entirely new program specifically addressing compensation for COVID-19 vaccine-related injuries or deaths should it so choose. Or, Congress could opt to leave COVID-19 vaccines out of the VICP and allow the traditional tort system to address any vaccine-related injuries, either now or after the public health emergency ends and CICP no longer applies.

Table 1. Comparison of Vaccine-Injury Compensation Programs: CICP v. VICP

	Countermeasures Injury Compensation Program (CICP)	Vaccine Injury Compensation Program (VICP)
Scope of Coverage	"Covered countermeasures" under the PREP Act, such as pandemic and epidemic products used to treat, mitigate, prevent, or cure COVID-19 (e.g., vaccines, PPE, treatments)	"Covered Vaccines" are those recommended by CDC for routine administration to children or pregnant women, subject to a federal excise tax, and included on the Vaccine Injury Table
Covered Injuries	Death, or serious physical injury that (1) warrants hospitalization or (2) led to a significant loss of function or disability	Death or an illness, injury, or condition that lasted more than six months or required inpatient hospitalization and surgical intervention and was associated with one or more vaccines in the Vaccine Injury Table, unless the cause was an adulterant or contaminant that was intentionally added to the vaccine
Process for Obtaining Compensation	Administrative Process: file request form and supporting documentation with CICP to prove eligibility and compensation amounts	Judicial Process ("vaccine court"): file a petition in the U.S. Court of Federal Claims
Available Benefits	Reasonable medical expenses, lost employment income, and death benefits	Non-reimbursed expenses related to the injury for the diagnosis, medical care, and various rehabilitation and recovery services; lost employment income; pain, suffering, and emotional distress damages; death benefits; attorney's fees
Unavailable Benefits	Attorneys' fees, pain-and-suffering damages, punitive damages	Punitive or exemplary damages
Benefit Caps	$50,000/year for lost employment income (lifetime cap is generally $379,000); standard death benefit of $370,376 for FY2021	$250,000 for death; $250,000 for pain and suffering and emotional distress
Filing Deadlines	Within one year of the administration of the covered countermeasure (or within one year of the issuance of a new Countermeasure Injury Table)	For injuries, within three years of the first symptom; for deaths, within two years of the death and four years of the first symptom
Standard of Proof	Must show the injury (1) meets the requirements on a Countermeasure Injury Table; or (2) was a direct result of the administration or use of a covered countermeasure	Must show the person (1) received a vaccine on the Vaccine Injury Table; (2) sustained or significantly aggravated an illness, disability, injury, or condition, or died; (3) the illness, disability, injury, condition, or death is either listed in the Vaccine Injury Table in association with the vaccine and occurred within a set time period as specified in the table or was caused by the vaccine; (4) suffered the effects for more than six months or required inpatient hospitalization and surgery or died; and (5) has not previously collected an award for the injury or death
Initial Decisionmaker	CICP (as delegate of the Secretary of HHS)	U.S. Court of Federal Claims special master
Appeals & Judicial Review	Claimant may seek reconsideration of CICP decision to a qualified	Claimant may seek review of special master decision by U.S. Court of Federal Claims within 30 days of decision; claimant may

	Countermeasures Injury Compensation Program (CICP)	Vaccine Injury Compensation Program (VICP)
	independent panel within 60 days; no further judicial or administrative review	seek review by the U.S. Court of Appeals for the Federal Circuit within 60 days of final judgment; claimant may accept the judgment or reject it and file a tort claim
Funding Source	Emergency appropriations to Covered Countermeasure Process Fund	Vaccine Injury Compensation Trust Fund based on excise tax of $0.75 per dose on "taxable vaccines"
Number of Claims Processed	Non-COVID-19 claims (2010-2021): 491 claims, of which 452 were determined ineligible and 29 compensated (6%) COVID-19 countermeasure claims (as of September 1, 2021): 2,392 claims, of which 1,031 claims (43%) relate to COVID-19 vaccines; most of these claims (99.9%) remain in or pending review	24,441 petitions as of 10/1/2021, of which 20,300 have been adjudicated, 11,947 were determined ineligible, and 8,353 compensated (41%)
Process for Adding New Vaccines	Scope of "covered countermeasures" is determined by Secretary of HHS's PREP Act declarations (within statutory limits)	Secretary of HHS may add vaccines to the Vaccine Injury Table that are (1) subject to the excise tax; and (2) recommended by the CDC for routine administration to children or pregnant women

Source: HRSA; CRS; 42 U.S.C. §§ 300aa-10–300aa-34; 42 U.S.C. § 247d-6d to -6e; 42 C.F.R. pt. 110.

Index

A

B

C

D

E

L

M

N

O

W